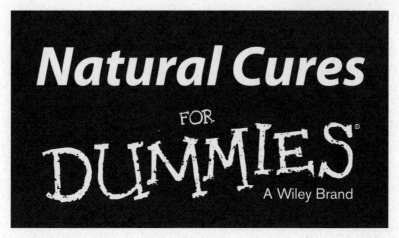

by Scott J. Banks, DC, IFMCP, CGP, PC, with Joe Kraynak

Natural Cures For Dummies®

Published by: **John Wiley & Sons, Inc.,** 111 River Street, Hoboken, NJ 07030-5774, www.wiley.com

Copyright © 2015 by John Wiley & Sons, Inc., Hoboken, New Jersey

Published simultaneously in Canada

No part of this publication may be reproduced, stored in a retrieval system or transmitted in any form or by any means, electronic, mechanical, photocopying, recording, scanning or otherwise, except as permitted under Sections 107 or 108 of the 1976 United States Copyright Act, without the prior written permission of the Publisher. Requests to the Publisher for permission should be addressed to the Permissions Department, John Wiley & Sons, Inc., 111 River Street, Hoboken, NJ 07030, (201) 748-6011, fax (201) 748-6008, or online at http://www.wiley.com/go/permissions.

Trademarks: Wiley, For Dummies, the Dummies Man logo, Dummies.com, Making Everything Easier, and related trade dress are trademarks or registered trademarks of John Wiley & Sons, Inc., and may not be used without written permission. All other trademarks are the property of their respective owners. John Wiley & Sons, Inc., is not associated with any product or vendor mentioned in this book.

For general information on our other products and services, please contact our Customer Care Department within the U.S. at 877-762-2974, outside the U.S. at 317-572-3993, or fax 317-572-4002. For technical support, please visit www.wiley.com/techsupport.

Wiley publishes in a variety of print and electronic formats and by print-on-demand. Some material included with standard print versions of this book may not be included in e-books or in print-on-demand. If this book refers to media such as a CD or DVD that is not included in the version you purchased, you may download this material at http://booksupport.wiley.com. For more information about Wiley products, visit www.wiley.com.

Library of Congress Control Number: 2014954669

ISBN 978-1-119-03022-5 (pbk); ISBN 978-1-119-03017-1 (ebk); ISBN 978-1-119-03019-5

Manufactured in the United States of America

10 9 8 7 6 5 4 3 2 1

Contents at a Glance

Table of Contents

Foreword

I learned firsthand about the power of natural cures when a hit-and-run driver struck my then-16-year-old son Grant in September 2012. Among his injuries were a torn aorta, spinal fractures, skull fractures, and bleeding throughout his brain. As Grant lay in a coma, doctors offered a grim prognosis; they told us they could do nothing and advised us to let Grant go.

Western medicine provides numerous valuable contributions, but it often fails to see the bigger picture for healing and health. That's where some of my closest friends — progressive doctors, nutritionists, and other healthcare professionals — selflessly provided their expertise to help heal Grant.

Bucking the status quo and implementing natural cures played a huge role in keeping Grant alive when doctors argued we had no hope. Eventually, he emerged from his coma and began to speak, every word becoming nothing short of a miracle. Grant not only survived; today he thrives. If I could glean a bright spot during that challenging time other than to never lose hope, I would emphasize how providing the right nutrients and other modifications can radically heal your body. That's where *Natural Cures For Dummies* comes in.

In this user-friendly reference, Dr. Scott J. Banks couples cutting-edge information about symptoms and root causes with science-supported, safe "prescriptions" — healing foods, natural supplements, and lifestyle modifications — that, unlike pharmaceutical drugs or potentially invasive therapies, assist rather than work against your body's natural ability to heal. Consider this comprehensive, expert-curated book your go-to guide to naturally heal numerous conditions that leave you tired, sick, overweight, and aging prematurely. *Natural Cures For Dummies* will empower you to take control and provide your body the nutrients it requires for healing and abundant health.

JJ Virgin

New York Times bestselling author of *The Virgin Diet* and *Sugar Impact Diet*

Introduction

· ·

Modern medicine has made amazing strides toward combating infectious diseases and improving the quality of human life. Sanitation has nearly rid humans in developed countries of exposure to a host of disease-causing bacteria, viruses, and nasty parasites. Vaccines have virtually eliminated many fatal or crippling diseases and have held many others at bay. Advances in medical imaging now enable doctors to look inside the body without opening it up. Anesthesia allows for pain-free surgeries. And through the miracles of modern medicine, many people have had their hearing and sight restored, limbs replaced with robotic prosthetics, and are even walking around with artificial hearts.

Yet something is missing. The steady decline of infectious diseases is matched with a comparable rise in chronic illnesses, including Alzheimer's disease, arthritis, asthma, autism, cancer, diabetes, fibromyalgia, heart disease, obesity, and osteoporosis. And the best that modern medicine can offer in fighting this rising epidemic is a whack-a-mole approach of treating symptoms with powerful prescription medications and surgeries that then trigger other illnesses that have other symptoms that must then be treated. Over time, many patients end up on a half dozen medications (or more), and they still feel lousy.

Natural medicine takes a different approach. Instead of treating symptoms or even illnesses, natural medicine focuses on identifying and treating underlying causes: nutritional deficiencies, hormonal imbalances, inefficiency in digestion and absorption of nutrients, the presence of heavy metals and other toxins, food allergies and sensitivities, structural imbalances, and dysregulation of the immune system, to mention a few. Natural medicine not only cures illness, but it also optimizes wellness.

About This Book

Fed up with conventional medical treatments? Welcome to *Natural Cures For Dummies*, your key to curing illness and optimizing wellness through nutrition, supplements, herbs, lifestyle changes, and other nonconventional treatments that harness the body's powerful self-defense and self-healing mechanisms.

Organized in an easy-to-access format and presented in plain English, this book introduces you to natural cures and takes you on a tour of common natural cures treatment approaches, including aromatherapy, Ayurveda, functional medicine, herbal medicine, homeopathy, and naturopathy. In addition, you'll find guidance on dietary and lifestyle changes you can make to instantly improve your health. I also provide natural prevention and cures for over 170 common ailments, explaining which nutrients, supplements, herbs, and other treatments are most effective in addressing the underlying causes of these ailments.

You'll also find appendixes that cover vitamins and minerals, nutritional supplements, natural hormones, herbs, homeopathic remedies, and essential oils. These vital references can be used time and again as you embrace natural remedies to protect and promote optimal health in yourself and your family.

Although I encourage you to read every single word of this book from start to finish, you're welcome to skip around to acquire your knowledge on a need-to-know basis and completely skip the sidebars (shaded gray) and anything flagged with a Technical Stuff icon. Although this information may be too fascinating to ignore, it's not essential.

During the writing of this book, I adopted a few conventions to help convey the content as simply and clearly as possible and highlight important information:

- ✔ All doses given are for adults unless otherwise specified. See Chapters 3 and 12 for guidance on converting to doses for children and for adults who weight less than 150 pounds.

- ✔ Doses appear in the unit most commonly used for each supplement, usually grams (g), milligrams (mg), micrograms (mcg), and United States Pharmacopeia (USP). Colony forming units (CFUs) indicate the number of live organisms (bacteria or yeast) in a probiotic that are capable of reproducing to form a group.

- ✔ When specified, the better form of a supplement appears in parentheses directly after the supplement; for example, "vitamin B12 (methylcobalamin, sublingually in a fast-dissolving tablet)." The better form is more easily processed and used by the body or is best for a specific condition.

Within this book, you may note that some web addresses break across two lines of text. If you're reading this book in print and want to visit one of these web pages, simply key in the web address exactly as it's noted in the text, pretending as though the line break doesn't exist. If you're reading this as an e-book, you've got it easy — just click the web address to be taken directly to the web page.

Foolish Assumptions

The fact that you're reading this book tells me that you're probably not feeling as well as you know you should feel and that you haven't had much success with conventional medical treatment. Maybe you're taking a prescription medication that's causing side effects that are worse than the illness itself. Perhaps you're worried about the long-term effects of being on multiple medications. Whatever the reason, you're not satisfied with what conventional medicine has to offer, and you're looking for a better way.

Other foolish assumptions I've made about you include the following:

- ✔ You want to optimize health and not merely rid yourself of illness.

- ✔ You're committed to making bold changes to your diet and lifestyle to achieve and maintain wellness.

- ✔ You're eager to transition from your passive role as patient to a more active role as doctor-patient.

- ✔ You're ready to start listening to and learning from what your body is telling you it needs and needs to avoid to function at its best.

- ✔ You recognize that conventional medical treatment is required for serious physical injuries and certain medical emergencies, including infectious diseases that threaten life or limb.

Icons Used in This Book

Throughout this book, icons in the margins highlight different types of information that call out for your attention. Here are the icons you'll see and a brief description of each.

I want you to remember everything you read in this book, but if you can't quite do that, then remember the important points flagged with this icon.

Tips provide insider insight. When you're looking for a better, faster way to do something, check out these tips.

"Whoa!" This icon appears when you need to be extra vigilant or consult your healthcare provider before moving forward.

Occasionally, I feel compelled to delve deeper into the biology or physiology of a given health condition or treatment. When I do so, I give you a heads up with this icon, so you can skip the details and head right to the cure.

Beyond the Book

In addition to the abundance of information and guidance on harnessing the power of nature and your body's self-protection and self-healing mechanisms, you also get access to even more help and information at www.dummies.com. Go to www.dummies.com/cheatsheet/naturalcures for a free cheat sheet that accompanies this book. It brings you up to speed on natural cure fundamentals, provides a list of junk foods to eliminate from your diet and healthy foods to eat more of, outlines a protocol for maintaining a healthy gut (the key to wellness), and tells you how to combat colds and other bacterial, viral, and fungal infections by enhancing your body's immune response.

You can also head to www.dummies.com/extras/naturalcures for a few free supplemental articles that I think you'll find helpful as you begin your journey to optimal health and well-being. Here you find out how to restore healthy gut bacteria after antibiotic treatment, discover ten key supplements to always keep on hand, and come to recognize why taking vitamins and minerals in their better forms is so important.

Where to Go from Here

I structured this book so you could use it in a couple different ways. To get the most out of it, read it from cover to cover so you don't miss out on any valuable information and insight. You may also use it as natural cures desk reference; when you're not feeling well, simply look up your illness in the table of contents or the index and flip to the designated page to find the cure for what ails you. The appendixes also provide several quick references to nutritional and natural remedies.

I do recommend, however, that you start with the chapters in Part I. Chapter 1 provides a brief overview of the natural cures approach to wellness and gets you up to speed in a hurry on the theory behind the practice. In Chapter 2, I recommend diet and lifestyle changes that form the foundation of good health. And in Chapter 3, I take you on a tour of the different treatment approaches that comprise natural medicine, including Ayurveda, chiropractic, homeopathy, and functional medicine.

As you embark on your journey to optimal health, keep in mind that you're a unique individual. Your DNA, body chemistry, and even the microbes living inside you are all very distinctive, so there is no one-size-fits-all path to wellness. I strongly recommend that you consult with a qualified natural medicine practitioner — a functional medicine practitioner, naturopath, osteopath, chiropractor, or other practitioner who has advanced training in functional medicine and natural cures — for an initial evaluation to identify any deficiencies or other conditions that may be getting in the way.

Part I
Stepping into the Wonderful World of Natural Cures

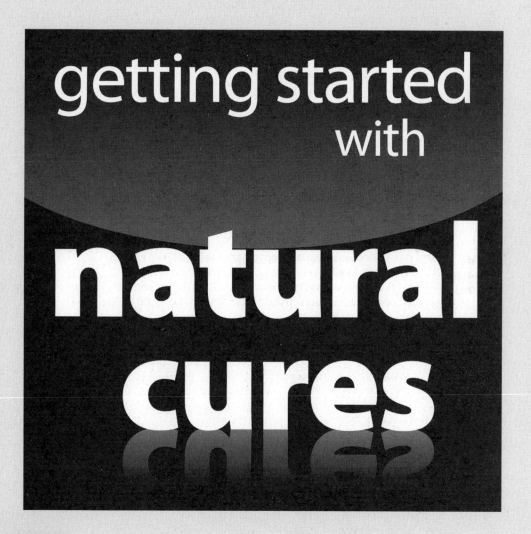

In this part . . .

✔ Get up to speed on the natural cures approach to curing illness and optimizing wellness through nutrition, lifestyle, herbal tonics, physical manipulation, homeopathic remedies, and other nonpharmaceutical treatments.

✔ Build a solid wellness foundation by eliminating junk "food" from your diet, stocking up on healthy foods, establishing a reasonable exercise routine, and making other adjustments to your diet and lifestyle that provide your body with everything it needs for self-defense and self-healing.

✔ Tour the various treatment approaches that make up natural medicine's healthcare model, including aromatherapy, Ayurveda, biofeedback, chelation, functional and herbal medicine, acupuncture, osteopathy, naturopathy, chiropractic, and nutritional medicine.

Chapter 1

Getting the Lowdown on Natural Cures

Modern medicine does a pretty good job fighting infections and acute illnesses. Unfortunately, its track record for preventing and treating chronic illness is abysmal. In fact, many chronic illnesses, including cancer, diabetes, heart disease, asthma, and arthritis, are now epidemics. According to the Centers for Disease Control and Prevention (CDC), people in the United States spend 86 percent of their healthcare dollars on chronic diseases — most of which are preventable through diet and lifestyle changes.

When you go to a conventional doctor, however, you rarely get educated or trained in proper nutrition or a healthy lifestyle. Instead, the doctor hands you a prescription for a medication that typically treats the symptoms and has a laundry list of very scary side effects, few of which are mentioned at the time.

There's a better way: Nature's way.

Wrapping Your Brain around the Concept of Natural Cures

Over the course of a couple million years, the human body has evolved to develop incredibly efficient self-defense and self-healing mechanisms. Yet when you visit a doctor complaining of an illness, the doctor typically disregards what nature has so carefully crafted and offers treatments cooked up in a laboratory, many of which degrade your body's own healing power. Consider the use of antibiotics, which kill not only harmful bacteria but also healthy bacteria in your gut — bacteria that are essential for proper digestion, nutrition, and immune response.

Natural medical practitioners take a different approach. They work with nature to strengthen the body's ability to fight infection and heal itself. In this section, I provide additional insight into the natural cures approach, provide some background on its history, reveal the science that supports it, and let you know what to expect from it as a patient.

Defining natural medicine

Natural medicine is any healing practice that harnesses the power of nature, including the human body's self-defense and self-healing mechanisms, to prevent and cure illness. Natural medicine includes the following practices:

- **Aromatherapy:** Essential oils extracted from plants are used in numerous preparations, including massage oils and bath salts, to enhance physical and psychological well-being.

- **Ayurveda:** This traditional Hindu system of medicine seeks to establish healthy balance in mind, body, and spirit through diet, herbal formulations, and yoga.

- **Biofeedback:** This healing technique helps you control bodily processes normally thought to be outside an individual's control. It does so by providing real-time monitoring and information about those processes as you perform techniques to regulate them.

- **Chelation:** Detoxification of heavy metals and other toxins from the body gets rid of harmful substances that your body isn't geared to eliminate on its own.

- **Functional medicine:** Functional medicine is personalized medicine that recognizes and addresses each person's individual genetic uniqueness and the complex interactions among genes, diet, and lifestyle.

- **Herbal medicine:** This practice treats illness with plants or plant extracts and is perhaps the oldest form of medical practice.

- **Homeopathy:** Homeopathy treats illness by giving the patient minute doses of natural substances that would cause the same symptoms in a healthy person. The concept behind homeopathic remedies is similar to the concept behind vaccination, which deliberately exposes people to dead or weakened bacteria or viruses to protect them from infections caused by those organisms.

- ✔ **Massage and bodywork:** Manipulation of the body, primarily the bones, muscles, and nerves, to relieve tension and pain, establish balance, promote detoxification, or treat specific conditions comes in many forms, including chiropractic adjustments, traditional massage, acupuncture, reflexology, rolfing, Reiki, and shiatsu.

- ✔ **Naturopathy:** The Swiss Army Knife of natural healing, naturopathy uses numerous alternative treatments to promote healing and health, including diet and lifestyle counseling, herbs, homeopathy, massage, aromatherapy, acupuncture, and biofeedback.

- ✔ **Chiropractic treatment:** Chiropractic treatment seeks to realign the spinal column and joints that cause pain and dysfunction related to the nerves, muscles, and organs of the body. Many chiropractors follow a functional medicine approach. Look for a chiropractor who's received advanced training in functional medicine.

- ✔ **Nutritional medicine:** This approach uses food along with vitamins, minerals, and other supplements as medicine to cure illness and optimize health.

For more about these natural healing disciplines, check out Chapter 3. Head to the chapters in Part II for details on treating specific health conditions.

No two individuals are alike; effective treatment requires a personalized treatment plan. Therefore, I strongly encourage you to visit an Institute for Functional Medicine Certified Practitioner (IFMCP) doctor or a naturopath for an initial evaluation to determine whether you have any food allergies or sensitivities, nutritional deficiencies, digestive disorders, or genetic vulnerabilities that need to be addressed. To find a practitioner who has trained with the Institute for Functional Medicine, visit www.functionalmedicine.org and click Find a Practitioner. To find a naturopath, visit www.naturopathic.org and click Find a Doctor.

Sifting through the science behind natural cures

Conventional science often questions the effectiveness of natural medicine by citing the dearth of well-designed clinical studies, but natural medicine actually has a growing body of scientific evidence to back it up. This evidence comes primarily in two forms:

- ✔ **Randomized, double-blind, placebo-controlled (RDBPC) clinical trials:** RDBPC studies, which test the effectiveness and safety of medications, are the gold standard in the pharmaceutical industry. More and more, these same studies are used to test the effectiveness of alternative treatments, including nutritional supplements. In the U.S., the National Institutes of Health's National Center for Complementary and Alternative Medicine (NCCAM) is devoted exclusively to studying and reporting on the safety and effectiveness of alternative and complementary treatments; visit nccam.nih.gov for details.

RDBPC studies aren't always suitable for testing natural treatments, however, because these treatments are often tailored to the individual patient's needs and involve a combination of interventions, including dietary changes, nutritional support, exercise, and physical manipulation.

✔ **Investigations into human biology and physiology:** Advances in technology are revealing more and more about how the human body functions and how genetic, environmental, and lifestyle variables alone and together influence health and illness. For example, a recent study published in the journal *Cell* found that some of the bacteria living in the human body produce antibiotics, which help prevent and fight infections from certain harmful bacteria. This study provides additional support for the natural cures approach of supporting a healthy immune system with probiotics and avoiding the overuse of broad-range antibiotics that kill beneficial as well as harmful bacteria.

Science not only supports the use of natural medicine, but it also drives its development. Many reputable nutraceutical manufacturers now have their own research departments to develop and test products. (A *nutraceutical* is a food-based product that's used as a medicine.) Among other advances, this research has helped to develop vitamins and minerals that are more easily and fully absorbed by the human body, probiotics that survive stomach acid exposure so more live microorganisms can populate the gut, and for-mulations that provide the right mix of nutritional supplements to support the proper function of various systems in the body, including the digestive, cardiovascular, and immune systems.

Buy products only from reputable manufacturers that have researched their products for effectiveness and that adhere to strict quality-control standards and practices; look for those that are Good Manufacturing Processes (GMP) certified. I've been treating patients for 33 years and practicing functional medicine for over 20 years. I've seen many fly-by-night nutraceutical com-panies and poor-quality products come and go. Take the supplements in the form I recommend from reputable manufacturers. Otherwise, your body may not absorb them properly, and they may simply not work.

Knowing what to expect from natural medicine

Natural medicine requires that you become an active participant in your own health. It requires commitment and sacrifice. You may need to eliminate from your diet some of your favorite foods and beverages. You need to exercise at least 30 minutes every other day. Most importantly, you need to invest time and effort in exploring what makes your body tick and figuring out what's causing certain symptoms or what your body needs and isn't getting to achieve optimum health.

The payoff is good health and vitality. Inflammation, at the root of many chronic illnesses, dissipates. You feel less congested and bloated and achy. You're less susceptible to infections and chronic illnesses, including heart disease, diabetes, and cancer. You add years — quality years — to your life. And if you do become ill, you know exactly what your body needs to kick its self-healing powers into high gear.

Recognizing Natural Medicine's Many Benefits and Its Few Drawbacks

Before investing time, effort, and money in any endeavor, it's a good idea to weigh the pros and cons so that you can make a well-informed decision regarding the type of healthcare you want. In this section, I highlight the potential benefits and drawbacks of natural medicine as compared to conventional medicine.

Highlighting the benefits

A natural cures approach to health and healing offers numerous benefits, including the following:

- ✔ **Provides a user-friendly alternative to the typical doctor-patient interaction.** Natural medicine practitioners tend to treat people instead of illnesses. You're more likely to get personalized care.

- ✔ **Treats the cause, not just the symptoms.** The natural cures approach attempts to identify and eliminate illness instead of merely suppressing symptoms. This approach is more likely to result in a cure.

- ✔ **Empowers you to take control of your own health.** A good natural healer is an educator, teaching you about your body and what it needs to be healthy. She doesn't just hand you a prescription and send you on your way.

- ✔ **Eliminates or reduces prescription medication side effects.** One goal of natural medicine is to reduce or eliminate prescription medications from your daily regimen. Less prescription medication means fewer medication side effects. No prescription medication means no medication side effects.

- ✔ **Improves your overall health.** Natural medicine doesn't merely eliminate illness; it strengthens the body overall. A body that's in optimal condition is better able to fight infection and cure illness. Being healthy is far more desirable than merely being not sick.

- ✔ **Strengthens your immune system.** Your digestive tract accounts for 70 percent of your immune system. Conventional treatments often undermine gut health by killing beneficial microbes that reside in the gut. Natural medicine promotes gut health by enhancing digestion and nurturing a healthy environment in which beneficial microbes thrive.

- ✔ **Enhances your mood, energy, and endurance.** Conventional medicine screens people for illness. Natural medicine screens for deficiencies, allergies, and sensitivities to find out what to eliminate that's making you sick and what your body needs for optimal function. As a result, natural medicine improves how you feel overall.

- ✔ **Saves money and time, due to fewer doctor visits.** Natural medicine teaches you how to be healthy so that you can develop the knowledge and skills to prevent illness and heal yourself. You may spend more time getting up to speed on the basics and more money on groceries and supplements, but preventing very costly chronic conditions that degrade your quality of life will likely save you much more in doctor bills, prescription costs, and time off work due to illness.

Acknowledging a few drawbacks

Admittedly, natural medicine has a few drawbacks, including the following:

- ✔ **It's not always easy.** Natural medicine isn't as easy as popping a pill. Overhauling your diet, exercising regularly, reducing stress, and learning about your body all require time and effort.

- ✔ **Sometimes, you have to fly solo.** If you can't afford a doctor and your insurance refuses to cover alternative healthcare options, you may need to fly solo with information in books and magazines and online.

Be careful when conducting online research. Snake oil salespeople run rampant on the Internet, and product reviews are often fictional. Stick to reputable sites run by reputable organizations, such as the Institute for Functional Medicine (www.functionalmedicine.org), the American College for Advancement in Medicine (www.acam.org), and Dieticians in Integrative and Functional Medicine (www.integrativerd.org).

✔ **Sometimes, natural treatments don't work.** Whether you're receiving conventional or alternative treatments, you may need more than one trip to your healthcare provider to narrow down the root cause(s) of an illness and find an effective treatment or combination of treatments. Don't let this discourage you; illness often involves complex interactions within the body, along with numerous environmental factors.

Keep a log of what works and what doesn't work for you so that you don't have to engage in a trial-by-error process the next time you come down with the same affliction.

✔ **Natural cures may take longer.** When treatment requires changes to diet and lifestyle, expect to see improvement in weeks and months, not overnight. Your body is composed of numerous interacting systems and billions of cells that need time to adapt to the changes you're making.

✔ **Insurance may not cover some treatments.** Natural medicine isn't cheap, and insurance may refuse to cover the costs of doctor visits and supplements. Paying a steep health insurance premium and then having to pay out-of-pocket for healthcare is enough to discourage just about anyone. Hopefully, enlightened lawmakers may someday require insurance companies to cover the costs of nutritional supplements and visits to natural medicine practitioners.

To take some of the sting out of the costs, look into whether you can pay for consultations, testing, and supplements with pre-tax dollars from a health savings account (HSA) or flexible spending account (FSA).

✔ **Some "natural" cures are scams.** Because dietary supplements aren't regulated as carefully by the U.S. Food and Drug Administration (FDA) as are pharmaceuticals, charlatans have an easier time producing and selling products with questionable benefits. To reduce your exposure to scams, I recommend that you purchase products only from reputable manufacturers and sellers. Visit my website, spinelife.com, for a list of reputable manufacturers.

Comparing Conventional and Natural Medicine

The good physician treats the disease; the great physician treats the patient who has the disease.

—Sir William Osler (1849–1919), pioneering diagnostician, author, and professor of medicine at the Johns Hopkins University School of Medicine

Throughout this book, I offer guidance on treating specific illnesses, but my approach to healing differs significantly from that of conventional medicine. In this section, I highlight the differences and point out situations in which conventional medicine is the better choice.

Comparing the illness versus the wellness model

The distinction between conventional and natural medicine boils down to the difference in their goals. Conventional medicine seeks to eliminate illness, while natural medicine seeks to optimize wellness. This is especially true for the type of medicine I practice — functional medicine. While conventional medicine focuses on battling infections and symptoms of illnesses, such as asthma, arthritis, cancer, diabetes, fibromyalgia, heart disease, and obesity, with symptom-suppression pharmaceuticals, functional medicine seeks to treat the imbalances or dysfunctions in the body that give rise to these illnesses.

The imbalances and dysfunctions that natural medicine treats include the following:

- Hormonal imbalances
- Mitochondrial dysfunction
- Overactive or underactive immune system
- Toxicity
- Vitamin and mineral deficiencies
- Food allergies, sensitivities, and intolerances
- Poor digestion and nutrient absorption

✔ Inflammation

✔ Obesity

✔ Structural imbalances, such as spinal misalignment

✔ Toxic emotions

✔ Sedentary lifestyle

Functional medicine seeks to restore health by giving the body what it needs for optimal function and removing anything that gets in the way. As a result, it leads to more durable, long-term solutions to chronic illness.

Taking a proactive instead of reactive approach

Preventive medicine is getting a lot of press these days, because even conventional medicine practitioners are realizing that an ounce of prevention is worth a pound of cure. Unfortunately, the prevention offered by conventional medicine typically comes in the form of early detection and treatment, and the treatment rarely targets the underlying cause of these illnesses.

Attend just about any hospital-sponsored health fair, and you'll see all sorts of screenings for cholesterol, atherosclerosis, blood pressure, diabetes, osteoporosis, colon cancer, lung cancer, breast cancer, and prostate cancer. What you don't see are screenings for many of the underlying causes of disease mentioned earlier in this section: vitamin and mineral deficiencies, impaired digestion and mineral absorption, and so on.

Conventional health screenings are great, but they're only the first step toward identifying and treating underlying conditions that give rise to illnesses. An enlightened physician may suggest making changes to diet and lifestyle, such as reducing the amount of salt you eat or cutting down on sweets, and your insurance company may offer discounts on gym memberships and exercise equipment, but without a treatment tailored to address deficiencies and dysfunctions, you're fighting a losing battle.

During a visit with a natural medicine practitioner, you can expect a much more thorough assessment of your health that's likely to include tests to detect vitamin and mineral deficiencies, hormone imbalances, food allergies and sensitivities, and gut health. And your treatment will focus on optimizing health so that your body has everything it needs to fight infection and heal itself and you have the information you need to remove anything that's getting in its way.

Weighing the side effects of each approach

No treatment is completely void of negative side effects, but natural treatments are much safer than those offered by conventional medicine, which usually involve prescription medications, risky medical procedures, and surgeries. The use of prescription medications is particularly dangerous, because many prescription medications cause side effects that require additional prescription medications to counter. Patients frequently end up taking a dozen medications or more and end up feeling as miserable as or worse than ever.

This never-ending cycle of diagnosis followed by prescription doesn't happen with a natural/nutritional approach to healing, because the natural approach treats the causes of illness instead of trying to play whack-a-mole with whatever symptoms happen to pop up during an office visit.

Natural cures are much safer than most treatments offered by conventional medicine, but natural herbs and supplements, even vitamins, carry some risks. Although I provide general guidelines on which supplements, herbs, probiotics, and other nutraceuticals to take and how much, I encourage you to consult a qualified natural medicine practitioner for guidance. If a supplement is powerful enough to heal you, it's powerful enough to harm you if you take too much or if it's something your body can't process.

Knowing when to seek conventional medical treatment

Conventional medicine isn't all bad. In fact, I recommend it over the natural approach for injuries, life-threatening emergencies, and acute illnesses, such as heart attack, lung infection (such as pneumonia), asthma or allergy attacks, renal (kidney) failure, gastrointestinal bleeding, certain bacterial infections, cancer, and alcohol or drug overdose.

Natural medicine is better suited to preventing and treating chronic conditions, including asthma, allergies, arthritis, diabetes, heart disease, fibromyalgia, and obesity. The increasing prevalence of chronic illnesses in the U.S. is sufficient proof that the current model for preventing and treating chronic illness not only doesn't work but also contributes to this trend. By exploring natural medicine as an alternative approach, you're taking a big first step in reversing this trend in your own life and the lives of the people you touch.

Chapter 2

Adopting a Natural Cures Diet and Lifestyle

In This Chapter
▶ Replacing junk with food
▶ Exercising and de-stressing

Most illness results either from a genetic susceptibility combined with physical or emotional stressor or from a weak immune system exposed to an infectious agent — a bacteria, virus, or fungus. You can't do anything to correct an underlying genetic vulnerability, but you can do a great deal to boost your immune system and avoid stressors that trigger illness — poor diet, emotional tension, and environmental toxins. In this chapter, I recommend changes to diet and lifestyle that strengthen your body's ability to prevent illness while reducing your exposure to common stressors that trigger illness.

Changing What and How You Eat: Using Food as Medicine

Scientists are beginning to discover that food is more than mere sustenance. Not only does food fuel the body and provide the basic building blocks for growth and development, but it also conveys information. Foods can flip switches in the DNA to trigger numerous illnesses and health conditions, including type 2 diabetes, obesity, inflammation, cardiovascular diseases, and neurocognitive disorders. To improve health and reverse the course of disease, treat food as medicine and start making better food choices. This section shows you how.

The standard American diet (SAD), heavy in sugars and grains, is highly inflammatory, which is why it's so bad for you. The foods I recommend constitute what could be considered an anti-inflammatory diet. Throughout this book, when I mention adopting an anti-inflammatory diet, I'm recommending the diet described in this chapter.

Eliminating the foods that ail you

Fewer than ten foods are responsible for triggering most cases of inflammation and numerous autoimmune disorders in humans: wheat, soy, dairy, sugar, corn, eggs, peanuts, artificial sweeteners, and trans fats. To find out whether any of the items on this list ails you, I encourage you to get tested for food allergies and sensitivities, as explained in Chapter 13, or perform a modified elimination diet. Table 2-1 lists the most common culprits to test.

You can do an elimination diet in a couple of different ways.

- ✔ Remove a suspect food from your diet for 28 days. If you feel better without it, you can eliminate that food from your diet for good, reintroduce it to see whether it really does cause problems, or get tested to confirm or rule out your suspicions. If you notice no difference whether you eat or abstain from eating the food, you can add it back into your diet.

- ✔ Eliminate for 28 days foods that are most likely to cause problems and then slowly re-introduce them, one every two to three weeks, until your symptoms return. Then eliminate any food(s) that triggered symptoms.

Don't eat even a small amount of the food you're testing for the entire duration of the 28-day period. If you're allergic to that food and you eat even a small amount, the antibodies to that food remain elevated in your system, and you may not notice an improvement in symptoms, defeating the purpose of the elimination diet.

Read on to discover more about the foods that commonly trigger inflammation, autoimmune illnesses, and other disorders and why each one is a trigger for illness in a large portion of the population.

Wheat and gluten

Today's wheat isn't the wheat your ancestors ate. It doesn't even resemble the wheat consumed during the 1980s. Modern wheat is grown and processed in ways that strip out vital nutrients and produce a high-starch flour that spikes blood sugar and insulin levels and triggers inflammation and immune reactions in many people.

Table 2-1	Performing a Modified Elimination Diet	
Category	*Include These Foods*	*Exclude These Foods*
Fruits	Fresh or unsweetened frozen fruits, unsweetened fruit juices, avocado	Oranges, orange juice, dried fruit
Vegetables	Raw, fresh, steamed, sautéed, juiced, or roasted vegetables, sweet potatoes, and yams	Corn, creamed vegetables If you have arthritis, also exclude nightshade vegetables and spices made from those vegetables: tomatoes, white potatoes, eggplants, peppers, paprika, salsa, chili peppers, cayenne, and chili powder
Starch, bread, cereal	Rice, millet, quinoa, amaranth, teff, tapioca, buckwheat, gluten-free oats processed in a plant that doesn't process wheat	Wheat, barley, spelt, khorasan, rye, triticale
Legumes	Any beans, lentils, peas, and hummus not listed in the "Exclude" column	Soybeans, tofu, tempeh, soy milk, soy sauce, edamame, other soy products
Nuts and seeds	Almonds, cashews, walnuts, Brazil nuts, sesame seeds (tahini), sunflower seeds, flaxseeds, pumpkin seeds; butters made from these nuts; seeds that do not contain added ingredients	Peanuts, peanut butter
Meat and fish	All canned (water-packed), fresh, or frozen low-mercury fish; wild game; pastured, hormone-free, antibiotic-free chicken, turkey, and grass-fed lamb	Beef, pork, cold cuts, frankfurters, sausage, canned meats, eggs, shellfish

(Continued)

Table 2-1 (Continued)

Category	Include These Foods	Exclude These Foods
Dairy	Rice, hemp, almond, or coconut milk — all unsweetened and without soy	Milk from animals; products made from milk or cream (cheese, cottage cheese, cream, yogurt, butter, ice cream, frozen yogurt); non-dairy creamers
Fats	*For cooking:* Coconut oil, palm oil, ghee, cold-pressed olive oil *No heat:* Flax, safflower, sunflower, sesame, walnut, pumpkin, and almond oils	Margarine, butter, shortening, processed (hydrogenated) oils
Beverages	Filtered or distilled water, herbal tea, seltzer, or mineral water	Soda, soft drinks, alcoholic beverages, coffee, nonherbal tea, other sweetened or caffeinated beverages
Herbs, spices, and condiments	Vinegar, any spices not listed in the "Exclude" column	Chocolate, ketchup, mustard, relish, chutney, soy sauce, teriyaki, tamari, Worcestershire sauce, mayonnaise, and sandwich spreads

Although you may be immune to the nasty side effects of consuming modern wheat, people with celiac disease can't consume a single morsel of wheat without experiencing a severe reaction resulting in abdominal pain, bloating, gas, diarrhea, cramps, malabsorption of nutrients, and weight loss. And for every person who has celiac disease, at least eight others suffer from nonceliac gluten sensitivity, which is often linked to inflammation, migraines, allergic reactions, eczema, cardiovascular events, and neurological disorders.

Regardless of whether you're experiencing symptoms, eliminate wheat/gluten from your diet for the next 28 days and take note of how you feel. I'd bet dollars to those donuts you're no longer eating that you'll feel better, eat less, and achieve a healthier, stable weight with lower body fat.

Here's a way to cut 400 calories from your diet: Eliminate wheat. Approximately 25 years ago, scientists discovered that wheat stimulates appetite. In fact, eating wheat makes the average person consume an additional 400 calories a day. Eliminate wheat from your diet, and you won't feel as hungry. You'll drop weight without even trying.

Don't simply go gluten-free. Many gluten-free products are nothing more than junk food, using various starches and guar gum as substitutes for white flour. These white-flour substitutes may spike blood sugar and insulin levels even more than does white flour. Go gluten-free, but at the same time avoid loading up on gluten-free starches, such as breads and pastas. These items should be a very small portion of your diet; eat a small serving only once or twice a week.

Soy

Soy is so abundant in "health foods" that most people actually think it's healthy. However, 90 percent of all soy in the United States is derived from genetically modified organism (GMO) crops and is overly processed. Soy messes with your hormones and often triggers thyroid disorders. If your thyroid antibodies are high, eliminating soy from your diet can bring them down into normal range. Soy is also rich in phytic acid, which blocks absorption of key minerals, including calcium, magnesium, and zinc. It also blocks *trypsin,* an important enzyme for digesting protein.

If you choose to consume soy, make sure it's verified organic (non-GMO) and eat soy only in the form of fermented products, such as tempeh, tofu, and miso. Unless you're born in a culture raised on soy products, eat it only once or twice a week. Soy lecithin is permitted, because it doesn't contain the allergenic protein.

Dairy

Regardless of how they're manufactured, all dairy products contain hormones and other potentially harmful substances, such as D-galactose, a carbohydrate associated with inflammation, oxidative stress, and neurodegeneration. Dairy can make you fat and may contribute to insulin resistance and *osteoporosis* (weak, porous bones). In addition, dairy is highly allergenic and addictive. Contrary to the ads, it doesn't do a body good.

Replace dairy with high-calcium foods that are actually good for you: Brazil nuts, broccoli, flaxseeds, kale, sardines, spinach, walnuts, and wild Alaskan salmon. Replace cow milk with unsweetened, fortified oat, almond, hemp, or rice milk. Try dairy-free coconut yogurt and kefir; look for products with less sugar and additives. Switch to vegan-style rice milk cheeses as substitutes.

Eggs

Eggs may be good or bad for you. To find out, take a break from eggs for 28 days and then start eating them again once or twice a week. (Be sure to read labels carefully, because many food products contain eggs.) Journal how well you feel on and off eggs. If you feel better without eggs, you may have an egg allergy or sensitivity and may want to avoid them entirely.

However, don't be too eager to eliminate eggs altogether from your diet. Eggs are a super food. The yolks, which many anti-egg people suggest you throw away, are a nutritional gold mine. And contrary to popular belief, eggs aren't the prime culprit in raising serum cholesterol or increasing the risk of heart disease.

If you can eat eggs, buy eggs collected from pastured chickens that haven't been fed a diet of corn and soy. Don't be fooled by eggs labeled "free-range" or "organic," because these labels are part of a marketing ploy by big agricultural producers. Although they might be allowed a small space to range and may be fed organic grain-based feed, these chickens are not pastured as nature intended. They're better than conventional in that they don't contain GMO-feed and hormones, but eggs from farm-raised pastured chickens are best.

Corn

Nearly 90 percent of all corn is genetically modified. The DNA in the corn marries the DNA of gut flora, contributing to microbial imbalance and leaky gut (see Chapter 13).

Corn also contains *aflatoxin*, a known carcinogen (cancer-causing agent); *lectins*, which can cause inflammation and interfere with absorption of nutrients; and *zein,* a kind of gluten that is okay for people with celiac disease but is still inflammatory to many and may also contribute to autoimmune and gut-related health issues.

Replace corn with healthier alternatives, including organic beets, green peas, snow peas, sweet potato, and winter roots or squashes (acorn or butternut squashes, parsnips, pumpkins, sweet potatoes, and turnips). If you do eat corn, eat it sparingly, and eat only non-GMO varieties. Eliminate from your diet high-fructose corn syrup, a known toxin that raises triglyceride levels and blood pressure; fails to stimulate insulin production, resulting in overeating and contributing to obesity; increases *intestinal permeability,* enabling food particles and other large molecules that are supposed to stay inside the intestines to leak out into surrounding areas; and causes inflammation.

Peanuts

Even if you're not allergic to peanuts, avoid them as much as possible. Peanuts and peanut butter are likely to contain *aflatoxin*, a carcinogen produced by the *Aspergillus flavus* and *Aspergillus parasiticus* molds, and *lectins*, indigestible proteins that commonly trigger an immune response. In addition, most commercial peanut butters are high in sugar and trans fats (see upcoming sections covering these items).

Replace peanuts with healthier alternatives: almonds, cashews, Brazil nuts, coconut (unsweetened), macadamia nuts, walnuts, and pecans (and butters made from these nuts), but read the labels carefully to make sure these healthy nuts don't contain unhealthy added ingredients, such as cottonseed oil.

Sugar

Sugar is a major factor contributing to obesity, diabetes, heart disease, and cancer, and the average person in the U.S. consumes a whole lot of it — 152 pounds of sugar and 146 pounds of flour (which quickly converts to sugar in the body) per year.

Don't add sugar to foods or beverages, and avoid foods or beverages with added sugar. Read labels closely to identify added sugar. Most ingredients that end in *-ose* are sugars, including sucrose, maltose, dextrose, fructose, glucose, galactose, lactose, high-fructose corn syrup, and glucose solids. Sugar goes by other names, as well: agave, barley malt, brown rice syrup, buttered syrup, caramel, carob syrup, corn syrup, dextran, dextrin, diatastic malt, ethyl maltol, fruit juice, golden syrup, honey, malt syrup, maltodextrin, maple syrup, molasses, refiner's syrup, sorghum syrup, and turbinado.

Taper sugar consumption gradually. Sudden elimination of sugar is likely to make you feel exhausted, irritable, and famished. To ease the transition, replace the worst sugars (agave, brown rice syrup, corn syrup, fructose, high-fructose corn syrup, and sucrose) with lower impact sugars — brown sugar, cane sugar, cane juice, coconut nectar, raw honey, grade B maple syrup, and stevia (not Truvia, which is primarily a GMO-corn-based sugar alcohol combined with a small amount of stevia extract and "natural flavors," whatever those are).

Be very careful of foods advertised as low-fat or nonfat. In almost all cases, the fats have been replaced with sugar.

Artificial sweeteners

Steer clear of artificial sweeteners, which stimulate insulin production, increase sugar cravings, and stimulate *glycation,* a major cause of premature aging and cognitive decline. Artificial sweeteners include aspartame, NutraSweet, saccharin, Splenda, sucralose, and acesulfame potassium (Acesulfame K or Ace K). Truvia is another sugar substitute to avoid.

Try using xylitol as your sugar substitute. Xylitol is a sugar alcohol extracted from birch trees and other plant sources. It helps prevent cavities and plaque formation on teeth and is used in nasal sprays to reduce ear infections in children. Start slowly (less than 15 g daily), because xylitol may cause gastric distress if you take too much too quickly.

Trans fats

Although some meat and dairy products contain *trans fats* (*trans fatty acids*), most trans fats are manufactured through a process that adds hydrogen to vegetable oil, creating a product that's solid at room temperature. Food producers love trans fats because they're inexpensive, improve the texture of food, and increase a food's shelf life.

Unfortunately, trans fats are linked to numerous chronic diseases, including cardiovascular disease, diabetes, and brain and cognitive disorders. In addition, trans fats replace the healthy fats that the body requires to function optimally. Your goal is to reverse this trend by reducing your consumption of trans fats and increasing your consumption of healthy fats — omega-3 fatty acids found primarily in fatty fish and in olives, nuts, and seeds.

Read labels closely and eliminate anything that contains trans fat, hydrogenated oil, or partially hydrogenated oil — even if the label claims "0 grams trans fats." (Government regulations allow manufacturers to claim that their products contain no trans fats if they contain up to 0.5 grams trans fat per serving.) Trans fats are often found in margarine, shortening, fried foods, peanut butter, store-bought snack items (cookies, crackers, chips, microwave popcorn), sweets (cakes, doughnuts, and other pastries, and chocolate candy), frozen pizzas, and coffee creamers. Microwaving certain foods may also form trans fats.

Genetically modified organisms (GMOs)

GMOs are foods that have been engineered by scientists who can't possibly predict the results of their experiments. As a result, more people are eating more foods that evolution hasn't prepared the human body to process, and many of these people are becoming very ill.

To steer clear of GMOs, look for the *Verified Non-GMO* seal on products that are commonly genetically modified. Currently, farmers are growing nine GMO crops: alfalfa, canola, corn, cottonseed, Hawaiian papaya (most), soybeans, sugar beets, yellow squash (small amount), and zucchini (small amount). Thankfully, wheat (hybridized but not genetically modified), potatoes, and tomatoes failed miserably in becoming GMOs.

Stocking up on healthy foods

Unless you eat out a lot (and if you do, that has to stop), you eat whatever you buy at the grocery store and then stick in your refrigerator and pantry. When you make the decision to eat healthier, the first order of business is to dump the junk food and stock up on healthy food.

Haul a large, empty trash container into your kitchen, go through your cabinets and refrigerator, and dump your junk foods:

- ✔ Foods you're allergic or sensitive to (see the earlier section "Eliminating the foods that ail you" for details)
- ✔ Sugar and anything that contains added sugar by any of its many names (see the earlier section "Sugar")
- ✔ White flour and cornstarch and anything made with white flour and cornstarch, because these ingredients are quickly converted to sugar in the body; this includes most breads and pastas
- ✔ Anything that contains trans fats (see the earlier section, "Trans fats")
- ✔ Cookies, candy, chips, cakes, pies, and most breakfast cereals

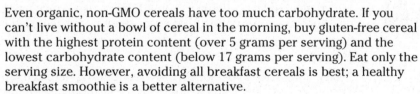

Even organic, non-GMO cereals have too much carbohydrate. If you can't live without a bowl of cereal in the morning, buy gluten-free cereal with the highest protein content (over 5 grams per serving) and the lowest carbohydrate content (below 17 grams per serving). Eat only the serving size. However, avoiding all breakfast cereals is best; a healthy breakfast smoothie is a better alternative.

- ✔ Soda pop and fruit juice (the diet stuff, too)
- ✔ Frozen prepared foods, including pizza, frozen dinners, pot pies, and burritos
- ✔ Anything that contains artificial flavoring, coloring, sweeteners, or preservatives

Also consider dumping anything that contains wheat/gluten, soy, or dairy. These three foods are at the root of many chronic illnesses. And if you really want to do yourself a favor, dump almost everything in your pantry and refrigerator/freezer with the exception of fresh vegetables, fruits, nuts, and seeds and any sources of quality protein, such as fish caught in the wild or products from pastured animals.

When the cupboards are bare, you're ready to restock them with healthy foods (I offer many suggestions in the upcoming sections). As you restock, buy organic fruits and vegetables whenever possible, because they're free of herbicides and pesticides and generally have a higher nutritional value. Wash fruits and vegetables thoroughly with a brush and nontoxic fruit and veggie wash.

Fruits and vegetables

Plant-based foods are chock-full of vitamins, antioxidants, and phytonutrients that keep your body strong and help fight infection and disease:

- ✔ **Fruits:** All fruits are healthy, but eat mostly those fruits that are relatively low on the glycemic index, including berries of all kinds, apples, cherries, coconuts, oranges, peaches, pears, and plums. Avoid dried fruits, because they contain much higher levels of sugar.

- ✔ **Vegetables:** When shopping for vegetables, choose different colors (green, red, orange, yellow, and purple) and rotate your selections. You can eat any and all vegetables raw, juiced, steamed, sautéed, or baked, but keep in mind that heating vegetables destroys some of their nutrients. Raw and juiced veggies are best.

Eat organic as much as possible, especially berries, apples, celery, and peaches, which are typically the most highly contaminated produce. Not only are organic foods pesticide-free, but they're also grown using farming methods, such as crop rotation, that produce more nutrient-rich foods.

Beans

Beans, both dried and canned, are a healthy staple to keep in your pantry. The only exception is soy beans, which you should eliminate from your diet; almost all soy products in the U.S. are genetically modified. Beans include foods actually called "beans" (lima beans, kidney beans, and so on), lentils (brown, green, and red), and split peas.

Grains: Breads, cereals, and pastas

When stocking up on grains, exclude wheat and other grains that contain gluten: wheat (spelt, khorasan, farro, durum, bulgur, semolina), barley, rye, and triticale. Instead, choose these grains, which are gluten-free: amaranth, buckwheat, millet, oats, quinoa, brown rice, white rice, wild rice, and teff. Limit your consumption of nongluten grains to no more than one serving daily.

Overcoming picky eating

If you're a parent of a picky eater and find it challenging to get your child to eat a variety of healthy foods, keep in mind that your child will eat whatever you buy. Stock the cabinets with healthy foods, and your child's choices are limited — eat healthy or starve. Your job is to put healthy food in front of your children and make it look appetizing. Leave the rest up to them in deciding what to eat (and whether or not to eat) and how much to eat.

Start young and set reasonable expectations. The average toddler consumes about 1,000 to 1,300 calories daily. He might eat a lot one day and next to nothing the next. That's normal. Don't freak out if your kid doesn't eat much for a day, but do make sure he stays hydrated. Focus on how well he eats over the course of a week. Here are some tips for encouraging your toddler to eat a healthy diet:

✔ Offer a nibble tray with a variety of different healthy foods in different, shapes, colors, and sizes. Use an ice tray or muffin tin or something similar and place in each compartment some avocados, banana, carrots, broccoli, egg, and apples. A child may need to be exposed to a new food 10 to 15 times before she tries it.

✔ Allow your child to dip foods into cottage cheese, guacamole, organic nut butters, Greek yogurt, or pureed veggies and fruits.

✔ Plant a garden. Involve your child in planting the seeds, watering the plants, and harvesting the crop.

✔ Mix veggies in with other foods (casseroles are great for hiding chopped vegetables) and instead of serving raw veggies, steam the veggies and use organic butter or organic coconut oil to flavor them.

✔ Don't make your child eat something he doesn't like or doesn't want to try. Doing so may set the stage for anxiety around mealtime. Likewise, don't bribe your child with dessert or anything else to encourage her to eat a particular food item or to eat more of something. And don't become a short order cook, because this encourages children to become picky eaters.

✔ Choose only foods that are nutrient dense; avoid processed foods that are empty calories — void of or low in nutritional value. In particular, avoid fruit juices, because most contain a high amount of sugar.

✔ Minimize distractions at mealtime (for example, turn off the TV) and set a good example by eating a variety of healthy foods yourself.

Oats are commonly contaminated with wheat. So when you're shopping for oats, read the label carefully and buy oats that are labeled "gluten-free" and are manufactured in a plant where wheat products are not processed or stored.

You typically consume grains in the form of cereals, pastas, and baked goods, including bread:

- ✔ **Cereals and pastas:** Too much carbohydrate spikes your glucose and insulin levels and triggers inflammation. For that reason, I don't advocate eating cereals and pasta routinely, but when you do have them, look for non-wheat varieties with a relatively high protein-to-carbohydrate ratio. Here's a list of acceptable cereals and pastas: Cream of Rice, oats (labeled "gluten-free" and processed in a wheat-free factory), puffed rice, puffed millet, quinoa flakes, rice pasta, 100 percent buckwheat noodles, and rice crackers.

- ✔ **Breads:** Even whole-grain, wheat-free, gluten-free breads are high in simple carbohydrates that spike blood glucose and insulin levels and have the potential to trigger inflammation. If you must eat bread, go gluten-free and look for breads stored in the freezer at the health food store or in the health food section of your grocery store, because these loaves are less likely to contain preservatives.

- ✔ **Flour:** If you do any baking, the good news is that you have plenty of options when it comes to choosing wheat-free, gluten-free flour, including amaranth, arrowroot, brown rice, chick pea (garbanzo bean), millet, potato, quinoa, sorghum, tapioca, teff, and white rice.

Grains are simple carbohydrates that spike your blood sugar and insulin and cause inflammation. If you have a health challenge, particularly an autoimmune disorder, then removing *all* grains from your diet may significantly improve your health. Many people do better on a totally grain-free diet. See the earlier section "Eliminating the foods that ail you" for details.

Herbs, spices, and extracts

Numerous herbs, spices, and extracts serve not only to flavor your food but also to improve absorption of nutrients in the foods you eat, reduce inflammation, and prevent and treat common illnesses. When stocking up on spices, be sure to include the following: basil, black pepper, cinnamon, cumin, dandelion, dill, dry mustard, garlic, ginger, nutmeg, oregano, parsley, pure vanilla extract, rosemary, sea salt, tarragon, thyme, and turmeric.

Animal proteins and fresh ocean fish

When you're in the market for meat, opt for organic, pastured animal products — from animals raised on a healthy diet free from antibiotics and growth hormones — and lean toward meat from the following animals: chicken, turkey, duck, lamb, and wild game.

Also, as you modify your diet, try to eat more cold-water, deep-diving, fatty fish mostly harvested in the wild. These types of fish are high in omega-3 essential fatty acids, which are crucial for overall health, especially a healthy brain, and help prevent and reverse inflammation. Good options include albacore tuna (packed in water, no added soy protein), cod, haddock, halibut, mahi-mahi, rainbow trout (farmed rainbow trout is okay), salmon (Alaskan or Pacific, not Atlantic), sardines, and sole.

Dairy substitutes

Milk and other dairy products trigger a host of illnesses for many people (refer to the earlier section "Eliminating the foods that ail you"), so I recommend that you eliminate it from your diet. Get your calcium from other sources, including fish, nuts, seeds, and dark green leafy vegetables. Replace milk with one of the following milk substitutes: unsweetened, fortified, full fat almond, coconut, oat, or rice milk

Avoid carrageen, which is added as a thickening agent to some major brands of milk substitutes. It can irritate the gastrointestinal tract and is a possible carcinogen. Under a microscope, it looks like charred glass.

Beverages

Avoid carbonated, caffeinated, sweetened beverages, and fruit juices. I recommend these beverages: unsweetened, caffeine-free green and herbal teas and spring water.

Vinegars and oils

Vinegar is great for seasoning salads and soups, but avoid standard white vinegar and opt for the following types instead: apple cider, balsamic, red wine, and rice.

Ditch the corn oil and canola oil and opt for one or more of the following oils for use on salads and when recipes call for oil or butter: almond, avocado, flaxseed, macadamia, olive, pumpkin, safflower, sesame, sunflower, and walnut. For high-temp cooking, use palm oil (organic or sustainably sourced) or coconut oil to prevent the formation of *atherogenic compounds,* chemicals that increase bad cholesterol and lead to clogged arteries. Use olive oil for medium-heat cooking.

Store vegetable oils in airtight, opaque containers.

Sweeteners

Buy natural, organic, verified GMO-free sweeteners and use them sparingly for treats and special occasions: brown sugar, cane sugar, coconut nectar, date sugar, organic raw honey (sourced locally), molasses, green leaf stevia (not Truvia), and xylitol.

Eliminate from your diet any and all artificial sweeteners, including sucralose, saccharine, and aspartame.

Nuts and seeds

Nuts and seeds make great snack foods. Just make sure you're buying raw, organic varieties. Many nuts have added cottonseed or canola oil, both of which are GMOs, and hydrogenated vegetable oil (trans fat). Organic is non-GMO. Add the following nuts and seeds to your pantry: almonds, cashews, flaxseeds, hazelnuts, pecans, pistachios, poppy seeds, pumpkin seeds, sesame seeds, sunflower seeds, and walnuts.

You may consume nuts and seeds as butters and spreads, but read the labels and avoid products that contain anything other than the nut or seed that the butter or spread is derived from, such as added sugar or molasses.

Adopting healthier eating habits

When and how you eat play important roles in how well you feel and how effectively your body can protect itself against infection and other illnesses. In this section, I recommend a few healthier eating habits.

Eat less, chew more

The average American adult consumes 3,700 calories per day. Ideally, daily caloric intake should be about 2,000 calories for the average woman and 2,500 for the average man. If you're overweight, one of the most effective steps you can take to improve health and increase longevity is to eat fewer calories, a strategy often referred to as *caloric restriction*.

When eating, chew your food to a liquid state before swallowing to more fully break the food up for your digestive system. Chewing food to liquid improves digestion and increases nutrient absorption.

Start the day with a healthy breakfast smoothie

Breakfast is the most important meal of the day, because it kicks your metabolism into gear. Within one hour of waking, drink a blood-sugar-stabilizing smoothie. Here's the recipe for my favorite breakfast smoothie; to make it, simply blend the following ingredients together:

   1 cup of liquid (water; almond, rice, soy, or skim milk; or diluted 100 percent juice made with ¼ cup juice and ¾ cup water)

   1 to 2 scoops of protein powder (I recommend VegaPro, a combination of hypoallergenic rice and pea protein, or a comparable product)

   ½ to 1 cup fresh or frozen fruit (no sugar added)

1 tablespoon ground or milled flaxseed or flax oil

1 tablespoon organic nut butter (optional)

Eat smaller meals more frequently

Eating smaller meals more frequently keeps your system working through-out the day so that it doesn't go into starvation mode and start to conserve energy. Therefore, instead of eating the traditional three square meals a day, eat every three to four hours. Eat before you're hungry and stop eating before you feel full. Stop eating for the day three hours before bedtime.

Ditch the fast food

Fast food is packed with trans fats, sugar, and simple carbohydrates that quickly convert to sugar after being eaten. In addition, you have no control over or knowledge of how the food was prepared or whether it contains genetically modified ingredients. Eat food you've prepared yourself, and if you must dine out, eat at a quality restaurant where the owners and staff are passionate about good nutrition.

Preparing healthy food is time-consuming and work-intensive. Set aside some time at the beginning of the week to chop vegetables and make sure you have plenty of healthy snack foods, such as nuts and fruit. Make grabbing healthy food as convenient as possible.

Stay hydrated

The average human body is mostly water, and everything in your body requires water to function properly and purge wastes. To keep your body hydrated, follow these tips:

- **Eat water.** Vegetables and fruits are mostly water, so upping your consumption of these healthy foods increases your water consumption.

- **Drink plenty of water.** Drink half your ideal body weight, in ounces, of water daily. If your ideal weight is 160 pounds, for example, you should drink about 80 ounces of water daily. Another option is to drink at least 8 ounces of water every two waking hours.

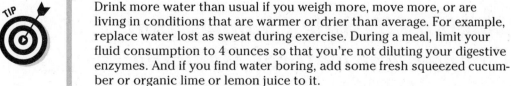 Drink more water than usual if you weigh more, move more, or are living in conditions that are warmer or drier than average. For example, replace water lost as sweat during exercise. During a meal, limit your fluid consumption to 4 ounces so that you're not diluting your digestive enzymes. And if you find water boring, add some fresh squeezed cucumber or organic lime or lemon juice to it.

- **Limit your consumption of carbonated or caffeinated beverages.** Carbonated and caffeinated beverages act as diuretics and tend to dehydrate you.

Getting quality water

Not all water is created equal. To ensure that you're getting quality water and no bad stuff, heed these suggestions:

- ✔ **Filter your tap water, which is likely to contain chemicals you shouldn't be ingesting.** Municipal water often contains chlorine and fluoride. Well water may contain pesticides, herbicides, industrial pollutants, runoff from nearby farms, and other toxins.

- ✔ **Don't drink from plastic water bottles, which contain *phthalates*, toxic chemicals that contribute to obesity and toxicity.** Use glass or stainless steel containers.

Fast occasionally

Fasting improves health: It increases brain-derived neurotrophic factor (BDNF), which supports the brain and reduces the risk of cognitive impairment, and it increases Nrf2, a protein in all cells that stimulates antioxidant activity. Fasting also stimulates the brain to use fat as fuel in the form of ketones. In mild ketosis, brain function improves, and the body taps its fat reserves for fuel. Antioxidant function improves, leading to an increase in mitochondria (the energy plants inside cells) and in production of new brain cells.

Fast four times a year, preferably when the seasons change, for optimal results. Stick with a 24-hour fast until you get the hang of it, and then gradually increase the time to 48 hours and then 72 hours. I recommend fasting on a day you don't have to work, because your brain is likely to get foggy and you may feel irritable. Have your last meal the night before the day of your scheduled fast and drink plenty of quality water on the day of your fast. Don't drink anything other than water. Continue taking any prescribed medications. Start the next morning with a healthy breakfast smoothie (refer to the earlier section "Start the day with a healthy breakfast smoothie" for a recipe).

Team up with your healthcare provider to develop a safe fasting regimen.

Making Lifestyle Changes That Complement Natural Medicine

While stress isn't inherently negative, prolonged emotional and environmental stress takes its toll on the immune, neurological, cardiovascular, reproductive, and endocrine systems and often triggers underlying genetic susceptibilities into becoming full-blown illness. In this section, I encourage you to evaluate four potential sources of stress in your life — exposure to toxins in your home, lack of quality sleep, lack of exercise, and home- and work-related stress — and I provide suggestions on how to reduce stress from these sources to improve overall health.

Detoxing your home

If you're like most people, your home is in dire need of detox. It's probably packed with toxic agents in the form of soaps, detergents, cosmetics, cleaning supplies, air fresheners, carpeting, certain types of furniture, non-stick and plastic cookware, and even the water you drink and bathe in. Following are some sources of toxins you may never have imagined as being hazardous to your health.

A good rule to follow is this: If the label instructs you to keep it away from children, you should probably keep it away from yourself, too.

Cleaning and laundry products

Most commercial cleaning and laundry products contain ingredients that are hazardous to humans and to the environment. As you use up your current cleaning and laundry supplies, replace them with safer alternatives. Look for products that carry the EPA's Design for the Environment (DfE) logo, which indicates that the product is formulated using the safest chemicals available in each category. Visit www.lesstoxicguide.ca for additional guidance. Also consider using natural cleaning agents in and around your home. When transitioning from commercial cleaning and laundry products, consider the natural cleaning agents listed in Table 2-1.

Don't use scented fabric softeners or dryer sheets. These products are loaded with harmful chemicals that trigger allergies, asthma, headaches, and a host of other ailments. Dry cleaning also leaves a toxic residue on clothes, so if you have any clothes dry cleaned, remove the plastic and then air out the clothes for 48 hours before bringing them into your home.

Air fresheners

Air fresheners contain many poisonous solvents, which can cause neurological and respiratory disorders. Many brands contain toluene and come with a drug abuse warning. Keep your house smelling fresh by opening the windows every so often to let the fresh air in or bringing nature inside in the form of plants and flowers. If you need something stronger, use essential oils, such as lavender, vanilla, and lemon oil to freshen the air.

Table 2-1	Natural Cleaning Agents
Cleaning Agent	*Use*
Baking soda	A great all-purpose cleanser.
Castile soap (made from olive and other plant-based oils)	An excellent alternative to harsh detergents and household cleaners.
Hydrogen peroxide	A great bleach alternative. Combine 1 cup hydrogen peroxide, 12 cups water, and ¼ cup lemon juice. Use 2 cups of the mixture per wash load or put it in a spray bottle to use as an all-purpose cleaner around the house.
Lemon juice	Effective for removing grease from stoves and countertops and for bleaching clothes.
Lemon oil	When mixed with a few drops of jojoba or olive oil, is great for dusting and polishing wood furniture.
Salt	Helpful for scouring cookware and removing stains from coffee pots. Combine with lemon or lime juice to remove rust stains.
Tea tree oil	When added to a vinegar and water solution, kills bacteria, mold, and mildew on kitchen and bathroom surfaces.
Vinegar	An excellent all-purpose cleaner and disinfectant. Cuts through grease and soap scum, removes stains, and is great for cleaning windows and linoleum floors.
Washing soda (a more concentrated form of baking soda)	Great for boosting the cleaning power of laundry and dishwashing soap and for cleaning sinks, countertops, and toilets.

Toxic mold

Examine your bathroom thoroughly for any water damage. Check to make sure the caulking is intact. If water gets behind the walls, toxic mold begins to grow. You probably won't smell it, but this is potentially the most toxic offense in your home. Call a professional to fix the problem immediately.

Flooring and furnishings

If you have a choice, go with genuine hardwood floors and area rugs instead of laminate and wall-to-wall carpeting. Wall-to-wall carpeting is loaded with toxic chemicals and collects allergens over time, so you're better off using area or throw rugs that you can shake out . . . outside. If you decide to install new laminate flooring or buy a house with laminate flooring, make sure the laminate is made without urea-formaldehyde glues.

Furniture and other home furnishings, such as plastic tablecloths and shower curtains, are also common sources of toxins and typically contain high levels of *pthalates,* hormone disruptors. Avoid these items altogether and choose furniture made from natural materials: solid wood (not pressboard or particle board), natural fabrics (such as cotton, wool, and linen), genuine leather, natural latex (unless you're allergic), and metal. Look for the Greenguard certification to find furniture with lower toxicity ratings.

Avoid pillows and mattresses made from foam, which *off-gases* (emits toxic gas) all night while you sleep. Purchase mattresses and pads made from natural latex (unless you're allergic) and bedding made from cotton. For healthier bedding options, check out www.ewg.org/pbdefree.

Cookware and food storage

To prevent toxins from leeching into your food, I recommend the following:

- ✔ Avoid canned foods from cans that contain bisphenol-A (BPA) linings.

- ✔ Cook in stainless steel, iron, glass, or porcelain- or ceramic-coated pots and pans rather than Teflon or aluminum.

- ✔ Store your food in glass or stainless steel containers instead of in plastic containers. If you use plastic wrap, buy products made with polyethylene, such as ClingWrap (Glad) and Handi-Wrap (Dow Chemical Company), or use wax paper as an alternative. Avoid products made with polyvinylidene chloride.

- ✔ Never microwave food in plastic containers or with plastic wrap.

- ✔ Use stainless steel or wood dish racks, not plastic.

Cosmetics and perfumes

Cosmetics, perfumes, soaps, shampoos, conditioners, sunscreen, and oral care products often contain harmful substances. Before you purchase products in any of these categories, search the Environmental Working Group's Skin Deep Cosmetics Database at www.ewg.org/skindeep. You can search for specific brands or browse product categories, such as makeup or sunscreen. You can also find out whether certain manufacturers have signed the Compact for Safe Cosmetics, a commitment to manufacture products without substances known to be or suspected of being toxic.

Airborne allergens

To clear the air of allergens, use a whole-house air filter or use room models for the rooms you spend the most time in, including your bedroom. Make sure the filter you use complies with High-Efficiency Particulate Air standards. I recommend products from IQAir (www.iqair.com) and Blueair (www.blueair.com).

Getting enough sleep

Sleep is essential for resting and rejuvenating the body. On average, you should be getting seven to eight hours of sleep daily (or nightly), and you should feel rested upon waking. If you're getting only four or five hours of sleep per day or wake up feeling tired, something's wrong. Head to Chapter 16 to find out how to deal with common sleep issues.

Depression and other mental health conditions may be at the root of a sleep disorder (sleeping too much or not enough). See Chapter 20 for details on how to address mental health conditions.

Developing a reasonable exercise routine

Regardless of your age or physical condition, you should engage in some sort of cardiovascular exercise for a minimum of 30 minutes every other day and an additional three days a week of strength training. Choose a cardiovascular exercise you enjoy, such as walking, biking, swimming, or rollerblading, and start doing it at least every other day. Your strength training may involve weight lifting, water aerobics, body-weight exercises (such as push-ups, pull-ups, and crunches), Pilates, or other exercises that challenge your strength and not necessarily your endurance.

If you just can't find the time to exercise, try anaerobic exercise (also called *high-intensity interval training, or HIIT*) for a few minutes a day. With *anaerobic exercise*, you push your body to the limit by going all out in one-minute bursts. Sprinting is a form of HIIT, and you can find plenty of HIIT routines that you can do at home or work. If you're looking for an exercise machine designed for anaerobic workouts, check out the X-iser (www.xiser.com), a mini stair-stepper that takes up very little space in your home or office. A *rebounder* (a mini trampoline) is also a great tool to get your blood circulating and improve balance and core strength with limited joint impact.

Before you begin any exercise program — and especially if you're older or have been inactive for some time — consult your healthcare provider to develop a program that's suitable for your current condition.

De-stressing at home and work

You may not have complete control over how much stress you feel at home or work, but you can reduce stress by learning communication and problem-solving skills, as well as by engaging in activities, such as yoga, tai chi, and meditation, that focus on mindfulness. Such practices are beyond the scope of this book, but you can find instructions and information about these in numerous other sources. I recommend these books by Wiley: *Meditation For Dummies,* by Stephan Bodian; *Yoga For Dummies,* by Larry Payne and Georg Feuerstein; *Relaxation For Dummies,* by Shamash Alidina; and *Mind-Body Fitness For Dummies*, by Therese Iknoian.

When it comes to diet, here are a few stress-reduction suggestions that you can implement now:

- ✔ **Stay hydrated, as explained in the earlier section "Stay hydrated."** Dehydrated, you're likely to feel tired and cranky, making you much less able to manage stress.

- ✔ **Decaf yourself.** Caffeinated beverages and energy drinks crank up your stress hormones — adrenaline and cortisone.

- ✔ **Take stress-reduction supplements to buffer your stress hormones.** Here is a list:

Supplement	Dosage
Magnesium (magnesium malate)	75 mg daily
Myo-inositol	2 g daily
Taurine	500 mg daily
GABA	100 mg daily
L-theanine (suntheanine)	50 mg daily

Chapter 3

Sampling Different Approaches to Natural Cures

*N*atural cures cover all healthcare approaches that fall outside the realm of conventional medicine: aromatherapy, Ayurveda, biofeedback, chelation, herbal medicine, and acupuncture, just to name a few. This book draws from all of these health and wellness *modalities* (treatment approaches) to provide the most effective alternative treatments for the most common ailments.

In my coverage of common illnesses and ailments in Part II of this book, I often mention one or more of these modalities as possibly effective treatments for specific conditions. In this chapter, I explain the philosophy behind each modality, offer insight into what each modality is generally best for, and provide basic how-to information for any modality you can practice on your own; for example, you probably can't give yourself acupuncture, but you can prepare an herbal tea or prepare and apply a homeopathic linament. A basic understanding of the modalities enables you to better understand the treatment options I discuss throughout this book. (*Note:* In certain sections, you may need to skip to the Appendixes for detailed information; for example, Appendix D provides details about commonly used herbs, and Appendix E covers homeopathic remedies.)

Aromatherapy

Aromatherapy is the art and science of using aromatic oils extracted from plants to improve and maintain the health, balance, and well-being of mind, body, and spirit. The theory is that the essential oils in certain plants help them to adapt to and thrive in a constantly changing environment, and these oils offer similar benefits for the human body.

Aromatherapy usually involves mixing an essential oil with a carrier oil, such as almond or avocado oil, to dilute the essential oil and make it easier to apply.

 Although aromatherapy is based on breathing in the aroma of essential oils, these oils permeate the body through the nose and nasal passages, the lungs, and the skin (when applied directly to the skin) and trigger numerous positive biological and emotional responses.

Shopping for essential oils and carriers

When shopping for essential oils, first consider the purpose of the oil. For example, lavender oil is good for treating anxiety, sleep issues, and skin conditions, including burns and insect bites. See Appendix F for a list of common essential oils and conditions each is used to treat.

The second consideration is whether you really need an essential oil or some other form of the essence:

- *Pure essential oils* are distilled from plants.

- *Hydrosols* are byproducts of the distillation process — typically diluted products, which are okay if you're just inhaling the aroma.

- *Absolutes* are highly concentrated forms for the pure essential oils. These generally enable you to use less of the product.

- *Oil/carrier mixes* are essential oils mixed with a carrier, which is fine if you don't want to mix these on your own. Just be sure to check the concentration.

- *Synthetic oils* are manufactured scents, sometimes called *fragrance oils* or *floral waters*. Avoid synthetic oils. Stick with genuine plant extracts, which contain trace elements not available in synthetic products.

A *carrier* is anything you mix with the essential oil (usually another type of plant-based oil or lotion) to dilute the essential oil and make application easier. In general, choose organic, cold-pressed, unrefined, vegetable oils that contain no additives. Refer to Table 3-1 for a list of common, recommended carriers.

Table 3-1	Aromatherapy Essential Oil Carriers	
Carrier	**Recommended for**	**Notes**
Almond oil	Body massage Relieving itching, dryness, and inflammation	Light, well-penetrating oil with a light aroma that doesn't over-power the essential oil *Warning:* Avoid if you're allergic to tree nuts
Apricot oil	Facial application	Leaves skin soft and supple and is better than almond oil for sensitive and prematurely aged skin
Argan oil	Body massage and facial application	Penetrates deeply to hydrate skin, hair, and nails
Avocado oil	Softening dry, mature, and damaged skin	Mixes well with other oils, penetrates deeply, and may help with eczema and psoriasis
Borage oil	Softening fine lines and wrinkles and possibly helping with joint stiffness and pain	Mix with a lighter carrier for massage
Canola oil (non-GMO)	Massage	Is light and offers good skin penetration
Coconut oil	Moisturizing hands, body, and hair	Is a good massage oil with antimicrobial properties *Warning:* Avoid if you're allergic to coconut
Flaxseed oil	Healing and regenerating skin	Is high in vitamin E
Grapeseed oil	Massage	Is light, satiny, and great for oily and acne-prone skin; offers good skin penetration
Hazelnut oil	Maintaining skin elasticity and firmness	Good choice for people with oily skin who want to use oils *Warning:* Avoid if you're allergic to tree nuts
Jojoba oil	Deep cleansing of blocked pores, moisturizing, and promoting healthy skin and complexion	Extends shelf life of other oils in mixture

(continued)

Table 3-1 *(continued)*

Carrier	Recommended for	Notes
Macadamia nut oil	Healing, regenerating, and conditioning skin	Deeply penetrates and mimics skin's own protective oils *Warning:* Avoid if you're allergic to tree nuts
Olive oil	Conditioning skin and hair	Mixes well with other oils
Sunflower oil	Nourishing and conditioning dry, damaged, weathered, and sensitive skin	Is high in vitamin E
Vitamin E oil	Repairing and conditioning skin	Mix with another carrier instead of using as sole carrier

When you purchase essential oils and carriers, keep these points in mind:

- Regardless of whether you're in the market for essential oils or carriers, buy from a reputable dealer — someone who's been in the business for many years and has a solid reputation among aromatherapy practitioners.

- Essential oils should be stored in dark glass bottles, which provide some protection from sunlight. Store them in a cool, dark place to maximize their shelf life. A refrigerator is ideal. Likewise, store your carrier oils in a cool, dark place.

Using essential oils

You can use essential oils with carrier oils and other substances in several ways, as this section explains.

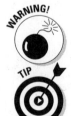

Essential oils are highly concentrated and can actually damage your skin if applied full strength. They're also highly volatile, meaning they evaporate quickly. Mixing the essential oil with a carrier oil gives the essential oil more time to do its magic before it evaporates into thin air.

Before mixing your oils, let your carrier oils warm up to room temperature and give them a good shake; these oils tend to separate when cooled, especially if you store them in a refrigerator.

Inhaling oils directly

One of the easiest and most direct ways to experience aromatherapy is to breathe the aroma of an essential oil. Rub a couple drops of the essential oil you want to use between your palms, cup your hands over your nose and mouth, and breathe in and out deeply several times. To open your sinuses, relieve headache, or steam-treat your face, place a few drops of essential oil in a bowl of steaming water and breathe in the steam; using a towel as a tent to cover your head and the bowl intensifies the treatment.

You can also dissolve a few drops in distilled water and spray it in a room, as you would an air freshener, or use various types of diffusers as essential oil air fresheners, including candle diffusers, electric heat diffusers, and cool-air nebulizers.

Consider making your own essential-oil perfume by mixing 10 to 20 drops of an essential oil with about $\frac{1}{8}$ ounce of a carrier oil and dabbing a little on each wrist or behind your ears.

Applying oils to your skin or hair

Depending on the desired effect and the type of essential and carrier oils you use, you can apply the oil to your skin as a facial or body lotion or to your hair as a conditioner. Certain essential oils combined with jojoba oil make great hair-conditioning treatments.

You can also purchase unscented varieties of shampoos, conditioners, and body and hand lotions and add your own essential oils to them. Add about 10 drops of essential oil per ounce of the other product.

Combining oils with massage

Essential oils are commonly used in massage as a one-two punch to knock out whatever ails you. Each — the oil and the massage — is therapeutic on its own. When combined, they magnify the effects of one another: Massage relaxes muscles and mind, detoxifies, and helps the essential oils penetrate the skin more deeply, and the essential oils have their own relaxation and healing properties that complement the massage.

Preparing a bath

Essential oils are great additions to a bath, where you can absorb the oils through your skin while breathing the steam:

1. **Choose essential oils that are mild and safe for bathing, such as lavender, clary sage, rose, geranium, frankincense, or cedar.**

   Avoid spicy oils, such as cinnamon, oregano, and thyme; citrus oils; and lemongrass.

2. **Mix 5 to 10 drops of essential oil with ½ to 1 cup of salts or an emulsifier, such as milk or sesame oil.**

   If you don't mix the essential oil with the salts or emulsifier, the oil simply floats on the water's surface and may be too concentrated for your skin.

3. **Add the mixture to your bathtub and fill with comfortably warm water.**

Preparing and applying compresses

To treat localized aches, pains, bruises, wounds, or skin conditions, place about 10 drops of essential oil in 4 ounces of warm water, soak a cloth in the solution, apply the cloth to the affected area, and wrap the area with an elastic or cloth bandage.

Using essential oils in mouthwashes

Essential oil mouthwashes are great for general oral hygiene, mouth ulcers, and gum disease. Combine 3 to 5 drops of essential oil, 1 or 2 drops of peppermint oil, 1 teaspoon of vodka, and ½ cup of warm distilled water. After brushing, swish the mixture around in your mouth for 30 to 60 seconds and then spit it out.

Ayurveda

Ayurveda (literally "the science of life") is one of the oldest forms of medicine, originating over 3,000 years ago in India. The approach, which parallels the approach presented in this book, relies heavily on diet, herbal remedies, exercise, and lifestyle recommendations as a way to achieve and maintain optimum health and well-being. In addition, many of the herbal remedies discussed later in this chapter and in Appendix D can be traced back to Ayurveda.

Biofeedback

Biofeedback is a mind-over-matter approach to treating common physical and mental health issues, including anxiety, asthma, attention deficit hyperactivity disorder (ADHD), chronic obstructive pulmonary disease (COPD), chronic pain, depression, epilepsy, headaches (including migraines), high blood pressure, post-traumatic stress disorder (PTSD), Raynaud's disease, sleep disorders, and urinary incontinence.

In a typical biofeedback session, a practitioner hooks you up to one or more monitors to measure heart rate, breathing, brain wave activity, muscle tension, skin temperature, and sweating. These monitors are connected to a feedback device that lets you know, via simple visual or auditory signals, when your bodily functions are revving up or slowing down. The practitioner engages you in one or more relaxation exercises, as explained in the following sections, and you practice using these techniques while monitoring your own progress. Over time, the positive physiological changes persist without the use of biofeedback.

A session typically lasts 30 minutes to an hour. The number of sessions required varies, depending on the condition and your progress in mastering the relaxation techniques. As you might guess, the cost can get pretty steep, and few insurance plans cover biofeedback. The good news is that you can practice many of these relaxation exercises at home.

To find a qualified biofeedback practitioner, visit the Association for Applied Psychophysiology and Biofeedback website at www.aapb.org and click Find a Practitioner. For home use, I recommend emWave2 manufactured by HeartMath (www.heartmath.com).

Practicing deep breathing exercises

With deep breathing exercises, you become more mindful of every inhalation and exhalation and the sensations of each part of your body in succession. You can find plenty of deep breathing exercises on the web; most of these exercises go something like this:

1. **Sit perfectly still and relaxed in a comfortable chair.**

2. **Take a slow, deep breath.**

3. **Exhale slowly and completely while concentrating on all the sensations you're feeling in your feet.**

   Focus on the sensations in your toes, heel, and arch: the temperature, the feel of any clothing or air, the pressure against the floor or chair, the feel of blood pumping.

4. **Breathe in slowly, imagining yourself breathing in all these sensations. Feel them flowing into and filling your lungs.**

5. **Exhale slowly, imagining your body releasing all those sensations. Continue to exhale until you've completely emptied your lungs.**

6. **Perform Steps 4 and 5 once or twice before proceeding to the next step.**

7. **Repeat Steps 2 through 6 with the next part of your body, and continue to repeat until you've attended to every part of your body.**

Qigong physical and breathing exercises are a great way to relax and revitalize your mind, body, and spirit. For additional information, visit www.robertpeng.com.

Engaging in progressive muscle relaxation

With progressive muscle relaxation, you focus your attention on a muscle group as you tense up and then relax the muscles in that group. I recommend starting at the top and working down, or starting at the bottom and working up. For a bottom-up approach, the sequence goes something like this: toes, feet, calves, thighs, buttocks, stomach, back, upper arms, forearms, hands, shoulders, neck, jaw, lips, cheeks, nose, eyes, forehead. Perform the sequence, tensing and then releasing tension of each muscle group, at least a twice.

You can do these exercises anywhere and in any position — sitting at your desk, standing on the bus, or sitting in your recliner after a long day at work or school, for example.

Using guided imagery

If you ever imagined the scent of a certain perfume or gotten goose bumps thinking about something that scared you in the past, you have a small taste of what guided imagery is all about. With guided imagery, you're led through a process of fully engaging your senses and your imagination to induce targeted physical or mental changes. For example, a cancer patient may be led through a process of imagining her immune system sending natural killer (NK) cells and T-cells into battle and destroying the enemy cancer cells.

You can harness the power of guided imagery with the help of a qualified practitioner or on your own, by using your imagination or by reading or listening to guided imagery scripts.

Practicing mindfulness meditation

Mindfulness is a meditation therapy that enables you to live in the moment and experience it more fully. With mindfulness, you observe thoughts just as you observe clouds passing overhead. You come to realize that thoughts and feelings are just as ephemeral and changing as clouds and, as such, have no control over you. They can't make you feel tense, depressed, or anxious. Thoughts and feelings no longer control you or your emotions.

To practice mindfulness meditation on your own, flip the switch from *doing* mode to *being* mode. For example, when you're washing your dishes, observe yourself and become more aware of how you're feeling right now — think about your emotional state, the warmth and texture of the water, the weight of the plate or pan you're washing, the sound of the water, the feeling of your clothes against your skin. If you're sad, simply acknowledge the feeling. Don't try to deny it or avoid it; simply observe it.

 Mindfulness is great for cranking down the volume on negative self-talk that can get you down. You crowd out your inner voices and any concerns about the future with thoughts and sensations. For more about mindfulness, check out *Mindfulness For Dummies,* by Shamash Alidina (John Wiley & Sons, Inc.).

Chelation

Chelation is used in conventional medicine to remove from the body toxic heavy metals, such as lead, mercury, aluminum, nickel, and arsenic, that the body itself can't otherwise excrete. Chelating agents, including EDTA (ethylene diamine tetraacetic acid) and DMSA (dimercaptosuccinic acid), bind chemically to the toxic metal molecules, so the newly formed compounds can be flushed from the system. In addition to its use in treating heavy-metal toxicity, chelation has shown some promise in treating cardiovascular illnesses and improving atherosclerosis (see Chapter 17). It may also be helpful in treating autism, ADHD, and a host of other conditions that may be related to heavy-metal toxicity.

 Chelation also removes beneficial nutrients from the body, including calcium, iron, and zinc, so proceed with caution (in many cases, chelation is administered with large doses of vitamins and minerals to replace those removed during chelation). Before undergoing any heavy metal detoxification program, have your healthcare practitioner test for metal toxicity and confirm the presence of heavy metals in your body and then obtain treatment under the supervision of a trained functional medical doctor. Make sure your doctor also monitors your kidney function.

 There are things that you can do everyday to assist your body in detoxifying heavy metals gently without undergoing heavy duty chelation. Adopt a healthier diet, as I explain in Chapter 2, and increase your intake of glutathione, magnesium, silymarin, calcium D-glucarate, quercetin, watercress, and milk thistle to start. Also be aware of how you can be exposed to heavy metals (pesticides, pressure-treated wood, paints, petroleum-based products, and environmental lead for example), and avoid these altogether or take reasonable precautions.

Functional Medicine

In functional medicine, knowing what kind of patient has the disease is more important than knowing what kind of disease the patient has.

With conventional medicine, health is the absence of illness. Your doctor diagnoses what ails you and then prescribes a medication to treat it. This approach is usually fine for acute illnesses, trauma, and infections, but it falls short in the treatment of chronic illnesses, including allergies, hormonal imbalances, heart disease, diabetes, metabolic syndrome, neurological conditions, and cancer. In these cases, conventional medicine usually provides only symptom relief.

In contrast, functional medicine views illness as a symptom of dysfunction. The goal is to restore function, not fight illness. Instead of following your doctor's orders, you build a collaborative relationship with your doctor and take ownership of your own health and well-being. You have a vested interest in your own health and are more motivated to make the sustained changes to diet and lifestyle required to achieve optimum health and vitality.

Following are the six principles of functional medicine:

- ✔ Nature and nurture are different for every individual, so treatment plans must be individualized.
- ✔ Evidence-based medicine supports a patient-centered rather than illness-centered approach to medical treatment.
- ✔ The treatment goal is to achieve a balance internally and externally with body, mind, and spirit.
- ✔ Internal function relies on a complex web of relationships that must be understood and nurtured to achieve optimum health.
- ✔ Health is vitality, not merely the absence of illness.
- ✔ Promoting healthy organ function enhances health span instead of merely extending the lifespan of each patient.

To find a functional medicine practitioner, visit www.functionalmedicine. org, click Find a Practitioner, and use the resulting page to conduct your search. When consulting a functional medicine doctor for the first time, don't expect a quick fix. The doctor will perform an examination and conduct an extensive interview first to get up to speed on your unique physiology and environment.

The first step in practicing functional medicine is to adopt a healthier diet and lifestyle, as explained in Chapter 2. Many of the treatments recommended in Part II rely heavily on functional medicine — providing your body with the nutrients it needs to restore function and eliminate ailments on its own.

Herbal Medicine

Herbal remedies represent one of the oldest forms of medicine, relying on certain plants or plant extracts to treat a host of ailments ranging from indigestion and athlete's foot to heart disease and cancer. In Part II, I highlight herbs that have shown some promise in treating specific ailments, such as turmeric for the prevention of Alzheimer's. Appendix D provides a list of commonly prescribed herbs along with ailments that each herb is used to treat.

In this section, I explain the basics of choosing, making, and using herbal remedies; offer some shopping tips and safety precautions; and provide general guidelines on adjusting dosages for children.

Choosing and using herbal preparations

Herbal remedies come in numerous forms and can be used in various ways to treat different conditions. For example, arnica is commonly packaged as a liniment to apply to bruises and sprains, whereas slippery elm bark, which is helpful in treating colds and sore throats, is commonly available in the form of lozenges or as a powder you use to create tea. Read on for guidance on choosing and using common herbal preparations.

Baths

Herbs are commonly added to baths in the form of bath salts combined with essential oils (refer to the earlier section "Aromatherapy" for more on essential oils). Lavender is one of the most commonly used herbs, because of its pleasant scent and relaxation properties, but chamomile, eucalyptus, basil, fennel, rosemary, and lemon balm are also popular choices. Placing your herbs in a cotton muslin bag and soaking the bag and its ingredients in your bath water is another option.

Compresses

Compresses are commonly used to alleviate pain and inflammation, clear congestion, relieve headaches, and promote relaxation. You can make a compress simply by making a tea out of selected herbs and then soaking a cloth in the tea and applying it to the affected area, usually for a minimum of 10 minutes and a maximum of 4 hours.

Another option is to sprinkle your herbs with water or rice vinegar and then steam them for 10 to 15 minutes, wait for them to cool enough so you don't burn yourself, and then apply them directly to the affected area. (Test the compress against your inner forearm to make sure it's not too hot.) In certain applications (for example, for treating headaches), refrigerate the steamed herbs to create a cold compress before applying it.

Wait at least 24 hours before using a warm compress to treat swelling or inflammation or to promote the healing of a wound. Applying heat too soon after injury intensifies the body's natural inflammation.

Creams

Many herbal remedies are available as creams, which penetrate the skin better than do salves and ointments. If you're a do-it-yourselfer, you can create your own herbal cream by following this simple recipe.

Ingredients

1 cup of oil (may be infused with herbs; see "Infused oil" to find out how to make herb-infused oil)

1 cup of water (may be infused with herbs; see "Decoction" and "Infused water" to find out how to make two types of water-based herbal solutions)

1 ounce of beeswax (an emulsifier that enables the oil and water to mix)

48 to 240 drops of essential oils or tinctures, optional (see "Tincture" to find out how to prepare a tincture); use 3 to 6 drops per ounce of cream for sensitive skin or 6 to 15 drops per ounce of cream for normal skin (¼ teaspoon = 25 drops, ½ teaspoon = 50 drops, 1 teaspoon = 100 drops)

Directions

1. Warm 1 cup of the infused oil in a double boiler.

A double boiler protects an ingredient from direct heat and prevents overheating. If you don't have a double boiler, you can make one by placing a bowl on top of a pot of boiling water so that the steam rises and heats the bowl.

2. Add 1 ounce of beeswax to the oil and stir until the beeswax completely dissolves.

3. Allow the beeswax/oil mixture to cool to lukewarm.

4. Slowly add any essential oils or tinctures to the beeswax/oil mixture and mix them in, using a handheld electric mixer.

5. **Continue mixing as you slowly add the cup of water (or water-based herbal solution).**

6. **Continue mixing until the mixture achieves a creamy consistency.**

Store your cream in a glass jar in the refrigerator to maximize its shelf life. Although shelf life varies depending on the ingredients you used, refrigeration typically extends the shelf life from one to three months.

Decoction

A *decoction* is a tea, usually made from the roots, seeds, berries, or bark of a plant. If you're using the leaves or flowers of a plant, create an herbal infusion instead (see the section "Infused water" for instructions).

To create a decoction, bruise and smash the herbs (use a mortar and pestle or a hammer for tougher parts of the plant). Place your herbs in a pan, cover them with water, bring the water to a boil, and then turn down the heat and let the herbs simmer for at least 20 minutes (longer if you want a more highly concentrated decoction). Strain the mixture through a cloth or coffee filter.

You can drink a decoction as a tea or use it to create creams, ointments, or salves. A decoction generally has a shelf life of about two days or four days when refrigerated.

Essential oils

Essential oils are highly concentrated oils extracted from plants. In herbal medicine, essential oils are commonly used to increase the potency of other herbal preparations, including creams, salves, and ointments. See "Aromatherapy," earlier in this chapter, for more about essential oils.

Fomentation

A *fomentation* is a cloth soaked in an herbal infusion or decoction and then applied to the affected area — usually a part of the body experiencing pain or inflammation. Fomentations are also commonly used to treat rashes and other skin ailments.

Glycerite

Glycerites are herbal extracts made using a United States Pharmacopeia (USP) food-grade, vegetable-based glycerin instead of alcohol. They're generally not as potent as their alcohol counterparts, but they're a good alternative for children and for adults who have alcohol sensitivities. To make your own glycerite, follow these steps:

1. Fill a clean jar with a fresh, chopped herb; if you're using dried herb, fill the jar halfway.

2. Fill the jar to about 1 inch from the top with about three parts glycerin to one part distilled water.

3. Using a chopstick or the handle of a wooden spoon, poke the plant material down into the glycerin-water mixture to cover the plant material with the solution and release air bubbles.

4. Add glycerin to bring the level back to about 1 inch from the top of the jar.

5. Cap and label the jar with the name of the herb and the date and store it in a dark location at room temperature for four to six weeks. Gently agitate it every few days and top off with glycerin as needed to keep the plant material covered.

6. Strain the mixture through cheesecloth and squeeze it tightly to get as much glycerite as possible.

7. Pour the glycerite into a jar, seal it, and label the jar with the name of the herb and the date. Store the glycerite in a cool, dark location.

Glycerites have a shelf life of one to two years.

You can use your glycerite as a tincture, typically adding ¼ to ½ teaspoon (30 to 60 drops) to water or tea. Glycerites are sweeter than alcohol-based tinctures, so you may not need to sweeten your drink with honey.

Infused water

Infused water is basically herbal tea that's allowed to steep for more time. To create an herbal infusion, place 2 to 4 teaspoons of dried herb (more if you're using fresh herbs) in a teapot or bowl, boil some water, and then pour about 1 cup of the boiled water over the herbs. Mix gently, cover the mixture, and let it steep for 10 to 15 minutes. Strain the mixture through a coffee filter or a cloth.

You can drink the herbal infusion as a tea or use it to create compresses, creams, ointments, salves, and other herbal preparations. The infusion has a shelf life of about two days when refrigerated.

Infused oil

Infused oil is vegetable oil that's been used to extract the active ingredients from herbs. Infused oil is great to use by itself in massage or topical applications. You can also use it to create creams, ointments, and salves.

To make infused oil, you need a vegetable oil (olive, sunflower, or almond oil are generally best) and dried or fresh herbs (I recommend using dried herbs to prevent moisture and mold). You can use the cold or the hot method to create your infused oil; choose the method you prefer or that is recommended for the particular herb you're using:

- ✔ **The cold method:** Fill a dry jar about halfway with dried herbs (or all the way with fresh herbs), add oil to about one inch from the top of the jar, stir the oil and herbs with a chopstick or the handle of a wooden spoon to cover all the herbs with oil and release any air bubbles, add oil to bring the level back up to about an inch from the top, seal the jar, label it with the herb's name and the date, and place it in the sun for three to six weeks, gently agitating it every few days.

- ✔ **The warm method:** This method requires a double boiler. Mix your herbs and oil in the inner portion of the double-boiler: for fresh herbs, the oil should just cover the herbs; for dried herbs, use more oil, because the herbs will expand. Bring the water to a boil, set the bowl with the oil and herb mixture on top, cover the bowl, turn down the heat, and let the mixture simmer for 2 to 3 hours. Remove the bowl and let the mixture cool until it's cool enough to handle.

Whichever method you choose, strain the oil-herb mixture through a muslin cloth and squeeze it to extract as much oil as possible. Pour the oil into a clean, dry jar; label it with the name of the herb and the date; and store it in a cool, dark location.

To increase the potency of your infused oil, stir in a few drops of essential oil from the same herb or repeat the infusion process, using the infused oil you made instead of starting with fresh oil.

Lozenge

Certain herbs, such as slippery elm bark, are often available as lozenges for treating coughs, sore throats, and congestion. You can create your own lozenges by combining 1 cup of water-based herbal infusion (see "Infused water") with 1½ cups of honey, heating the mixture while stirring until it reaches 300 degrees Fahrenheit/148.9 degrees Celsius (use a candy thermometer), and then pouring it into candy molds or on a baking sheet that's been greased with coconut oil. Toss the cooled lozenges in slippery elm bark powder and xylitol to keep them from sticking together.

Pill

Almost all herbs come in a pill form, typically a capsule or caplet that you can swallow. This provides a convenient way to take herbs, especially those that have an unpleasant smell or taste. If you're giving the herbs to a child who can't swallow pills, opt for capsules, because you can usually open them and pour the contents into water or juice or sprinkle it on food.

Poultice

An herbal *poultice* is simply mashed herbs spread on a cloth and applied directly to the skin. If you use dried herbs, grind them with a mortar and pestle, place them in a bowl, and add enough hot water to make a thick paste. Spread the paste on a cloth and apply it to the affected area. If you use fresh herbs, bruise/soften them with a mortar and pestle and perhaps simmer them in a little water for a couple minutes, and then spread them on a clean cloth and apply them to the affected area.

After you apply the poultice, you can then cover the it with a warm, moist cloth and wrap it with a long piece of cloth or an elastic bandage to keep it contained and avoid making a mess. You usually leave the poultice on for 1 to 24 hours and may change the warm, moist cloth several times to maximize the benefits of heat application.

Salves

Herbal salves are great for topical applications that don't require deep penetration. To make a salve, combine about 5 parts infused oil with 1 part beeswax beads or shavings, and warm the mixture in a double boiler, stirring until the beeswax is completely melted. You may add certain ingredients, including essential oils (to contribute medicinal scents), vitamin E (to condition the skin), glycerin (to improve shelf life), and lanolin (unless you're allergic to wool, to make the salve creamier).

Steam

For upper-respiratory ailments and certain other conditions, add herbs to boiled water and breathe in the steam. Placing your head over the water and tenting a towel over your head to keep the steam in maximizes the effect, but be careful not to get so close to the steaming water that you burn your face.

Suppository

Herbal suppositories are frequently used to treat hemorrhoids and vaginitis. You can purchase these or make your own, using this recipe.

Ingredients

> 1 ounce decoction or infused water of the herb you want to use
>
> 1 ounce pure vegetable glycerin
>
> 2 ounces distilled water (or for hemorrhoids, 1 ounce water and 1 ounce witch hazel–infused water)
>
> 1 envelope (about 7 grams or ¼ ounce) of gelatin

Instructions

Combine and heat all the ingredients in a double boiler. Then pour it into molds and cool the suppositories in the refrigerator or freezer.

To make your own mold for anal suppositories, wrap aluminum foil around a fat pencil (about a half inch in diameter), pull out the pencil, and pinch one end of the foil cylinder closed or fold it over so that the finished product is bullet-shaped. Vaginal suppositories are usually more egg-shaped; use a mini-ice cube tray that makes rounded cubes.

Syrup

For coughs and colds, herbal syrups are just what the doctor ordered. Combine 2 ounces of concentrated herbal infusion or decoction with 1 quart of distilled water; add 1 cup of honey, maple syrup, or vegetable glycerin; and heat on a low setting, stirring until the honey combines with the liquid (at about 110 degrees Fahrenheit/43.3 degrees Celsius). You can add a few drops of an essential oil or a small amount of brandy to improve the flavor and smell. The brandy also extends the shelf life.

Tea

Herbal teas are essentially water-based herbal infusions that may not be steeped quite as long as traditional infusions. Simply place your herbs in a tea pot, pour in boiling water, and let the mixture steep for at least a few minutes. Strain and drink.

Tincture

A *tincture* is typically an herbal extract in which alcohol is used to extract the active ingredients from the herbs. To make a tincture, here's what you do:

1. **Place your herb in a jar, filling the jar about half way with dry herbs or nearly to the top with fresh herbs.**

   Dry herb expands.

2. **Pour 80 to 100 proof vodka or grain alcohol over the herbs to fully cover them.**

3. **Mix with a chopstick or the handle of a wooden spoon to remove air and ensure that all the herbs are soaked in alcohol. Add alcohol, if necessary, to cover the herbs.**

4. **Seal the jar and label it with the name of the herb and the date.**

5. **Store the jar in a cool, dark place, gently agitating it every two to three days and adding alcohol as needed to keep the herbs covered. Do this for six to eight weeks.**

6. **Strain the mixture through a cheese cloth, capturing the filtered tincture in a clean, dry jar or bowl; squeeze the remaining mixture in the cheese cloth to extract as much tincture as possible.**

7. **Pour the tincture into dark, glass dropper bottles and label them with the name of the herb and the date.**

   Tinctures have a very long shelf life, lasting for several years.

To use tinctures, simply apply the drops under your tongue in the recommended dosage. If the alcohol is too strong, add the tincture to hot water or tea and allow the alcohol to evaporate before drinking.

Gathering herbs and using them safely

The best herbs are fresh. You can grow them yourself; get them from friends who grow herbs; buy them at the grocery store, health food store, or farmer's market; or find them growing in the wild. If you buy herbs, look for certified organic products or those that are *wildcrafted* — harvested from wild stands. You can also purchase dried herbs, but if you do, purchase them from a reputable dealer and look for packaged herbs (not loose) that are stored in airtight packaging that protects the herbs from sunlight. Commercial herbs sold in grocery stores are okay in a pinch, but they tend to be overfertilized and water-heavy.

Any substance that's powerful enough to cure you is usually powerful enough to make you sick, so when using herbs, follow these precautions:

✔ Research any herb thoroughly before using it to create an herbal preparation (see Appendix D).

✔ Follow instructions, especially recommended dosages. More isn't necessarily better and may actually make you ill.

✔ If you take any medication, prescription or over-the-counter, consult your doctor or pharmacist before adding an herbal remedy to the mix. Herbal remedies may complicate treatment by increasing or reducing the effectiveness of the medication you're taking or by causing a dangerous interaction. Certain herbs are also contraindicated (not to be used) for certain conditions.

✔ If you're pregnant, planning a pregnancy, or nursing, consult your doctor before taking any herbal remedies.

If you feel worse after you start taking an herbal remedy, stop taking it or take less of it. Common side effects of taking the wrong herb or too much of an herb are stomachache, cramps, and diarrhea.

Adjusting dosages for children

To use herbal remedies safely with children, use less concentrated forms of the herbal remedy, give less of it, or do both. Although there are all sorts of methods that help you convert adult dosages to children's dosage — things like Clark's rule (divide the child's weight by the weight of an average adult (150 pounds) and then multiply that by the adult dosage), or Cowling's rule (divide the child's age at his next birthday by 24 and multiply the result by the adult dosage) — an easier approach is to follow this chart, which I repeat in Chapter 12:

Weight (in Pounds)	Dosage
5 to 29	⅕ the adult dosage
30 to 59	¼ the adult dosage
60 to 89	⅓ the adult dosage
90 to 119	½ the adult dosage
120 to 150	¾ the adult dosage

Note: If you are an adult who falls into the 120 to 150 pound range, you should also follow the dosage outlined in this chart.

Consult a doctor before giving any herbal remedy to a child under the age of six months. Also, don't use honey to sweeten an herbal tea or other preparation for any child under 1 year old. Honey may contain a certain bacterial spore that can cause infant botulism, which can be fatal.

Homeopathy

The principle that drives homeopathy is this: *Like cures like.* Like vaccines, homeopathy challenges the body with a substance to trigger a reaction that helps the body fend off disease. In the case of a conventional vaccine based on the like-treats-like theory, weak or dead viruses or bacteria are typically injected into the body to provoke a response from the body's immune system. Homeopathic remedies are rarely injected, and instead of bacteria and viruses, they contain minute doses of natural substances — mineral, plant, or animal — that, if given to healthy people in larger doses, would cause the symptoms of a particular illness. The homeopathy remedy that's most similar to a conventional vaccine is a *nosode*, in which the active ingredient is a diseased tissue or an entity that causes the disease (bacteria, parasite, virus, and so on) that has been rendered sterile.

Unlike conventional vaccines that can cause undesirable side effects, homeopathic remedies are extremely dilute, at some potencies, so dilute that no molecule of the original substance is likely to be left in the solution. As a result, homeopathic remedies can't harm you and won't cause any dangerous drug interactions. They're also pain-free, usually taken by mouth, *sublingually* (under the tongue). Skeptics argue that the remedies are so dilute they're ineffective.

Homeopathic remedies are provided at different potencies expressed in terms of *x* and *C*. 3x, for example, is 10^3 or 1,000; and 3C is 100^3 or 1,000,000. You generally take lower potencies (3x or 6x) for acute illness and higher potencies (up to 30C) for chronic illness. Just be aware of the different potencies and take the potency that's recommended for the condition you have.

Don't use homeopathy to treat acute, life-threatening illnesses, such as deadly viral or bacterial infections. Conventional medicine is the approach of choice for battling these illnesses.

Taking homeopathic remedies

In most cases, you take a homeopathic remedy 20 minutes between eating or drinking, and you take them *sublingually* — under your tongue. If you're taking pills or pellets, hold them under your tongue until they dissolve.

You can find homeopathic remedies at nearly any health food store and online. I use a company called Deseret Biologicals (DesBio, for short) (www.desbio.com). Homeopathic remedies generally come packaged as liquids in dropper bottles or as tiny, round pills, or pellets. Turn to Appendix E to find the substance for the ailment you need to treat.

Don't take a homeopathic remedy for more than two weeks, because at that point your body has become accustomed to it and will no longer react to the substance.

Treating specific imbalances with cell salts

Homeopathic cell salts are intended to treat mineral deficiencies. They usually come in 6x potencies in liquid or pill form. You take them as you take any homeopathic remedy — sublingually 20 minutes before or after eating or drinking. Table 3-2 lists commonly used cell salts along with conditions they're used to treat.

Certain substances, such as mint, coffee, and some essential oils, are considered antidotes for homeopathic remedies and are thought to negate the effects of treatments. Some homeopathic companies such as Energetix use a method of production intended to make homeopathic preparations less vulnerable to the antidotes.

Table 3-2	Homeopathic Cell Salts
Cell Salt	*Use for These Conditions*
Calcarea fluorica	Weak tooth enamel, cracks in the lips and palms of the hands, ligament/tendon weakness or sprains, hemorrhoids
Calcarea phosphorica	Weak bones and fractures, teething and dentition (arrangement of teeth), growing pains, osteoporosis, upset stomach, post-nasal drip, chronic cold feet
Calcarea sulphurica	Abscess, boils, acne, herpes blisters, sores that heal poorly
Ferrum phosphoricum	Inflammation, fever, earache, sore throat, anemia, bleeding
Kali muriaticum	White mucus, swollen glands, sore throat, fluid in ears, indigestion from rich food
Kali phosphoricum	Anxiety, brain fatigue, irritability, temper tantrums
Kali sulphuricum	Yellow mucus, cough and congestion that's worse at night, yellow crusts on eyelids, gas, poor digestion
Magnesia phosphoricum	Cramps (muscle, stomach, menstrual), seizures, hyperactivity, hiccups, cold-sensitive teeth
Natrum muriaticum	Clear thin mucus (from hay fever or early stage common cold), itching hair at nape of neck, insect bites (applied topically), dry skin, cold sores
Natrum phosphoricum	Morning sickness, heartburn, vaginitis, teeth grinding at night
Natrum sulphuricum	Newborn jaundice, hepatitis, colitis, green stools, sensitive scalp
Silica	Acne, boils, sinusitis, sty in eye, tonsillitis, brittle nails

Bodywork (Massage)

Bodywork covers numerous approaches to healing and wellness that are based on external manipulation of the body, including the skin and underlying muscles, soft tissue, and nerves. In this section, I describe the more common forms of bodywork so that you can make well-informed decisions on what you think may be best for you.

Acupuncture and acupressure

Acupuncture and acupressure are rooted in traditional Chinese medicine. The theory is that the human body contains 12 primary channels, called *meridians*, through which vital energy called *qi* or *ch'i* (pronounced "chee") travels. When one of these channels is blocked or out of balance, illness occurs. Acupuncture and acupressure manipulate specific points along the meridians to restore energy flow and balance. For example, to increase energy flow to the liver, an acupuncturist may insert a needle at point LR-3 (Liver-3), located in the soft flesh between your big toe and your second toe. The needles are very thin and inserted in a way that you may not even feel.

To find a National Certification Commission for Acupuncture and Oriental Medicine (NCCAOM) certified practitioner, visit www.nccaom.org and click Find a Practitioner.

Chiropractic

Chiropractic is based on the notion that the body's structure (primarily the spine) affects its function (through the nervous system). The theory is that many illnesses stem from pressure on the nerves caused by *vertebral subluxation* (misalignment of the bones that make up the spinal column). Pressure on the nerves disrupts the communication network throughout the body that connects the brain to the body's various organs. Realigning the bones relieves pressure on the nerves and restores healthy neural communication and proper functioning of all organs. Realigning bones may also improve circulation and speed the body's natural healing process. Chiropractic is especially useful for treating back and neck pain, headaches, and pain in the arms or legs.

The best way to find a qualified chiropractor is by asking your primary care doctor or your friends and family to recommend one. All states require chiropractors to be licensed. When you have a few names, contact your state's licensing board to find out whether the person is licensed to practice in your state. You may need to visit a few chiropractors to find the right match. Chiropractors vary in the techniques they use; some techniques are gentler than others. Some chiropractors use their hands only, while others use additional instruments and therapies, such as hydrotherapy and even acupuncture or acupressure.

Hydrotherapy

Hydrotherapy uses water as a liquid, solid (ice), or gas (steam) to improve circulation and stimulate healing. You have no doubt performed your own hydrotherapy at some time in your life by taking a hot bath to soothe sore muscles or applying ice to a strained muscle to reduce swelling. Physical therapists often use or recommend hydrotherapy as part of a treatment regimen, often to promote the healing of sports injuries.

Massage

Massage consists of applying pressure to the skin and underlying muscles, soft tissues, and nerves to improve circulation, reduce stress, alleviate pain, and calm the mind. Massage is often combined with aromatherapy and other treatment modalities to optimize its effect.

To find a qualified massage therapist, conduct your search at the American Massage Therapy Association website at `amtamassage.org` or the National Certification Board for Therapeutic Massage and Bodywork website at `ncbtmb.org`.

Osteopathy

Osteopaths (often referred to as *doctors of osteopathy [DOs]*) receive conventional medical training along with additional specialized training in osteopathic medicine. Like chiropractors, osteopaths believe that a healthy spine and healthy bone structure are essential for overall health. Osteopaths use spinal manipulation as one technique for restoring and optimizing health and well-being.

You can find a licensed osteopath using the online search forms provided by many insurance companies — added assurance that the osteopath is covered by your insurance plan. You can also conduct your search through the American Osteopathic Association's website at `www.osteopathic.org`.

Reflexology

Reflexology is sort of a cross between massage and acupuncture that's intended to complement other medical treatments. A reflexologist applies pressure to specific points and areas on the feet, hands, or ears that correspond to certain internal organs and systems. For example, for sinus problems, the reflexologist is likely to apply pressure to the tips of your toes. You can find numerous reflexology maps online that illustrate the pressure points and corresponding internal organs.

A couple national and several state organizations maintain directories of certified reflexologists. Visit the American Reflexology Certification Board website at arcb.net to search for a reflexologist near you. You may also want to conduct your search at the Reflexology Association of America website at reflexology-usa.org or pull up a list of state reflexology associations at www.holisticwebworks.com/Reflexology-Associations.htm.

Naturopathy

Naturopathy offers natural healthcare within the realm of conventional medicine. Naturopathic physicians are trained in the art and science of various natural healthcare modalities at accredited medical colleges and often establish partnerships with conventional medical doctors to provide patients with the best of both worlds. Naturopathic physicians commonly use nutrition, herbal remedies, homeopathy, natural hormones, hydrotherapy, and even pharmaceutical medications and minor surgery in the arsenal to battle illness and restore health. Many are also trained in functional medicine.

If you're interested in receiving treatment from a naturopathic physician, ask your doctor to recommend one, or use the physician search features on your insurance company's website to find a naturopath who's covered by your insurance plan. The American Association of Naturopathic Physicians (www.naturopathic.org) also has an online directory you can search to find a qualified physician in a number of (but not all) states. As of the writing of this book, fewer than half of the United States and its territories had licensing or regulation laws for naturopathic doctors.

Nutritional Medicine

According to nutritional medicine practitioners, food is the best medicine. Providing the body with the nutrients, including essential micronutrients, it requires for the many biochemical processes that are constantly occurring not only equips the body to fight infection and other illnesses but also supports optimum health and well-being.

The role food plays in restoring and maintaining health isn't exactly a secret. Everyone knows that eating junk food puts your body on a physical and emotional rollercoaster ride of highs and lows. Eating a well-balanced diet of organic whole foods that are free of processed sugar, artificial colors and flavors, preservatives, pesticides, herbicides, and other poisons and synthetic compounds makes you feel better throughout the course of a day.

In this book, I recommend good nutrition as the foundation of good health and vitality. For more about proper nutrition and how to adopt a natural cures diet and lifestyle, check out Chapter 2.

Part II

Curing Common Maladies: Trustworthy Treatments at Your Fingertips

Immune-Booster Supplements

Supplement	Dose*
Colostrum	10,000 mg daily
Andrographis	400 mg daily
Whole beta glucan	700 mg once daily upon waking or before bed with 8 ounces of water
Probiotics	Twice daily before or during meals: 4 billion CFUs of *Lactobacillus acidophilus* Rosell 1 billion CFUs of *Bifidobacterium longum* Rosell
Vitamin D3	2,000 to 10,000 IUs daily
Vitamin C (mineral ascorbates)	1,000 to 10,000 mg daily
Proline-rich polypeptides	Four sprays in mouth, hold for 30 seconds, and swallow, twice daily early morning and before bed, for a total of 16 mg daily
Zinc glycinate chelate	20 mg twice daily
Vitamin B12 (methylcobalamin, sublingual fast-dissolving tablet)	5,000 mcg one to two times daily
Folate (5-MTHF)	2,000 mcg one to two times daily
Olive leaf extract	50 mg daily

Dosages are for adults.

For a bonus article on restoring healthy gut bacteria after antibiotic treatment, visit www.dummies.com/extras/naturalcures.

In this part . . .

✔ Prevent and cure the common cold, the flu, and other infections by enhancing your body's own immune system response.

✔ Significantly reduce the occurrence of ear infections and dental cavities through the use of a natural sugar substitute extracted from birch trees and other plants.

✔ Minimize or eliminate the need for antihistamines and decongestants in the treatment of allergies and asthma by providing your body with the nutrients it needs to self-regulate its immune response.

✔ Improve digestion and nutrient absorption while reducing indigestion and supporting a healthy immune response with the use of probiotics, digestive enzymes, and betaine hydrochloride (HCl).

✔ Sample a variety of herbs and other sleep-enhancing supplements that work as well as or better than prescription sleep aids and are much healthier alternatives.

✔ Discover natural treatments for a wide range of chronic illnesses that conventional medicine struggles to cure, including cardiovascular disease, diabetes, osteoporosis, and Parkinson's disease.

Chapter 4

Treating Injuries and Minor Ailments

. . . .

In This Chapter

▶ Soothing bee stings and insect and spider bites

▶ Healing cuts, bruises, and burns, including sunburn

▶ Speeding recovery from hangovers, headaches, heartburn, and hiccups

▶ Alleviating sprains, strains, and other swelling

▶ Curing motion sickness and poison ivy

. . . .

*E*very day, you expose your body to conditions and activities that are likely to hurt. Bees, bugs, and spiders seem to be ready and waiting to inflict pain, and every day the sun blasts you with wonderfully warm but potentially harmful ultraviolet radiation. And if nature doesn't get you, you're almost sure to experience some sort of self-inflicted malady by eating or drinking too much of the wrong things and not enough of the right things, playing or working too hard, or just being careless or falling victim to the occasional unavoidable accident.

Whether you experience one of life's minor mishaps or suffer from some other common affliction, such as a headache, hiccups, or motion sickness, this chapter shows you how to harness the power of your own secret weapon — your body — to speed your recovery.

Doses in this chapter are for adults, not children. For guidance on how to adjust dosages for children (and adults under 150 pounds), turn to Chapter 12.

Making Bruises Disappear

Bruises are often uglier than they are painful. To treat a bruise, elevate the bruised area, if possible, and apply ice immediately for 20 minutes every hour for the first 24 hours. Continue to apply ice for 20 minutes several times over the course of the next two days. In addition to ice, apply arnica gel to the bruise several times daily or take arnica pellets orally.

You can also take bromelain (150 mg) several times a day, 20 minutes before or 2 hours after eating. Don't use bromelain if you have gastritis or ulcers or are taking a blood thinner, such as warfarin or Coumadin. Another option is to take the enzymes chymotrypsin and trypsin immediately after the trauma to reduce swelling and discoloration; take 600 USP several times daily, 20 minutes before or 2 hours after eating.

Eliminate the standard American diet (SAD), which is loaded with processed foods high in sugar and the wrong type of fats, because they promote inflammation. Instead consume quality vegetables and fruits, and grass-fed animal products and healthy oily fishes. This simple step reduces bruising and speeds recovery.

Extinguishing Burns

For severe burns that damage the skin (blisters or charring), seek immediate medical attention. For minor burns, try any of the following home remedies:

- ✔ **Ice:** Run cool (not cold) water over the area for up to 20 minutes. Don't go any longer than 20 minutes, however, because doing so is counter-productive, restricting blood flow to the burned skin. Don't use ice, which can cause frostbite and further damage the skin.

- ✔ **Honey:** Apply honey to a gauze pad and tape it over the burned area. Honey draws out fluid, cleansing the area. Change the pad several times daily.

- ✔ **Oatmeal:** Soak in a lukewarm bath with 1 cup of oatmeal for 20 minutes, and don't rinse afterward. The oatmeal bath leaves a thin film of oatmeal on your skin, which continues to draw heat out from the burn. (Oatmeal can be slippery, so be careful not to slip and fall in the bath or when getting out.)

- ✔ **Black tea:** Soak several tea bags in cold water; then soak the affected area in the water or dab the water on the affected area. The tannic acid in tea tends to draw heat out of the burn.

✔ **Vinegar:** Mix equal parts white vinegar and water together and apply the mixture to the burn. Vinegar is an astringent that tightens the skin and reduces the chance of infection.

✔ **Milk:** Apply milk to a wash cloth and dab the affected area.

✔ **Salt:** For mouth burns, rinse with a salt-water solution (½ teaspoon salt in 8 ounces of water) several times daily.

Here are some additional herbal remedies for burns:

✔ **Aloe plant:** Break off a piece of aloe plant and gently dab the broken end on the affected area several times daily.

✔ **Lavender oil:** Apply a small amount of lavender oil to the burn several times daily.

✔ **Comfrey, witch hazel, and elder flowers:** Create an infusion (refer to Chapter 3) and apply it to the burned area.

✔ **Vitamin C (mineral ascorbates):** Speed recovery by taking 1,000 to 3,000 mg daily. Children 6 years old and younger can take half the adult dosage.

Immediate medical treatment is required for severe burns, but you can complement treatment and speed recovery by doing the following:

✔ **Shift to a high-calorie diet with an emphasis on high-quality protein.** People with extensive burns are at risk for serious weight loss and malnutrition, increasing the risk of infection.

✔ **Supplement your diet with zinc, copper, and selenium.** Your body loses zinc, copper, and selenium in response to more intensive burns. Supplementation with these minerals can reduce infection and speed tissue recovery. Take up to 20 mg zinc twice daily with 1 mg copper per every 10 mg zinc, and take 200 mcg selenium daily.

✔ **Take vitamin E.** You can apply vitamin E oil to the burn (with your doctor's permission) and take it internally at 400 IU daily. (Take vitamin E in its better form; see Appendix A.)

✔ **Apply clean potato peels to the affected skin and wrap with gauze.** Potato peels speed recovery but are not antibacterial. (Again, get your doctor's approval before applying this treatment.)

Curing Cuts

If you get a cut, the first step is to evaluate how serious it is. If it's deep enough that you see fat, muscle, or bone; it's spurting blood; or it has jagged edges or edges that are far apart, seek immediate medical attention. In the meantime, use a clean rag to apply pressure to the wound. If the cut occurred on outside equipment or rusted, old, or dirty metal, you may also need to get a tetanus booster vaccine if you haven't gotten one in the past five years or can't recall the date of your previous booster.

Use a tourniquet *only* if you're in real danger of bleeding to death; improper use of a tourniquet can cause loss of limb.

For less severe cuts, here's what you do:

1. **Wash the cut with soap and water.**

2. **Apply hydrogen peroxide.**

   You can dunk the wounded area in a cup or bowl of peroxide, pour the peroxide over the cut, or apply the peroxide with cotton. Repeat several times until the bubbling effect slows down.

3. **Dry the area thoroughly.**

4. **Apply iodine or an over-the-counter antibiotic ointment, such as Neosporin.**

   Use iodine for superficial cuts that don't require a bandage; if you use iodine, don't cover the cut, because covered iodine tends to burn the skin. Also keep in mind that iodine stings. Use antibiotic ointment for deeper cuts that require a bandage.

   Here are some alternatives to iodine and Neosporin:

   - **Garlic:** Chop 3 cloves of garlic and mix with 1 cup of water. Let the mixture stand for several hours and then strain. Apply the solution to the cut several times daily. (Garlic acts as an antimicrobial but may irritate the skin.)

   - **Honey:** Apply honey to a gauze pad and tape it to the cut, changing the bandage several times daily. Honey dehydrates the skin and pulls out the bad bacteria.

   - **Onion:** Crush onion with the side of a knife or place it in a blender. Apply the crushed onion to a gauze pad and tape it to the cut, changing the bandage several times daily. You can also mix the onion with honey. (Onion acts like garlic but is less irritating to the skin.)

   - **Broadleaf plantain (*Plantago major*):** Crush or squeeze the leaves of this common weed to extract the liquid and then apply the liquid to the cut.

   - **Aloe:** Break off a piece of aloe plant and gently rub the broken end over the cut.

5. **Apply a bandage or gauze to keep the cut covered.**

   Don't cover the cut if you applied iodine.

6. **Reapply fresh iodine, Neosporin, or other antimicrobial agent until the cut is healed, and change the bandage if you're covering the cut.**

   As the cut heals, protect it from direct sunlight and apply a high SPF sunscreen to prevent darkening of the scar after the cut heals.

If a scab forms, don't pick it. Instead, mix 1 tablespoon of white vinegar in 1 pint of water and soak the scab in this solution for 10 to 20 minutes several times daily. Vinegar stings, but it removes the scabs without your picking at them.

Handling Hangovers

A hangover is your body's way of telling you not to drink so much, so the best cure is prevention. Drink in moderation and alternate your alcoholic beverages with at least the same amount of water. Avoid drinking on an empty stomach, and make sure you have a belly full of food if you do indulge. The morning after, eat light and drink plenty of water.

Don't take acetaminophen before, during, or after drinking because it can cause serious liver damage. Avoid aspirin and ibuprofen, as well, because they can irritate an already irritated stomach and perhaps give you an ulcer. Instead, take 500 to 1,000 mg of curcumin with food; curcumin is a natural anti-inflammatory.

I'm a big fan of rehydration formulas that are high in electrolytes, including magnesium and B vitamins. Those without artificial coloring, sweeteners, and added sugar (the ones that taste bad, that is) are best. Replacing lost electrolytes can make you feel much better. Here are some additional suggestions:

- Get plenty of sleep.
- Eat a banana to replace lost potassium.
- Drink a cup of ginger-root tea (good for nausea and sea sickness).
- Drink a virgin hot toddy: 1 cup hot water flavored with lemon and honey (not sugar).
- Place an ice pack on the area of your head that hurts.

Heading Off Headaches

If you rarely get headaches, stretching and pain relievers generally do the trick, but if headaches become a regular occurrence, look for the cause and remove it instead of masking it with pain relievers. To track down the causes and cures, you can divide headaches into the following categories:

- ✔ **Tension headache:** Tightness and throbbing in the head usually accompanied by tightness and tension in the muscles of the upper back, neck, and scalp.

    Bodywork, including massage, acupuncture, acupressure, hydrotherapy, reflexology, and chiropractic and osteopathic adjustments are all effective in treating tension headaches (see Chapter 3). If you suspect eyestrain to be the cause, head to Chapter 9 for suggestions. Here are a few additional therapies that may help:

    - Menthol cream applied to the temporal bones

    - Stress reduction through meditation and biofeedback (see Chapter 3)

    - Exercise, especially yoga

    - Deep-breathing exercises

    - Treatment for temporomandibular joint (TMJ) or clenching of teeth (see Chapter 10)

- ✔ **Sinus headache:** Pain and pressure in and around the sinuses, in the forehead, or between the eyes and above the nose, typically from congestion. See Chapter 6 for more about treating sinus congestion. If the sinus congestion is caused by infection, see Chapter 5. If the congestion is due to an underlying allergy, head to Chapter 13.

- ✔ **Migraine:** Severe, debilitating pain generally on one side of the head, light sensitivity, and nausea or vomiting. Unlike typical tension headaches, migraines are caused by alterations in blood flow to the brain. See Chapter 17 for guidance in treating migraines.

- ✔ **Cluster headaches:** Intense headaches that affect one side of the head and can last for weeks only to disappear for months and then reappear again.

    At the first sign of a cluster headache, take 3 to 5 mg of melatonin and apply 0.025 percent capsaicin cream preparation (Zostrix) intranasally (inside your nostrils) to relieve pain. Treating underlying food allergies or sensitivities (especially to wheat) is likely to provide long-term relief (see Chapter 13).

- ✔ **Rebound headache:** Headaches caused by the overuse or sudden discontinuation of pain medication. To treat rebound headaches, wean yourself slowly off pain medications and treat pain with natural alternatives.

✔ **Headaches related to foods, deficiencies, or toxins:** Headaches that don't respond to massage and stress reduction can usually be traced to digestive disorders, a food allergy or sensitivity, caffeine withdrawal, poor diet, nutritional deficiency, blood sugar fluctuations, heavy-metal or chemical exposure, or liver toxicity. Identify and treat the underlying cause:

- **Digestive disorders:** If constipation is an issue, address it first. See Chapter 14 for details and Chapter 2 for diet and lifestyle recommendations that also support healthy digestion.

  Improve bowel function with plenty of fiber from either foods or supplements. Drink half your desired body weight in ounces of water daily; for example, if you weigh 160 pounds, drink 80 ounces of water daily.

- **Food allergies or sensitivities:** Totally eliminate gluten and wheat from your diet, both of which are potent triggers for headaches in many people. If that doesn't resolve the problem, head to Chapter 13 for more about testing for and treating food allergies and sensitivities.

- **Magnesium deficiency:** Increase your daily magnesium intake (see Appendix A). If you need a supplement, I recommend magnesium in the form of a magnesium glycinate chelate for maximum absorption: 125 mg twice daily. This form will not cause diarrhea.

- **Blood sugar and insulin spikes:** To maintain blood sugar balance, start the day off with a balanced smoothie (see Chapter 2). Avoid all breakfast cereals and carbohydrate-rich foods, such as donuts, bagels, rolls, muffins, and pancakes. Eat balanced meals consisting of quality protein, complex carbohydrates, and healthy fats.

If your headaches don't respond to other treatments, try the following:

✔ Take 75 mg of butterbur twice daily to prevent and reduce the severity of chronic headaches. Use half this dosage for children under 6 years old.

✔ Take 100 mg of 5-HTP (5-hydroxytryptophan) in a controlled release formula twice daily to balance the serotonin levels in the brain, thus reducing headache severity, intensity, and frequency. Don't take 5-HTP if you're on an antidepressant or anti-anxiety medication.

✔ Certain homeopathic remedies are very effective for treating headaches. See Chapter 3 for homeopathic basics and Appendix E for specific remedies.

If these remedies don't put an end to your chronic headaches, consult a functional medicine practitioner, who can get to the root of what's ailing you. A functional medicine practitioner is likely to perform numerous tests to evaluate for conditions such as leaky gut syndrome, hormone imbalances, vitamin and mineral deficiencies, blood sugar dysregulation, and heavy-metal toxicity. After identifying the cause, you have a clearer idea of what to do to eliminate it and fix the problem.

Preventing and Treating Heartburn

If you're experiencing occasional, minor heartburn, you've come to the right place. Here are some natural remedies to relieve heartburn:

- Eliminate common trigger foods, including wheat, dairy, mint, and spicy and fried foods. (If symptoms don't resolve, consider being tested for food allergies, as explained in Chapter 13.)

- Eat smaller meals, mostly vegetables.

- Stop eating three hours before bed. (In a reclined position, acid from your stomach has an easier time rising up into your esophagus.)

- Try the following nutritional supplements:

Supplement	Dosage/Amount
Glutamine (best in a powder form)	3 g, mixed with water and taken on an empty stomach, one to three times daily for several months
Aloe (best in a powder form)	100 mg mixed in liquid, one to three times daily for several months
DGL (deglycyrrhizinated licorice, best in a powder form)	500 mg, one to three times daily
Digestive enzymes (acid resistant, broad spectrum containing 50,000 to 100,000 USP protease; 50,000 to 100,000 USP amylase; and lipase)	8,000 to 15,000 USP, with meals
Probiotics containing at least two strains: *Lactobacillus* and *Bifidobacterium*	At least 5 billion CFU (see note following table)
Zinc carnosine	75 mg twice daily between meals
Oregano oil	0.5 ml one to three times daily
Berberine HCL	400 ml two to three times daily
Betaine HCL	1,300 mg with each meal
Pepsin	90 mg with each meal
Chinese herbs (a proprietary blend of corydalis, astragalus root, and tienchi ginseng root)	400 mg twice daily

Not all probiotics are created equal, nor is the probiotic with the higher number of CFUs necessarily the better choice. A good probiotic adheres to the intestinal tract wall, colonizes, and multiplies. So purchase from a reputable source. Quality, proper storage, and shipping can make all the difference in whether the probiotic works.

If your heartburn is severe and chronic, head to Chapter 14, where you'll find treatments for acid reflux, also known as *gastroesophageal reflux disease* (GERD).

Don't get into the habit of popping a little purple pill or guzzling some pink liquid to reduce stomach acid. This strategy does more harm than good. Turn to Chapter 14 to find out why and to explore healthier options for curbing heartburn.

Quieting Hiccups

A *hiccup* is an involuntary spasm of the diaphragm — the muscle that separates the chest and abdominal cavities. A split second after the spasm, the glottis (vocal cords) closes. The spasm triggers an intake of breath that's stopped suddenly when the glottis slams shut, causing the characteristic and very annoying "hic" and making your upper body jerk.

You can try a few of the classic cures (see the nearby sidebar for some suggestions), but prevention may be the best cure. If you frequently get hiccups after you eat, try slowing down and eating less. If you get them when you're overstimulated due to anxiety, fear, or euphoria, you may want to consider adopting a calmer lifestyle or demeanor.

The good news is that most hiccups resolve on their own regardless of what you do or whether you do anything at all. If, however, your hiccups become a chronic condition, something more serious may be going on, such as infection, stroke, multiple sclerosis (MS), or a lesion on the brain stem.

For chronic hiccups, rule out those other possible conditions and then try the following remedies:

- ✔ Apply lidocaine gel 2 to 3 percent solution into each ear canal. The lidocaine numbs the eardrum for only a couple hours, but it may provide long-term relief. Avoid loud noises and don't put anything in the ear canals for a couple hours after treatment.
- ✔ Sip a small amount of apple cider vinegar.

Classic cures for hiccups

Everyone has a favorite hiccup remedy. Here are a few of my favorites, although they're not backed up by any reliable medical research:

✔ Hold your breath for as long as you can — the classic hiccup cure.

✔ Stand on your head.

✔ Drink an entire glass of water upside down — good luck, by the way.

✔ Breathe into a paper bag.

✔ Try really hard to make yourself hiccup.

✔ Get someone to scare or tickle you silly.

✔ Place a finger in each ear.

✔ Pinch the skin that covers your deltoid muscles (shoulders).

✔ Slowly swallow a teaspoon of honey or dill seed.

✔ Drink some chamomile tea.

✔ Dissolve ¼ to ½ teaspoon of sugar in 1 teaspoon of water and ¼ teaspoon of apple cider vinegar, apply intranasally (inside your nostrils), and inhale gently to stimulate nerves inside your nose and pharynx — the membranes behind your nose and mouth.

✔ Get a chiropractic adjustment. Pressure on the phrenic nerve from a *vertebral subluxation* (a vertebra that's shifted out of position) may cause hiccups. (The phrenic nerve originates in the neck and extends to the diaphragm.)

Alleviating the Pain and Swelling of Insect and Spider Bites and Stings

Determining the right treatment for an insect or spider bite or sting hinges on knowing what bit you. Treating a mosquito bite differs a great deal from treating a bee sting or a bite from a black widow spider. If you don't know what bit you, you may need to take an educated guess and try a few different remedies or head to the doctor (or emergency room) for help in identifying the critter that bit you and getting treatment for it.

If you know what bit or stung you and can capture the critter without getting bitten or stung again, place it in a jar and hang on to it. That way, you can get help identifying it in the event that any symptoms you have become more serious.

In this section, I offer guidance first on treating bee, wasp, and hornet stings and then on treating insect and spider bites.

Treating bee, wasp, and hornet stings

If you're stung by a bee, the first order of business is to pull out the stinger. (Wasps and hornets don't leave their stingers, so you can skip this step if you're stung by one of those.) To remove the stinger, don't grab it between your fingers! That'll just squeeze more toxins into your system. Instead, use your fingernail, a nail file, a credit card, a coin, or a key to gently scrape the stinger away from your skin. Do this right away, because within 20 seconds, 90 percent of the venom is released, and the more venom, the more severe the reaction.

If you've ever had an allergic reaction to a bee sting, even a minor reaction, consider the possibility of *anaphylaxis* — a life-threatening allergic reaction characterized by severe itching, rash, welts, tightening of the chest, and closing of the airways. Carry a fresh EpiPen with you during bee season and use it immediately. If you don't have an EpiPen, call 911 or have someone nearby rush you to the nearest emergency room.

For normal reactions, after removing the stinger, or first thing if you were stung by a wasp or hornet, apply ice for 20 minutes every hour for the first six hours. Take *Apis mellifica* (homeopathic) pellets orally and apply it topically as a gel. Pain relievers, including acetaminophen, ibuprofen, and aspirin, can help with any associated pain, and antihistamines (orally and topically), such as Benadryl, can help reduce the swelling.

If you're treating a child, don't use aspirin, which can cause Reye's syndrome — a serious condition that causes swelling in the liver or brain.

Broadleaf plantain *(Plantago major)*, a common North American weed, may also be used as a remedy for stings. From April to October, you can find it growing in nearly any yard, field, or vacant lot (look it up online to find a picture of it). This plant contains *tannin*, an astringent that helps draw tissues together and stops the itching. Gather up some of the leaves, break them in half and scratch the ends vigorously to release a pulp that you mix with saliva and then apply to the sting. Do this once daily until the pain, swelling, and itching subside.

Treating insect and spider bites

Here are some general recommendations for treating minor bites from mosquitos, bedbugs, ticks, flies, ants, fleas, chiggers, mites, and nonvenomous spiders:

- ✔ If you're treating a tick bite, remove the tick first. Use fine-tipped tweezers to grasp the tick as close to the skin's surface as possible; then pull gently and steadily upward. Twisting or jerking the tick risks breaking off parts of the tick's mouth inside you.

✔ Wash the area with soap and water and apply rubbing alcohol to prevent infection.

✔ Don't scratch. Scratching makes the bite more prone to becoming infected. If you're treating a child, you may want to trim his or her fingernails.

✔ Bathe in apple cider vinegar. If you have several bites, take a bath in cool or lukewarm water with 2 to 3 cups of apple cider vinegar mixed in.

✔ Break off a piece of aloe plant and gently rub it across the bite(s), or apply raw honey to the bite.

✔ Make a paste of baking soda and water, apply it liberally to the bite(s), and let it dry.

✔ Dab some lime or lemon juice onto the bite to alleviate itching.

✔ Apply a dilute solution of water with tea tree, lavender, witch hazel, or rosemary essential oil to alleviate itching. A few drops of oil per ounce of water should do the trick.

✔ Apply witch hazel or deodorant to the bite.

If you were bitten by a spider, keep a close eye on the site of the bite and monitor your symptoms carefully. If the bite site swells, blisters, or otherwise gets a lot uglier, or if you experience fever, chills, stiffness, sweating, abdominal pain, or nausea, seek immediate medical attention, because you may have been bitten by a venomous spider.

The treatments provided here are solely for the bite itself. Many insects carry more serious viral and bacterial illnesses, including encephalitis, Lyme disease, Rocky Mountain spotted fever, and malaria. If you suspect that you've contracted an insect-borne virus, seek medical attention.

Moderating Motion Sickness

If you feel queasy while riding in a car, sailing the seas, or flying in an airplane, chances are good that you're susceptible to motion sickness. Conventional medicine treats motion sickness with antihistamines, such as Dramamine (dimenhydrinate), and anticholinergics, which slow message transmission along the nerve system that controls involuntary bodily functions. The side effects associated with these two classes of drugs include visual disturbances and sedation. Here are a few natural cures for motion sickness:

✔ Watch where you're going. Motion sickness is often caused by the balancing mechanism of the inner ear sending false signals to your brain. Watching where you're going enables your vision to override some of this misinformation. Sitting in the front seat of a car or in a window seat of an airplane, or keeping your eyes on the horizon while cruising in a boat can help.

✔ Drink plenty of water and eat small meals prior to and during the trip.

✔ Avoid alcohol and caffeine, which tend to dehydrate.

✔ Take 1 g of ginger before and during the ride as needed.

✔ Take DHEA (dehydroepiandrosterone) before and during the ride: Start with 10 mg daily and increase slowly as needed to 25 mg daily. (You can take DHEA for a few days or weeks without testing or medical supervision, but if you plan to take it any longer, consult your healthcare provider.)

✔ Drink freshly squeezed lemon juice (about ⅛ to ¼ of a lemon) diluted each morning in hot water.

✔ Wear an acupressure bracelet that applies pressure to specific points on your wrist.

Soothing Poison Ivy, Oak, and Sumac Reactions

In people who are allergic to these plants, poison ivy, oak, and sumac cause an intensely itchy rash called *allergic contact dermatitis*. If you have the misfortune of being one of these people and you're currently itching in misery, here are a few suggestions that can relieve the itching and help you not make the rash any worse:

✔ Don't scratch. Scratching can lead to infection, and if you still have oil from the plant on your skin, itching may spread the rash.

✔ Wash immediately with cool water and soap. Warm water opens the pores and increases penetration of the toxic oils.

✔ Apply calamine lotion. Don't apply antihistamines, benzocaine, or topical antibiotics, because they can worsen the rash.

✔ Apply baking soda. You can take a cool or lukewarm bath with ½ cup of baking soda mixed in with the water, or make a baking soda paste (3 teaspoons baking soda per 1 teaspoon of water) and apply it to the affected area.

✔ After washing the toxic oil off your skin, cook some oatmeal mixed with a teaspoon of baking soda. Then, when the oatmeal is cool to the touch, apply the warm oatmeal to the affected areas. Leave it on for at least 20 minutes before rinsing it off.

Preventing poison ivy, oak, and sumac

Prevention is the best medicine for poison ivy, oak, and sumac. Learn to identify these plants (you can find plenty of photos and identification guides online) and steer clear of them. If you're in areas where you're likely to come into contact with these plants, wear long pants, a long-sleeve shirt, and gloves. When you're done, remove and wash your clothes immediately and then take a cool or lukewarm shower — soap up and rinse off at least twice. Washing is key to removing any oil before it can trigger a reaction and keeping the oil from getting on other parts of your body.

CorteX makes a product called IvyX — a pre-treatment solution that's effective in preventing a reaction when you come into contact with poison ivy, oak, or sumac. You still need to wash your clothing and take a cool or lukewarm shower after working outside.

Keep in mind that the plant's oil causes the reaction. You can't catch poison ivy from someone who has it unless, of course, the oil from the plant is still on that person's (or pet's) body.

 ✔ Apply the following directly to the affected area: aloe (break off a piece of an aloe plant and gently rub the broken end over the affected skin), organic apple cider vinegar, witch hazel (use a cotton ball to dab the witch hazel on the affected area), mashed or sliced cucumber, or the inside of a banana peel.

Monitor your condition closely. If the rash blisters and continues to spread, seek medical attention sooner rather than later, because it *will* get worse.

Relaxing Sprains and Strains

Sprains and strains are common, especially for athletes and others who lead an active life. What's the difference? A *sprain* is a stretch or tear of a *ligament* — a fibrous band of tissue that connects two bones. A *strain* is an injury to a muscle (a pulled muscle) or tendon. In either case, the injury usually results in swelling and pain, and the pain tends to subside within 24 to 48 hours. If the pain or swelling gets much worse over that time, you may have suffered a fracture, which requires medical attention. If the pain is severe and the area exhibits discoloration, get to a doctor as soon as possible.

For sprains and strains, the standard treatment is RICE:

 ✔ **Rest:** Don't use the injured appendage; for example, stay off your feet as much as possible if you sprained or strained a part of your leg.

✔ **Ice:** Apply ice, alternating 20 minutes on and 20 minutes off, for the first 24 hours.

✔ **Compression:** Keep the area firmly wrapped to keep the swelling down. You want the wrap snug but not so tight that it cuts off blood circulation.

✔ **Elevation:** Elevate the injured appendage to reduce blood flow to it, which is likely to increase swelling.

In addition to RICE, diet can make the difference between a speedy recovery and a long one. Dump the trans fats found in processed foods, sugar, and the standard American diet. Eat fish high in omega-3 essential fatty acids, vegetables rich in antioxidants, and high-quality grass-fed protein. These foods decrease inflammation and give you the raw materials needed to build new, healthy tissue. For additional nutritional support, supplement your diet with one or more of the following:

Supplement	Dosage/Amount
White willow extract	120 mg, two to three times daily between meals for several days; decrease dosage as you see improvement
Boswellia extract	50 mg, two to three times daily between meals for several days; decrease dosage as you see improvement
High ORAC berry blend	Follow label instructions
Chymotrypsin	6,000 USP, two to three times daily between meals for several days; decrease dosage as you see improvement
Trypsin	6,000 USP, two to three times daily between meals for several days; decrease dosage as you see improvement
Bromelain	150 mg, two to three times daily between meals for several days; decrease dosage as you see improvement
Arnica	Apply arnica ointment several times daily to the injured site

For long-term nutritional support, take the following daily in three divided doses: MSM (methylsulfonylmethane), 1,000 mg; glucosamine sulfate, 1,500 mg; and chondroitin sulfate, 1,200 mg. You can purchase formulations that combine glucosamine, chondroitin, and MSM. (Don't go cheap; quality trumps price.)

Snuffing Out Sunburn

If your skin has been seared from too much sun, here are some natural cures to alleviate the pain and repair damaged skin; take these natural cures until the sunburn is healed:

Remedy	Dosage
Beta-carotene	5 to 180 mg daily
Lycopene	10 to 20 mg two times daily
Aloe vera	Apply aloe to the burned skin several times daily
Lavender oil	Apply lavender oil lotion to the burn several times daily (see Chapter 3 for the basics of working with essential oils)
L-glutamine	500 to 1,000 mg three times daily
Zinc and copper	20 mg zinc with 2 mg copper, twice daily
Antioxidant blend (vitamins C [mixed mineral ascorbates] and E [mixed tocopherols] with minerals including selenium and magnesium)	1,000 mg vitamin C and 400 IU vitamin E (see appendix A for more about the better forms of vitamins)
Bee propolis (spray or lotion)	Apply several times daily
Raw unprocessed honey	Apply to burned skin several times daily
Hypericum	10 drops of tincture under tongue, hold for 30 seconds, and then swallow; take three to four times daily
Calendula	Infuse 1 heaping teaspoon of herb in 1 cup of water; strain, allow to cool, and then apply as a lotion to the affected skin

What you eat has a profound impact on healing. Your body needs the right raw materials to build new healthy tissue. Eliminate sugar, wheat, potatoes, juice, trans fats, and artificial sweeteners. Eat high-quality proteins and fats and a variety of vegetables in an array of colors.

Reducing Swelling

Swelling is inflammation, and inflammation is the root cause of a host of chronic illnesses that afflict primarily western cultures. Most inflammatory conditions can be traced back to diet or digestion. Western diets that are high in sugar, highly processed carbohydrates, and trans fats are highly

---

How much sun is healthy?

Some sun is essential for good health, but how much is enough and how much is too much? As with most things in life, that depends. Some people have pale skin that's susceptible to burns. Others have more melanin in their skin, which improves their ability to tan, which protects the skin from burns and decreases the risk of skin cancer. Also, the closer you are to the equator, the more intense the sunlight.

Current thinking around sun exposure has changed since people learned that vitamin D is produced with some sun exposure. Therefore, a small amount of sunlight is recommended. The recommendation is that you now get sun on 6 percent of your body for 15 to 20 minutes three times a week without sunscreen.

---

inflammatory and don't supply the sufficient nutrients, such as omega-3 fatty acids, that calm inflammation. In addition, an imbalance of micro flora in the gut and leaky gut syndrome (Chapter 13) contribute to creating a highly reactive immune system that causes inflammation throughout the body.

The suffix *itis* means "inflammation," so every illness with a name that ends in *itis* involves inflammation — arthritis, bronchitis, diverticulitis, meningitis, sinusitis, tonsillitis — you name it!

Adopt a modified elimination diet (see Chapter 2) that includes fiber, antioxidants, and other nutrients. Such a diet permits a healthy immune response and enables you to identify specific foods that may be worsening your condition. Eliminating foods that stimulate an immune response reduces swelling and inflammation. Also consider supplementing your diet with the following nutrients:

- **Turmeric:** 300 mg once or twice daily

- **Ginger:** 100 mg once or twice daily

- **Omega-3 essential fatty acids (EFAs):** Get as much as possible through your diet and then follow up with supplementation: 1 g yielding 180 mg EPA (eicosapentaenoic acid) and 120 mg DHA (docosahexaenoic acid) three times daily.

- **Quality protein:** Consume wild fish several times per week. Reduce consumption of grain-fed livestock and replace with grass-fed animal proteins. Protein from grass-fed livestock costs significantly more, but it's worth the price. Consume vegetable protein from rice, pea, and hemp sources instead of animal protein.

For chronic swelling, consult a qualified physician to rule out other possible causes, including kidney and cardiovascular problems and leaky gut syndrome. For more about leaky gut syndrome and other digestive disorders, see Chapters 13 and 14.

Avoid long-term use of medications commonly used to treat the pain associated with chronic inflammation. These medications interfere with underlying human physiology and often cause serious adverse events. Talk to your doctor about the possibility of weaning off of these medications and replacing them with alternative pain-relief treatments.

Chapter 5

Coughing and Sneezing? Curing Nose and Throat Conditions

In This Chapter

▶ Quieting coughs

▶ Alleviating laryngitis

▶ Clearing congestion and postnasal drip

▶ Soothing a sore throat

Your upper respiratory tract, consisting of your nose, nasal passages, mouth, and throat, is your first line of defense against many airborne irritants and illnesses. Each day, you probably breathe in about 400 cubic feet of air, all of which is filtered, to some degree, through the upper respiratory system, so it's no wonder that this area is so prone to illness. In this chapter, I describe several conditions that afflict the upper respiratory system and recommend natural cures for each condition.

If you turned to this chapter to find out about natural cures for the common cold, you're in the wrong place. Turn to Chapter 6, where you'll find remedies for colds, flus, and other common infections.

Doses in this chapter are for adults, not children. For guidance on how to adjust dosages for children (and adults under 150 pounds), turn to Chapter 12.

Combatting a Cough

Coughing is your body's way of clearing the lungs and airways of infection and irritants, so it's not an illness requiring a cure; it's a symptom requiring a diagnosis. Common causes include the following:

- **Infection:** Coughing is a common symptom of cold, flu, bronchitis, sinusitis, or tuberculosis. See Chapter 6 for more about fighting viral and bacterial infections.

- **Allergies or asthma:** Nasal allergies increase production of mucus, which can drain into the throat or lungs and trigger a cough. If the cough is associated with wheezing or difficulty breathing, asthma is the likely culprit. See Chapter 13 for details.

- **Postnasal drip:** Excess mucus draining down the back of your throat, for any number of reasons, may cause a constant need to clear your throat, or the mucus may get into your lungs and trigger a more dramatic cough. See the later section "Treating Sinus Congestion and Postnasal Drip" for details.

- **Medication side effects:** If you're taking any pharmaceuticals, particularly beta blockers for high blood pressure, check its side effects or ask your doctor or pharmacist whether coughing is a side effect. If it is, consult your doctor for options.

- **Smoking and airborne irritants:** Cigarette smoke irritates the upper respiratory system and lungs, often triggering a cough. Similarly, secondhand smoke, air pollution, dust, and pollen commonly trigger coughs.

- **Gastroesophageal reflux disease (GERD):** Indigestion often triggers an immune response in the throat that leads to overproduction of mucus, resulting in a cough. To find out what to do about GERD, see Chapter 14.

- **Heart disease:** With heart disease, fluid may accumulate in the lungs, causing coughing and wheezing. See Chapter 17 for more about treating cardiovascular illness, including heart disease.

- **Cancer:** A lingering cough may be an early sign of lung cancer, requiring prompt medical intervention. See Chapter 17 for more about treating cancer and other chronic conditions.

  If you're coughing up blood, seek immediate medical attention. If the cough persists despite your best efforts to cure it, consult your health-care provider for a diagnosis and treatment recommendations.

Tracking down the root cause of a cough isn't always easy. If you're not sure what's causing your cough, try adopting an anti-inflammatory diet. Eliminate sugar, dairy, and wheat/gluten (Chapter 2 has details on elimination diets). Drink 8 ounces of quality water every two waking hours. To thin mucus secretions and soothe any throat irritation, eat homemade chicken soup made with organic ingredients and without noodles (brown rice is okay). Use as much garlic and onion as you can stand, both of which boost the immune system.

Support your dietary changes with one or more of the following supplements (the more the better) in the recommended dosages, to break up phlegm, reduce inflammation, support respiratory health, and more:

Supplement	*Dosage*
N-acetyl cysteine	600 mg twice daily on an empty stomach
Mullein	500 mg twice daily
Proteolytic enzymes (combination including pancreatin, papain, rutin, bromelain, trypsin, serrapeptase, and chymotrypsin)	Between meals, according to label instructions
Perilla seed extract	100 mg twice daily
Quercetin	250 mg twice daily
Echinacea	500 mg twice daily
Astragalus	500 to 1,000 mg twice daily

After waking in the morning and using the restroom, drink two glasses of quality, filtered water and repeat daily until your cough clears. This is a very simple way to detox your system.

Clearing Up Laryngitis

Laryngitis, more a symptom than an illness, is inflammation of the larynx, resulting in a hoarse voice or inability to speak and difficulty swallowing. Common causes include acid reflux (Chapter 14), nasal or food allergies (Chapter 13), smoking, coughing (see the earlier section on coughs), overuse of vocal cords, burns from hot foods or drinks, and infection (see Chapter 6). Attend to any of these underlying causes as you implement the treatment options I present here.

Whatever the cause, rest your vocal cords. The vast majority of laryngitis cases clear up on their own with no other treatment.

Use eucalyptus oil to reduce inflammation. Mix a few drops of eucalyptus oil in a cup of tepid water, and use the solution to gargle (don't swallow) every two or three waking hours until symptoms fade.

For laryngitis from hot foods or drinks, sip on cool liquids and follow the pain and inflammation protocol:

Supplement	Dosage
White willow bark extract	600 mg once or twice daily between meals
Boswellia	100 mg once or twice daily between meals
Turmeric	200 mg once or twice daily between meals

For laryngitis caused by viral or bacterial infections, follow the acute cold protocol presented in Chapter 6.

Treating Sinus Congestion and Postnasal Drip

Sinus congestion occurs when the nasal passages get stopped up, and it's usually due to a combination of inflammation and excess mucus production. *Postnasal drip* is a condition in which excess mucus or excessively thick mucus flows down the back of the throat, causing coughing, sore throat, or a constant need to clear the throat.

Conventional medicine treats both conditions with antihistamines and decongestants, which can cause chronic sinus problems. Instead of taking that route, I recommend that you identify and treat the underlying cause: the common cold (Chapter 6), sinus infection, allergies (Chapter 13), tobacco smoke, overuse of nasal medication (antihistamines and decongestants), or nasal polyps (see a doctor). Here are some additional treatments to help cure the root cause of sinus congestion and postnasal drip:

✔ For sinus congestion in children, use a soft rubber bulb syringe to suck out mucus.

✔ Remove wheat (gluten) and dairy from your diet, even if you haven't tested positive for allergies to these foods.

✔ Drink 8 ounces of water every two waking hours.

✔ Place proline-rich polypeptides (PRPs) in a nasal mister and use several times daily: 2 shots up each nostril, lie down for several minutes, and breathe the spray into your sinuses.

✔ Use a xylitol nasal spray, such as Xlear (`www.xlear.com`), three to five times daily to wash your nasal passages and keep them hydrated.

✔ Gargle with a salt-water solution (½ teaspoon of Celtic sea salt dissolved in 1 cup of quality water).

✔ Irrigate your nasal passages using a neti pot and saline solution three times daily until the congestion clears. To make the saline solution, dissolve 1 teaspoon of sea salt and ⅛ teaspoon of baking soda in 1 cup of warm (body temperature) distilled water.

✔ After brushing your teeth at bedtime, chew slowly and completely and swallow a chewable preparation of the probiotic *Streptococcus salivarius* DDS 18, 1 billion CFU.

✔ Use a HEPA air filter to remove airborne allergens and other irritants from the air at home and work.

Snuffing Out Sneezing

If you're sneezing and have nasal congestion, skip back to the preceding section and address the nasal congestion first. An allergy or infection is probably causing both symptoms. If you're sneezing and don't have nasal congestion, then you're probably dealing with an airborne irritant. To provide your nasal passages with the support they need to remove irritants, do either of the following:

✔ Use an over-the-counter xylitol nasal spray, such as Xlear several times daily.

To make your own xylitol nasal spray, dissolve 1 teaspoon of sea salt, 1 tablespoon of xylitol, and ⅛ teaspoon of baking soda in 1 cup of warm, distilled water; add four drops of grapefruit seed extract as a preservative.

✔ Irrigate your nasal passages with a neti pot and xylitol-saline solution three times daily until symptoms subside (use the recipe in the preceding paragraph but leave out the grapefruit seed extract, and discard any unused solution). Don't irrigate your nasal passages for more than a few days, because excessive irrigation may irritate the sensitive nasal passages and wash out beneficial microbes.

Filtering the air with a HEPA filter at home and work also helps reduce airborne irritants before they reach your nose.

Soothing a Sore Throat

A sore throat *(pharyngitis)* is a symptom of the common cold (Chapter 6) and other viral infections, postnasal drip (covered earlier in this chapter), nasal allergies (Chapter 13), and bacterial infections such as strep throat.

Don't take antibiotics unless your doctor tests for infection and the test indicates that bacterial infection is the cause. Antibiotics are often prescribed for sore throats caused by viruses, and in these cases, the antibiotics do more harm than good because they don't kill the virus; instead, they wipe out many of the beneficial bacterial in your gut, increasing your risk of developing leaky gut and autoimmune disorders. Take antibiotics only if you have a severe bacterial infection, and if you take antibiotics, take a quality probiotic four hours after each antibiotic dose to help restore the beneficial flora in your gut.

For immediate relief of sore throat pain, try Biocidin TS Throat Spray. Spray one to three times toward the back of your throat as needed.

Most sore throats are caused by viral infection, such as the viruses that cause the common cold. For virus infections, eat lightly. Consume plenty of steamed vegetables, chicken, and miso soups. Stay well-hydrated by drinking plenty of quality water and herbal teas. Eliminate sugar (it suppresses your immune response) and dairy (it thickens mucus) and support your dietary changes with the acute cold protocol I recommend in Chapter 6.

Chapter 6

Combating Flus, Colds, and Infections

* *

In This Chapter

▶ Turbocharging your immune system to fight infection

▶ Battling bronchitis, pneumonia, and the common cold

▶ Fighting fever, flu, and other viruses

▶ Healing hepatitis and related conditions

▶ Defeating parasites and drug-resistant bacteria

▶ Curing shingles

* *

Your body is engaged in an unrelenting battle with environmental threats, many of which you can't even see with the naked eye. Bacteria, viruses, fungi, parasites, and other life forms are competing with you for survival and using your body as their battleground. In this chapter, you find out how to fight back . . . and win!

All doses of oral preparations are for adults. See Chapter 12 for guidance on adjusting dosages for children (and adults under 150 pounds).

Boosting Your Immune System

If you suffer from chronic infections — yeast overgrowth; a long history of bacterial or fungal infections; constipation, diarrhea, and bowel irritation; or chronic sinus infections — or if you've had to take several doses of antibiotics over the years, your immune system has probably been compromised. In most cases, this means that the bad bugs living in your gut are winning the battle against the good bugs.

Your doctor can order blood tests with an immune panel to determine whether your immune system is functioning within range.

Your digestive tract is responsible for about 70 percent of your immune response, serving as a key barrier to prevent bad things from entering into your *systemic* (whole body) circulation. To restore the delicately balanced ecosystem within your gut and boost your immune system, take any or all of the following key nutrients (the more the better) in the recommended doses:

- ✔ **Colostrum:** Bovine colostrum, derived from pre-milk that a cow secretes to feed a newborn calf, provides a rich source of immunoglobulin G (IgG, the most abundant antibody) and proline-rich polypeptides (PRPs, which modulate the immune system). Numerous scientific studies have shown that colostrum supports the human immune and *cytokine* (immune cell signaling) systems. (Bovine colostrum is 40 times richer in immune factors than human colostrum.) *Dosage:* 10,000 mg daily.

- ✔ ***Andrographis:*** *Andrographis* extract supports the body's natural defenses against viruses in the respiratory tract. *Dosage:* 400 mg daily.

- ✔ **Beta glucan:** Numerous clinical trials show that beta glucan, a unique complex carbohydrate, is a powerful immune system modulator. It directs immune cells to the infection site and facilitates the removal of infectious agents. *Dosage:* 700 mg daily first thing in the morning or last thing at night with 8 ounces of water.

- ✔ **Probiotics:** Probiotics protect the intestinal tract and restore beneficial intestinal flora. Choose a probiotic blend containing live organisms of 5 billion CFU (colony forming units) *Lactobacillus acidophilus* Rosell and 1 billion CFU *Bifidobacterium longum* Rosell. Buy from a reputable company that takes great care in the manufacturing, storage, and shipping of its probiotics. Take twice daily, before or during meals.

- ✔ **Vitamin D3:** Look for a product that uses extra virgin olive oil as its carrier. Many companies use soy oil, typically derived from genetically modified organisms. *Dosage:* 1,000 to 10,000 IU, depending on your blood levels (see Appendix A).

- ✔ **Vitamin C (mineral ascorbates):** A product that combines vitamin C with black pepper extract may increase vitamin C bioavailability as much as 40 percent. *Dosage:* 1,000 to 10,000 mg daily, depending on bowel tolerance, in divided doses. If you experience diarrhea, take less.

✔ **Other nutrients:** The following supplements also support a healthy gut and digestion. Take the dosage specified.

Nutrient	Dosage
Bee propolis	100 mg daily
Cinnamon bark extract	100 mg daily
Grapefruit seed extract	100 mg daily
Grapeseed extract	100 mg daily
Olive leaf extract	50 mg daily
Monolaurin	200 mg daily

Battling Bronchitis

When you have bronchitis, the lining of your bronchial tubes are inflamed, and you cough up thick, possibly discolored mucus. To relieve symptoms and speed healing, drink 8 ounces of water with fresh lemon every two hours, eat grandma's penicillin (chicken soup), drink peppermint and/or ginger tea, and take as many of the following as possible to boost lung function and immunity:

Natural Cure	Dosage
N-acetyl cysteine	600 mg twice daily taken on an empty stomach
Tylophora asthmatica extract (root)	15 mg two to three times daily
Boswellia serrata	150 mg two to three times daily
Picrorhiza extract (root)	75 mg two to three times daily
Quercetin	500 mg two to three times daily
Lobelia herb and seed	1,000 mg one to two times daily
Echinacea root	250 mg twice daily
Ginger	250 mg three to four times daily
Andrographis leaf extract	200 to 400 mg daily

Follow this regimen for a week, and your bronchitis should improve, but your cough may linger for about a month, which is natural.

TIP

If your symptoms don't improve, you may have chronic bronchitis, which usually requires medical intervention. If your doctor puts you on an anti-biotic, take a probiotic four hours before or after taking the antibiotic, and when your prescription runs out, continue taking probiotics and eat plenty of fermented foods, such as kimchi, sauerkraut, and yogurt or kefir (a yogurt-like drink), which are good sources of probiotics. If you have recurrent bouts of lung congestion, get tested for food allergies. See Chapter 13 for details.

Curing the Common Cold

You're coughing and sneezing, your nose is running, your throat is sore, and maybe you're running a fever. Those are all symptoms of the common cold. Colds generally last seven to ten days, and symptoms may linger for a couple weeks. To speed your recovery, hit back with the following acute cold protocol when you first notice symptoms:

Supplement	Dosage
Colostrum	10,000 mg one or two times daily
Proline-rich polypeptides	4 sprays in mouth, hold for 30 seconds and then swallow, twice daily early morning and before bed for a total of 16 mg daily
Probiotics (*Saccharomyces boulardii;* multistrain containing *Lactobacillus acidophilus, Bifidobacterium longum,* and *Lactobacillus plantarum;* and *Bifidobacterium lactis* [HOWARU Bifido]	250 mg *Saccharomyces boulardii;* 15 billion CFU multistrain probiotic, and 15 billion CFU HOWARU Bifido twice daily
Vitamin C (mineral ascorbates)	1,000 to 3,000 mg daily
Whole beta glucan	500 mg twice daily
Vitamin A	10,000 to 25,000 IU daily (see Appendix A for precautions)
Vitamin D3	5,000 to 10,000 IU daily, depending on blood levels (see Appendix A)
Zinc (lozenges and pill form)	Lozenges several times daily plus 20 mg in pill form twice daily during acute illness, not to exceed 40 mg total daily (see Appendix A for precautions)
Andrographis	200 mg twice daily
Isatis extract	150 mg twice daily
Licorice extract	80 mg twice daily
Olive leaf	1 to 2 g daily

The best cure for the common cold is not to get one. Keep your immune system strong to fight off infection. Minimize stress, get plenty of sleep, and wash your hands after being out in public places and before eating or touching your nose or mouth.

Fighting Fever

If you have a temperature above 99.5°F (37.5 °C), associated perhaps with chills and shivering, you have a fever. With the exception of high fevers (above 102°F [38.9 °C]), the best course of action is to let the fever run its course so that your immune system can fight what's ailing you. If the fever starts to climb above 102°F (38.9 °C), however, try to lower it by using ibuprofen; follow the label instructions for proper dosage. If the fever doesn't respond to medication or lasts longer than three days for an adult or one day for a child, consult your doctor.

Speeding your recovery

Regardless of the fever's severity, you can speed recovery by taking several herbs, including angelica, elderberry, rosemary, and yarrow as follows:

When	What
For the first 1 to 2 days	1 teaspoon of a tincture, or 1 to 2 capsules every one to three hours
For the next 5 days	2 teaspoons of tincture or 6 capsules daily

You may take each of these herbs separately or in combination; doses represent the total amount of herb to take.

All of these herbs make you sweat. See Chapter 3 for more about herbs and tinctures and Appendix D for details about these specific herbs.

Giving your immune system extra support

Fever is a sign that your body is actively fighting intruders, so when you have a fever, give your immune system some extra support. Take Echinacea (300 mg), vitamin C (1,000 mg), vitamin D3 (5,000 to 10,000 IU), and zinc (20 mg) several times daily for the first day or two and then decrease your dosage as the fever subsides.

For aggressive immune support, take mushroom extracts — reishi, shitake, maitake, or cordyceps — as a tonic: 15 to 30 drops two to three times daily.

Purging the Flu and Other Viruses

Like the common cold, the flu attacks your respiratory system, but it hits harder and faster. Symptoms include fever over 100°F (37.8 °C), severe muscle ache, chills, sweating, fatigue, and congestion.

If you or the person you are caring for has a severe case of the flu and is in a high-risk category — a young child, an older adult, a pregnant woman, or someone with a compromised immune system — see your doctor immediately. Flu can quickly turn into pneumonia, which can be fatal.

In the beginning stages of the flu, you have little appetite. Focus on drinking water, teas, and healthy green drinks loaded with antioxidants. Avoid dairy products, animal protein, sugar, and refined processed foods. Stick with low-glycemic fruits and vegetables. Chicken soup with extra onion, garlic, ginger, and lemon works wonders.

To boost your immune system, take the following supplements:

Supplement	Dosage
Vitamin C (mineral ascorbates)	Up to 10,000 mg daily (**Note:** If you develop diarrhea, reduce the dosage.)
Vitamin D3	2,000 to 10,000 IU daily, depending on your blood level (see Appendix A) (**Note:** The lower your vitamin D level, the more benefit you'll see.)
N-acetyl cysteine	600 mg twice daily, on an empty stomach
Selenium	200 mcg daily
Sambucol	1 tablespoon four times daily
Green tea (aqueous extract containing EGCG)	600 mg daily
Lomatium dissectum (capsule form or tincture)	500 mg in capsule form or 2 to 4 ml of tincture four times daily

Healing Hepatitis

Hepatitis refers to a group of inflammatory diseases of the liver. Symptoms of acute hepatitis include fatigue, vomiting, nausea, fever, loss of appetite, dark urine, yellowing of the skin (jaundice), enlarged and tender liver, and elevated liver enzymes. If you have these symptoms, see your doctor because pharmaceutical approaches for treating hepatitis are often necessary and beneficial. Note, however, that these treatments usually come with numerous side effects and lack the ability to prevent cirrhosis, further liver damage, and even liver cancer. Therefore, in addition to the conventional treatments and at the earliest stages of the disease, use natural cures to prevent the virus from replicating, reduce the severity of the illness, and repair liver damage. Here are some suggestions:

✔ **Start with your diet, which is fundamental in the healing process.** Everything you eat, breathe, touch, and smell is detoxified through your liver. If you consume alcohol, stop. Eat unprocessed or minimally processed whole foods in moderation and make sure that most are plants (fruits, vegetables, nuts, and seeds):

- Eat cruciferous vegetables — cauliflower, cabbage, cress, bok choy, broccoli, brussels sprouts, and others — many of which have the correct B vitamins, minerals, and sulfur-based amino acids that the detox process relies heavily on.

- Consume green tea and plenty of quality water.

- Reduce foods that are toxic to the liver, such as alcohol, refined sugar, processed carbohydrates, fried foods, caffeine, trans fatty acids, and unnecessary medications.

- Eliminate or severely reduce consumption of meat and dairy. If you do have meat, make sure it's of the highest quality available from pastured animals raised organically and fed non-GMO products.

- Look for dairy alternatives, such as nut milk, sheep, or goat sources and choose products from only free-range, pastured, well-cared-for animals.

You can also support your liver's recovery with one or more of the following supplements (the more the better) at the recommended dosages:

Supplement	*Dosage*
Vitamin C (mineral ascorbates)	1 to 2 g three times daily for several weeks
Vitamin E (mixed tocopherols)	400 IU per day
Selenium	200 mcg per day
Alpha-lipoic acid	300 mg twice daily
Vitamin K2	45 mg daily
Thiamine	100 mg daily
Phosphatidylcholine	1.8 g daily for hepatitis C (not hepatitis B)
Acetyl-L-carnitine	2 g daily on an empty stomach
Zinc	20 mg daily (see Appendix A for precautions)

(continued)

(continued)

Supplement	Dosage
Vitamins B12 (methylcobalamin, sublingual fast-dissolving tablet) and folate (5-MTHF)	5,000 mcg B12 and 2,000 mcg folate one to two times daily
Licorice root (*Glycyrrhiza glabra*)	500 mg three times daily (***Note:*** Monitor blood pressure; at high doses, licorice root may elevate blood pressure.)
Turmeric (*Currcuma longa*)	500 mg three times daily
Green drinks (high quality)	1 or more daily

You may take any or all of these supplements for the rest of your life. In fact, if you have hepatitis, I recommend it.

Celiac disease and nonceliac gluten sensitivity have been associated with inflammatory liver disorders, so get tested for gluten sensitivity. See Chapter 2 for more about gluten in your diet and Chapter 13 for guidance in treating gluten sensitivity.

Mending MRSA (Methicillin-Resistant Staphylococcus Aureus)

Methicillin-resistant Staphylococcus aureus (MRSA, pronounced "mersa") is an infection caused by a strain of *Staphylococcus* bacteria that's become resistant to antibiotics. If left untreated, MRSA may lead to loss of limbs or even death. MRSA first appears as small red bumps that look like pimples and may quickly turn into painful abscesses.

If you suspect a MRSA infection, seek immediate medical attention. Certain powerful antibiotics have been developed to fight this infection. Special medical-grade manuka honey has been shown to be highly effective in curing MRSA — more effective than even antibiotics.

The natural cures approach is best for prevention and early treatment. Start with the anti-inflammatory diet (see Chapter 2) and drink half your body weight in ounces of water daily. Avoid sugar and refined processed carbohydrates, which lower your immune response. Consume high-quality organic vegetables and a small amount of low glycemic fruits. Support diet with one or more of the following supplements or topical applications:

Supplement	Dosage/Application
Oil of oregano	Take 50 mg with meals and before bed; you can also apply the oil topically
Tea tree oil	Apply oil to affected area several times daily
Thyme oil	Apply oil to affected area several times daily
Bioactive silver hydrosol (Argentyn 23)	Take 1 dropper full three times daily and apply gel to the infected area

You can use any one of the topical treatments listed in the preceding or alternate any two or all three. Oil of oregano, which has been shown to kill MRSA, has the most research backing up its effectiveness.

Take all of the following supplements to boost your overall immune response to the infection:

Supplement	Dosage
Whole beta glucan	500 mg twice daily
Vitamin C (mineral ascorbates)	1,000 mg two to three times daily
Probiotics (high-quality multistrain)	30 to 100 billion CFU once daily (**Note:** If you're taking an antibiotic, separate your probiotic from your antibiotic by at least four hours.)

Flushing Internal Parasites Out of Your System

Unlike the beneficial microorganisms of probiotics, parasites are microorganisms that live off nutrients in your body and usually compromise your health. Parasite infections can cause numerous and varied symptoms, including diarrhea, constipation, abdominal bloating, gas, indigestion, heartburn, inflammatory fever, suppressed appetite, skin conditions, behavioral changes, anal itching, weight loss, rectal bleeding, and bowel disease, including colitis and Crohn's disease.

If you have these symptoms and suspect that the cause may be related to internal parasites, see your natural cures provider, who can order a digestive stool analysis with parasitology test. With the results, you can pinpoint exactly which parasite you have so that your treatment can be tailored specifically to that parasite.

The key to getting rid of parasites is to starve them out (they eat whatever you eat) while simultaneously nurturing the good bacteria in your digestive tract so they can wage an effective fight against the bad guys. Eliminate sugar, high-fructose corn syrup, heavily processed foods (especially refined carbohydrates), and trans fatty acids. Consume a low carbohydrate diet and take the following supplements:

Supplement	*Dosage*
Monolaurin	200 mg twice daily
L-lysine	150 mg twice daily
Bee propolis	100 mg twice daily
Cinnamon bark extract	100 mg twice daily
Grapefruit seed extract	100 mg twice daily
Grapeseed extract	100 mg twice daily
Olive leaf extract	50 mg twice daily
Oil of oregano	500 mg up to four times daily
Ginger	Drink several cups of ginger tea daily or take 500 mg in capsule form two to three times daily
Black walnut	250 mg three times daily or 30 drops of a black walnut tincture
Probiotics (*Saccharomyces boulardii* and a multistrain of *Lactobacillus* and *Bifidobacterium*)	250 mg *Saccharomyces boulardii* twice daily; 5 billion CFU multistrain two to three times daily

Recognizing the importance of a healthy gut

People generally don't want to think about the critters living inside of them, feasting on their food and leaving toxic waste behind. The good news is that some of these microorganisms live symbiotically with your body, performing essential biological processes that keep you healthy. The bad news is that some of these microorganisms are *parasites* — living in you at the expense of your health. So how do you kill the bad guys without hurting the good guys, when they all live in such close proximity?

The answer lies inside your gut. Numerous factors affect your intestinal tract's overall health. Being breast-fed, being born vaginally, and avoiding exposure to antibiotics in prescription medications and in the animal products you consume promote a healthy gut. However, today, many people are bottle-fed, born via cesarean section, have taken numerous rounds of prescribed antibiotics, and have eaten animal products of livestock given loads of prescription antibiotics to prevent infection. This sets the stage for parasitic overgrowth by killing off your good bacteria.

Maintaining the healthy and sensitive balance of the ecosystem living inside your gut is the single most important step you take in defeating parasites and warding off a host of other illnesses.

Clearing Your Lungs of Pneumonia

Pneumonia, an inflammation of the lungs, is a common lung infection. Whether the infection is viral or bacterial, it causes cough, chest pain, fever, and difficulty breathing. Other symptoms may include headache, excessive fatigue, loss of appetite, and confusion (especially in older adults).

Pneumonia is a major cause of death worldwide and the sixth leading cause of death in the United States. If you have symptoms of pneumonia, consult your doctor, especially if you or the person you're caring for is in a high-risk category — a child under 2 years old, an adult over 65 years old, or a person with a compromised immune system. Pneumonia can progress quickly and become life-threatening, so aggressive conventional treatment may be required.

If you're diagnosed with pneumonia, rest as much as possible. Drink plenty of water and herbal teas (no sugary or diet drinks). Take antibiotics or antivirals as prescribed by your doctor. Because your diet can profoundly affect the speed of your recovery, change to the anti-inflammatory diet (see Chapter 2) and eliminate animal protein. The protein you get from vegetables such as artichokes, spinach, peas (fresh or frozen), eggplant, beets, and cauliflower is fine.

Creating your own spa

Some spas feature a eucalyptus steam room or sauna to help patrons with respiratory issues clear their lungs. If your local spa doesn't offer this feature, gather the supplies you need to create your own mini eucalyptus steam room: eucalyptus and tea tree oil, hot water, a heat-resistant bowl, and a towel large enough to fit over your head and the bowl. (Eucalyptus breaks down mucus, and tree oil is antimicrobial.) Then follow these steps:

1. Place hot water in the bowl, enough to produce steam but not hot enough to burn you.

2. Placed several drops of eucalyptus and tea tree oil in water.

3. Place the towel over your head and lean your head down over the bowl, so the towel forms a tent over your head and the bowl.

4. Breathe deeply through your nose, allowing steam to enter deep into your lungs for about two to four minutes.

5. Repeat Steps 1 to 4 three or more times daily (the more the better).

See Chapter 3 for more about preparing and using herbal remedies.

If you take antibiotics, take probiotics during and after treatment to maintain healthy bacteria in your gut, but be sure to take your antibiotics and probiotics at least four hours apart so that they don't interfere with one another. The exception is *Saccharomyces boulardii,* a beneficial yeast, which you can take at any time, preferably with meals.

Supplement your diet with one or more of the following:

Supplement	Dosage
N-acetyl cysteine	600 mg twice daily, on an empty stomach
Pleurisy root	20 drops of tincture two to three times daily
Garlic	300 mg in capsule form, or 5 ml garlic extract diluted in water or juice, twice daily
Turmeric	400 mg daily in capsule form; added as a spice to meals; or 5 ml turmeric extract diluted in a small amount of water or juice twice daily
Ginger	2.5 ml diluted in water or juice, or 300 mg in capsule form, two to three times daily
Vitamin C (mineral ascorbates)	1,000 mg two to three times daily
Oil of oregano	5 ml oregano oil mixed with coconut oil and dissolved in mouth several times daily
Astragalus	500 mg in capsule form two to four times daily, or 5 ml diluted in water or juice two to three times daily
Echinacea root	150 mg in capsule form or 5 ml diluted in water or juice, two to three times daily
Eucalyptus and tea tree oil	Inhale as steam or rub a preparation made from these oils on your chest and back

Shedding Shingles (Herpes Zoster)

Shingles is the sequel to chicken pox. It causes pain typically followed by blisters that appear on either the left or right side of the body. It may also cause headache, fever, chills, and fatigue. Although the rash typically clears up in two to four weeks, nerve pain *(post-herpetic neuralgia)* may last for several weeks or months afterwards.

To prevent and treat shingles, adopt a natural foods diet, as explained in Chapter 2. If infected, supplement your diet with the following nutrients:

Nutrient	Dosage
Whole beta glucan (whole glucan particle derived from *Saccharomyces cerevisae*)	500 mg three times daily during active lesions; decrease dosage as lesions heal
Proline-rich polypeptides	4 sprays in mouth, hold for 30 seconds and swallow, twice daily in the early morning and before bed for a total of 16 mg daily
Vitamin C (mineral ascorbates)	1,000 mg every two to three hours (or as much as you can tolerate without developing diarrhea); decrease dosage as symptoms improve
Olive leaf extract	100 mg three times daily
Vitamin E (mixed tocopherols)	400 IU daily
Zinc glycinate chelate	20 mg twice daily (see Appendix A for precautions)
Vitamin A (retinyl palmitate and beta-carotene)	2,500 IU retinyl palmitate and 2,500 IU beta-carotene daily (see Appendix A for precautions)
Andrographis	400 mg two to three times daily

You can also ask your doctor for vitamin B12 injections, which can accelerate recovery from an outbreak: 1,000 mg daily injected intramuscularly for five days, followed by 500 mg every other day until the lesions heal.

Deseret Biologics (desbio.com) has a two-kit homeopathic treatment that's safe and effective for shingles. The kit contains ten vials, each containing a different dilution of the actual deactivated virus. You take the vials of the first kit in ascending order over the course of a month to boost your active immune response and then you take the vials of the second kit in descending order to support passive immune protection. You can't buy the kits directly; you must obtain them through a healthcare provider.

To fight the infection from the outside in and relieve pain, apply the following to the affected area at the first sign of outbreak:

- ✔ **Capsaicin:** Found in plants including chili pepper, red pepper, cayenne, and paprika. This burns initially, but it quickly reduces inflammation and dries the lesion.

- ✔ **Peppermint oil:** Apply liberally as an effective treatment for post-hepatic neuralgia

Chapter 7

Healing Skin, Hair, Scalp, and Nail Conditions

*W*hen your skin, scalp, hair, or nails succumb to illness, you have two problems: the condition itself and how it makes you feel about yourself and your appearance. That doesn't make you vain; it makes you normal. Whether you find out that lice have infested your locks, you break out in acne, or your fingernails turn yellow, you want a cure, and you want it *now!* Although I can't promise immediate results, in this chapter, I offer guidance on what you can do right now to turn the tide on the most common ailments affecting your skin, scalp, hair, and nails.

Doses in this chapter are for adults, not children. For guidance on how to adjust dosages for children (and adults under 150 pounds), turn to Chapter 12.

Getting the Skinny on Skin Conditions

Skin conditions may or may not be only skin deep. Certain skin conditions, such as blisters, corns, calluses, and ringworm, are obviously caused by external irritants and respond to topical treatments. Other skin conditions are caused by underlying, often *systemic* (body-wide) issues, such as food allergies and intolerances, or missing nutrients. In these cases, the skin condition is merely a symptom of a deeper illness. In this section, I provide a host of natural remedies that target the root cause of the ailment and help make the symptoms disappear.

Eradicating abscesses, boils, and carbuncles

An *abscess* is an inflamed, pus-filled mass surrounded by pink or red. Abscesses typically occur in the armpits; in the groin, anal, or vaginal areas; near the base of the spine; on the face; and inside the mouth. Abscesses are caused by bacterial infection usually made possible by a weakened immune system. An abscess around a hair follicle is a *boil*. A *carbuncle* is a cluster of boils affecting more than one hair follicle. Boils and carbuncles are commonly caused by a compromised immune system, diabetes, contact with a boil, skin conditions such as acne and eczema, or poor hygiene. This section explains how to remedy abscesses and boils.

When you notice an abscess, boil, or carbuncle, first do no harm. Resist the temptation to press down on it, which can drive the infection deeper into the skin. Nor should you try to lance it with a needle, because that may worsen the infection. Instead keep the area clean, using soap and water. Seek medical attention if you have a fever approaching 102°F (38.9 °C), the abscess is bigger than two inches in diameter, is in the groin or rectal area, or has red streaks leading away from it.

Treating abscesses

For an abscess up to a half inch in diameter, apply a warm, moist compress for 30 minutes four times daily and then apply a topical antiseptic.

To make your own antiseptic wash, follow these steps:

1. **In a glass container, mix the following herbs:**

   1 to 2 teaspoons of barberries

   1 tablespoon of white oak bark

   1 teaspoon of Echinacea root

   1 teaspoon of granulated Oregon grape root

2. **Pour 2 cups of boiling water over the herbs and allow the mixture to sit for three to four hours.**

3. **Pour the mixture through a strainer, keeping the liquid and discarding the rest.**

Apply the antiseptic wash topically with a gauze pad. To treat dental abscesses, swish this mixture in your mouth for several minutes and then spit it out.

Boost your immune system with 30 drops each of Echinacea and yerba mansa tincture mixed into 1 cup of warm water. Drink a cup of this tonic three to five times daily. For additional immune support, adjust your diet, as necessary, following the guidelines in Chapter 2, and take one or more of the following nutritional supplements until your abscess heals:

Supplement	Dosage
Echinacea root (4:1 extract)	150 mg three times daily for up to two weeks
Whole beta glucan particle	500 mg twice daily
Proline-rich polypeptides	4 sprays in mouth, hold for 30 seconds and swallow, twice daily early morning and before bed for a total of 16 mg daily
Vitamin C (mineral ascorbates)	1,500 mg three times a day
Argentyn 23 bioactive colloidal silver hydrosol	1 dropper full in mouth for 30 seconds and then swallow, two to three times daily

Most abscesses progress to a head and then spontaneously rupture. If the infection becomes more severe, it may spread into deeper tissue and a fever may ensue. If symptoms worsen or don't improve in a couple of days, consult your doctor, who may lance the abscess to promote drainage and prescribe antibiotics. If you're given a prescription for antibiotics, take a quality probiotic containing 5 billion CFU (culture forming units) of *Lactobacillus acidophilus* and *Bifidobacterium* Rosell four hours after each dose of antibiotic.

People with immune systems weakened by diabetes, AIDS, cancer, or chemotherapy are more prone to abscesses than others. In addition, alcohol abuse and intravenous drug use increase the risk for developing an abscess. Additional risk factors include skin-to-skin contact with an abscess, poor hygiene, and compromised peripheral circulation.

Treating boils and carbuncles

You can treat small boils at home by applying warm compresses to relieve pain and promote drainage. The key to healing a boil is to soften it so that the bacteria and infection can drain out of the inflamed area. Apply the warm compress 20 minutes four times daily. Use a clean towel or compress each time to avoid spreading the infection. After touching a boil, wash your hands and launder any clothing or linens that come in contact with it.

Here are some additional natural cures for boils:

- **Neem (Indian lilac):** Grind a handful of neem leaves to form a paste and apply to the boil several times daily.

- **Black seed:** For a painful boil, grind black seeds to form a paste and apply to the infected boil several times daily.

- **Tea tree oil:** Using a cotton swab or cotton ball, apply tea tree oil several times daily until the boil heals.

- **Turmeric:** Take 1.5 g by capsule twice daily.

- **Turmeric and ginger paste:** Make a paste with ¼ teaspoon fresh ginger and ¼ teaspoon turmeric, apply it to the boil, and cover with a breathable bandage. Change several times daily.

- **Onion:** Place a slice of onion over the boil, cover it with a breathable bandage, and let it dry out the boil. (Onions have antiseptic as well as antimicrobial properties.)

- **Whole beta glucan:** Take 500 mg twice daily to prime and mobilize the cells that support the body's first line of defense.

- **Vitamin C (mineral ascorbates):** Take 1,000 mg two to three times daily.

In rare instances, a boil infection can spread to the blood, causing *sepsis* — a whole-body infection. Sepsis can affect your heart as well as every organ system in your body and needs to be taken seriously. Seek medical care if the boil appears on your face, is extremely painful, is accompanied by fever, is larger than two inches in diameter, or has lasted longer than two weeks.

Clearing up acne

Acne is related more to what you put into your body than what you put on it. Therefore, the most effective approach to treating acne is to adjust your diet. Here are some suggestions:

- Lower the glycemic load in your diet by avoiding sugar, bread, rice, cereal, pasta, and all flour products.

- Stop drinking cow milk, because it has high levels of androgens, which have been linked to acne outbreaks. (*Androgens* are hormones produced in both male and females that cause the sebaceous glands to produce more oily secretions.)

- If you eat chocolate (some is okay), opt for dark chocolate over milk chocolate and look for a variety of dark chocolate that contains the lowest amount of sugar.

✔ Eat a healthy, plant-based diet rich in phytonutrients and antioxidants along with lean animal protein. Increase your consumption of vegetables and low glycemic fruits (eight to ten servings daily).

✔ Supplement your diet with the following:

Supplement	Dosage
Evening primrose oil	1,000 to 1,500 mg twice daily
Zinc glycinate chelate	20 mg twice daily (see Appendix A for precautions)
Vitamin A (retinyl palmitate and beta-carotene)	2,500 IU daily (see Appendix A for precautions)
Vitamin E (mixed tocopherols)	400 IU daily
Probiotics (quality multistrain consisting of *Lactobacillus acidophilus* and *Bifidobacterium*)	5 billion CFU

✔ Increase the ratio of omega-3 to omega-6 fats you consume. Omega-6 fats, found in meat, dairy, and shellfish, are pro-inflammatory. A small amount of omega-6 benefits your health; however, the standard American diet now has a much higher ratio of omega-6 to omega-3, putting the entire body, including the skin, into an inflammatory state. The majority of inflammatory omega-6 comes from the oils used in packaged snack foods and chips. Instead, consume a diet high in omega-3 essential fatty acids (EFAs), found in deep-sea, cold-water ocean fish and in flax oil.

A latent food allergy may also contribute to acne. The biggest offenders are wheat, corn, soy, eggs, dairy, and yeast. See Chapter 13 for more about diagnosing and treating food allergies and sensitivities. Several medications, including corticosteroids, lithium, and androgens are also known to cause acne.

Avoid using long-term antibiotics and Accutane to treat acne. These prescription medications are associated with significant harmful side effects that can last for many decades after you stop using them.

Ditching jock itch

Jock itch is a fungal infection that affects the groin area. Symptoms include itching and burning around the affected area along with red, flaking, peeling, and cracking skin. Common causes of jock itch include a lowered immune system; tight, restrictive clothing; fungal contact through shared showers, locker rooms, clothing, or towels; and being overweight. The most effective cures begin with addressing the common causes first:

- ✔ Shower immediately after athletic activities.

- ✔ Stay clean and dry.

- ✔ Apply antifungal powders after showering (don't use antifungal powders that contain cornstarch, which feeds the fungus; use a powder with baking soda instead).

- ✔ Don't share clothing or towels.

- ✔ Avoid tight-fitting clothing.

If you get jock itch, try one or more of the following natural cures:

- ✔ **Tea tree oil or oil of oregano:** If your skin is cracked and irritated, proceed with caution because tea tree oil and oil of oregano can sting. Soak a cotton ball in the oil and apply several times during the course of the day. For severe cases, mix tea tree oil or oil of oregano with coconut oil and apply several times during the course of the day.

- ✔ **Apple cider vinegar:** Mix 2 tablespoons of apple cider vinegar in 2 cups of warm water. Soak cotton balls in the solution and apply liberally to the affected area. Let the area dry on its own. Apply during the day and before going to sleep.

- ✔ **Rubbing alcohol or Listerine:** Soak a cotton ball in rubbing alcohol or Listerine (the dye-free version) and apply several times during the course of the day, letting the area dry on its own (rubbing alcohol evaporates quickly). *A **word of caution:*** If your skin is severely cracked, the rubbing alcohol burns, so don't use rubbing alcohol unless you want to hit the ceiling. Listerine also burns initially but not as intensely, and it burns less with continued treatment.

- ✔ **Salt bath:** Use Epsom salts, or plain or iodized salt. Fill a bathtub with warm water and mix in a generous amount of salt. Soak in the tub for 20 minutes twice daily.

- ✔ **Manuka honey with minced garlic:** Make a paste of 2 teaspoons of honey and a small amount of minced garlic. Apply the paste to the infected skin, leave it on for a few minutes, and then wash it off. This may burn at first, but the cure is worth the pain and effort.

In severe or stubborn cases, consult your doctor; you may need to use a conventional antifungal medication.

Bearing down on blisters

Blisters result from friction, chemical exposure, or infection and are the body's way of protecting the underlying skin as the body grows new skin. Therefore, you don't want to pop a blister; instead, let it heal naturally. The following natural cures may help in the meantime:

- ✔ **Aloe vera:** Break off a piece of the plant, rub the broken end gently over the blister, and cover with a breathable bandage. Do this several times a day.

- ✔ **Apple cider vinegar:** Place a small amount on a cotton swab and apply it around the blister. Be aware that this is likely to sting.

- ✔ **Green tea:** Green tea has anti-inflammatory properties. Boil a cup of green tea, let it cool, and then use a cotton swab to apply the tea to the blister several times daily.

- ✔ **Tea tree oil ointment:** Apply this ointment several times daily and cover with a breathable bandage.

Softening corns and calluses

Corns and *calluses* are thick, hardened layers of skin that develop as your skin tries to protect itself from excess friction or pressure. A corn is smaller than a callous, usually appears on the top or side of the foot or toe, and is characterized by a hard center surrounded by inflamed skin. A callous is larger but rarely painful and usually forms on the palms of the hands or soles of the feet. Although they may be uncomfortable or unsightly, corns and calluses rarely pose a serious danger to your health, unless they become infected. Complications are more likely to arise in individuals with compromised immune systems or poor circulation, such as certain people with diabetes.

Don't cut to remove a corn or callous because doing so can cause infection or bleeding. Instead, treat corns and calluses with a two-pronged approach: removing the cause of the problem and then treating the corn or callus itself.

Removing the source of the problem

First, relieve the pressure or friction that caused the corn or callus. Avoid repetitive actions that caused the corn or callus to form and be sure that you're wearing the right shoe for your foot. Check your foot size periodically (your foot grows as you age) and shop for shoes at the end of the day when your feet are swollen. Doing so prevents you from buying shoes that are too small. For corns, you can also try nonmedicated corn pads, available in most stores to relieve pressure.

Consult a podiatrist or chiropractor to obtain *custom orthotics* — inserts designed specifically to support the three arches of *your* feet. Don't settle for over-the-counter shoe inserts. I recommend Foot Levelers; visit www. footlevelers.com to find a practitioner in your area. Get two or three pairs — one pair each for your work, dress, and exercise shoes — to provide custom support for that particular shoe type and activity.

Removing the corn or callus

After you do what you can to avoid corns and calluses, then turn your attention to removing the corn or callus by following these steps (if you have diabetes, consult your doctor prior to trying any of the home remedies outlined in these steps):

1. **Soak your hands or feet in warm water or apply over-the-counter patches that contain 40 percent salicylic acid, as instructed on the label.**

   This step softens the corn or callus.

   Soak your feet in warm water with Epsom salt, apply moisturizer, and wrap each foot in a plastic bag. Keep the bags on for at least one hour. You can do this while reading or watching TV.

2. **Use a nail file, emery board, or pumice stone to gently scrub away the dead skin.**

   Scrub away only the dead skin. Dead, softened skin rubs off easily; if you need to scrub hard to remove the skin, either it's not soft enough or you're removing live skin and will end up with a painful raw area if you continue.

3. **Apply an antibiotic cream to prevent infection.**

4. **Repeat Steps 1 through 3 one or two times daily until the skin feels normal.**

Dealing with dermatitis and eczema

Dermatitis is an inflammation of the skin, which typically causes the skin to be red, dry, and itchy. There are several forms of dermatitis, including *contact dermatitis* (for example, poison ivy, which I cover in Chapter 4), *atopic dermatitis* (such as eczema), and *seborrheic dermatitis,* which I cover in the later section "Scrubbing Away Hair and Scalp Conditions").

The first step in treating dermatitis is to identify and remove whatever's causing it. If you've been playing in a patch of poison ivy, you probably know the cause. If not, you need to do some detective work. Several factors are known to contribute to various skin conditions, including dry skin from extended baths or showers, stress, soaps, wool clothing, tobacco smoke, air pollution, food allergies, leaky gut (see Chapter 13), and essential fatty acid deficiencies. In this section, I provide guidance on investigating some of the less obvious causes.

Throw yourself a tea party. In one study, a majority of participants who drank oolong tea saw improvement in their symptoms within a few weeks. Drink a liter of tea daily — steep a 10-gram tea bag in 1 liter of boiling water for five minutes.

Retooling your diet

The standard American diet (SAD) is the root cause of many health conditions, including those that affect the skin. Remove *all* sugar, dairy, and wheat products from your diet for a minimum of three weeks and note any effect on skin inflammation. If you notice a difference, either remove these items from your diet permanently or reintroduce them slowly, one at a time, to determine which one is causing the problem, and then eliminate that item from your diet.

Exploring the food allergy and sensitivity connection

A large body of evidence indicates that many patients with atopic dermatitis benefit from identifying and removing symptom-causing foods. See Chapter 2 for more about following an elimination diet to identify food allergies and sensitivities.

Food challenges — that is, eliminating and then reintroducing suspected problem foods — may cause severe reactions in highly sensitive individuals. If you're at risk for severe reactions, either conduct food challenges only under the close supervision of an experienced practitioner in a setting that's properly equipped to deal with severe allergic reactions, or don't conduct food challenges. *Anaphylaxis* (a life-threatening reaction) is uncommon, but it has been reported when reintroducing trigger foods.

Considering nickel and fluoride as possible contributing factors

In certain people, ingesting nickel or fluoride may trigger dermatitis. Nickel occurs naturally in certain foods or leaches into food from stainless steel cookware. Foods that often contain nickel include wine, beer, chocolate, herring, tomato, onion, whole-grain bread, carrots, and peas. Leaky gut is common in people with dermatitis and may be the reason why nickel absorption appears to be increased in certain people.

Several studies identify fluoride as a contributory factor. Try using only fluoride-free toothpaste and water.

Eliminating trans fatty acids

Trans fatty acids, a common ingredient in processed foods, are a "Frankenfood," an artificial food that has no place in the human diet. By ingesting trans fatty acids, you displace healthy essential fats from the cell membranes; these essential fats are key to preventing dermatitis.

If you see "partially hydrogenated oil" on a food label, you know that you're holding a food that contains trans fatty acids. Even some foods that claim to have zero trans fats may contain trans fatty acids, because the government allows any food that contains less than 0.5 mg trans fatty acids to be labeled as having no trans fatty acids — a practice that is harmful to your health. The only way to avoid trans fatty acids is to consume only real, whole foods and to not deep fry with most vegetable oils.

Taking in good fatty acids

The majority of evidence indicates that fatty acid supplementation helps individuals with skin conditions. Prior to supplementing your diet with fatty acids, ask your healthcare provider to order a fatty acid profile, which shows you which fatty acids, if any, you're deficient in. If you find that you're deficient, here are some general dosage guidelines:

Fatty Acid	*Dosage*
EPA	2 g daily
DHA	1.5 g daily
Evening primrose oil	2 g twice daily
Flaxseed oil	10 to 30 ml daily (2 teaspoons to 2 tablespoons)

Supplement long-term use of essential fatty acids with 400 IU vitamin E in the form of mixed tocopherols.

Supplementing your diet

Additional supplementation may help with various types of dermatitis. Try adding the following supplements to your diet:

Supplement	*Dosage*
Colostrum	10,000 mg daily
Vitamin A (retinyl palmitate and beta-carotene)	2,500 IU retinyl palmitate and 2,500 IU beta-carotene daily (see Appendix A for precautions)
Vitamin C (mineral ascorbates)	1,000 mg two to three times daily
Vitamin D3	2,000 to 10,000 IU daily, depending on blood levels (see Appendix A)
Vitamin E (mixed tocopherols)	400 IU daily

Supplement	Dosage
Coconut oil (organic)	1 teaspoon one to two times daily (***Tip:*** Swallowing a teaspoon of thick oil isn't the most pleasant experience, but you get used to it. If you can't get used to it, try adding your daily dose to cooked vegetables or rice.)
Apple cider vinegar	2 teaspoons daily (***Tip:*** Mix it into a warm cup of water and add honey to make a palatable tea.)

In addition to these supplements, take pancreatic enzymes, betaine HCL, and probiotics to stimulate digestion. See Chapter 14 for details.

Boosting your zinc intake

Zinc deficiency has been linked to dermatitis. Ask your healthcare provider to order an RBC zinc test on a blood sample to determine whether you have a zinc deficiency.

Alternatively, you can perform the following at-home test: Place 2 teaspoons (about 2 mg) of zinc sulfate in your mouth. If you taste the distinctive flavor of zinc, your zinc level is probably okay. If you don't taste anything or have a delayed taste perception, you're probably deficient in zinc.

If you're deficient in zinc, supplementing your diet with zinc may help clear up your dermatitis. Take up to 20 mg zinc glycinate chelate twice daily. Supplement long-term use of zinc with 1 mg copper for every 10 mg zinc daily.

Soothing your skin

To reduce inflammation and soothe your skin, try one or more of the following topical treatments (avoid coconut oil or oatmeal if you're allergic to these foods):

- Apply warm coconut oil (not too hot) to the affected areas before bed.
- Mix 1 cup of oatmeal in your bathwater and soak in it daily for several weeks.
- Mix 1 part apple cider vinegar with 1 part water and apply the solution to your skin twice daily.

 ✔ Apply aloe vera gel to the affected skin several times daily until the dermatitis is healed.

 ✔ Combine equal amounts of manuka honey, beeswax, and olive oil. Heat the mixture in a double boiler to make an ointment and then allow it to cool. Every day for several weeks, apply the mixture to your skin, allowing it to remain there for several hours.

Handling herpes simplex 1

Herpes simplex is a highly contagious virus that causes blisters or lesions. Herpes simplex virus 1 (HSV-1) typically appears above the waist (in and around the mouth) in the form of cold sores. Herpes simplex virus 2 (HSV-2) typically appears below the waist (in and around the genital area; see Chapter 19). The virus can spread through direct contact with an infected person who is producing or shedding the virus — whether or not the person is experiencing an active outbreak.

After the herpes virus infects someone, it remains with that person for life, becoming latent and hiding in the cell bodies of nerve cells. After primary infection, some people never experience another outbreak; others experience sporadic episodes of viral reactivation. In a reactivation, the virus is transported to the skin, where it replicates, and new lesions appear. Reactivation often occurs when the immune system is compromised by cold, flu, eczema, fatigue, lack of sleep, sunburn, or physical or emotional stress.

The herpes virus can't yet be eradicated from the body. Conventional medicine uses antiviral drugs to hinder replication of the virus and prevent or treat outbreaks. Medical research shows that daily use of antiviral medications, such as acyclovir and valacyclovir, significantly reduce recurrences of infection.

The natural cures approach focuses on boosting the body's immune system to keep the virus in check:

 ✔ Avoid refined sugar, which weakens the immune system.

 ✔ Identify and avoid any allergenic foods (see Chapter 13).

 ✔ Avoid high arginine foods that can cause the virus to replicate. These foods include peanuts, pecans, almonds, Brazil nuts, and cashews, as well as grains that are higher in arginine and lower in lysine.

 ✔ Take 1,000 mg vitamin C (as mineral ascorbates) three times daily to prevent outbreaks. For an acute episode, take up to 10,000 mg daily for five to ten days (as much as you can take without getting diarrhea).

✔ Take 500 to 3,000 mg L-lysine daily to prevent outbreaks.

✔ Apply vitamin E oil three to six times daily for the first three days of an acute episode.

✔ Take 20 to 40 g zinc glycinate chelate daily. (Supplement long-term use of zinc with 1 mg copper for every 10 mg zinc daily.)

✔ Take 250 mg whole beta glucan twice daily to prevent outbreaks. During an acute episode, take 500 mg twice daily.

✔ Take 1 dropper full colloidal silver daily to prevent outbreaks. During an acute episode, take 1 dropper full three times daily. You may also apply colloidal silver topically as a gel.

To retrain your immune system to keep infection in check, try Deseret Biologicals Herpes Simplex Series kit. Use two kits over the course of two months — one vial every third day.

Honing in on hives

Hives (also known as *urticaria*) is a skin rash with raised itchy bumps. It often occurs as a result of a food allergy, nervous condition, or change in temperature, and is often treated with antihistamines and corticosteroids. These medications may help reduce symptoms in the short run, but they fail to address the root causes, which commonly include food allergies, especially to shellfish, dairy, nuts, yeast, and wheat; food additives, including preservatives and artificial colors and flavors; medications, especially those that are high in salicylates, such as aspirin and other nonsteroid anti-inflammatory drugs (NSAIDs); leaky gut; physical irritants, including friction, pressure, heat, cold, exercise, and sunlight; fluoride in municipal drinking water, children's multivitamins, and toothpaste; penicillin in commercially prepared milk and milk products; candidiasis (yeast overgrowth); insufficient chewing or low stomach acid; aspartame, an artificial sweetener; and autoimmune thyroid, a condition in which the immune system attacks the thyroid gland.

Ask your doctor to order tests for leaky gut and food allergies and sensitivities (Chapter 13). The results can help your doctor determine a treatment protocol that can have a profound effect on reducing hives.

While you're waiting for the test results, start a modified elimination diet (see Chapter 2) with an emphasis on removing common trigger foods, including dairy, eggs, yeast, nuts, sugar, and wheat. Supplement your diet with one or more of the following nutritional supports (the more the better) at the recommended dosages:

Nutrient	Dosage
Colostrum	10,000 mg once daily
Proline-rich polypeptides	4 sprays in mouth, hold for 30 seconds and swallow, twice daily early morning and before bed for a total of 16 mg daily
Probiotics (multistrain of *Lactobacillus acidophilus* Rosell and *Bifidobacterium* Rosell)	5 billion CFU daily
Vitamin B12 (methylcobalamin, sublingual fast-dissolving tablet)	5,000 mcg twice daily
Vitamin C (mineral ascorbates)	1,000 mg two to three times daily
Vitamin A (retinyl palmitate and beta-carotene)	2,500 IU retinyl palmitate and 2,500 IU beta-carotene daily (see Appendix A for precautions)
Vitamin D3 (cholecalciferol)	1,000 to 10,000 IU daily, depending on your blood levels
Betaine HCL	300 mg with meals
Quercetin	1,000 mg three times daily with meals
Milk thistle extract and N-acetyl cysteine	250 mg milk thistle extract and 200 mg N-acetyl cysteine twice daily

Subduing psoriasis

Psoriasis is a chronic recurring autoimmune skin condition characterized by raised, inflamed lesions covered with silvery white scales. In psoriasis, skin cells replicate rapidly, giving the new cells no place to go, thus creating mounds of skin. Psoriasis is associated with inflammatory arthritis affecting the fingers and toes.

Conventional therapy focuses on reducing lesions from the outside in but doesn't address the fundamental underlying root cause of psoriasis — bad genes along with one or more of the following: delayed food allergies, leaky gut, inadequate protein digestion, *Candida* yeast overgrowth, inadequate liver detox, unbalanced essential fatty acids, unhealthy intestinal microbes, vitamin D or zinc deficiency, poor lifestyle choices, and alcohol abuse. The most effective approach to treating psoriasis generally focuses on diet and nutrition. Focus first on your diet:

✔ Adopt a modified elimination diet, as discussed in Chapter 2, to identify any potential problem foods. Some people with psoriasis do well on a vegan diet (no animal products).

✔ Consume eight servings of colorful vegetables and two servings of fruit daily. Eat more veggies in the cabbage family, including cabbage, brussels sprouts, cauliflower, broccoli, watercress, and bok choy.

✔ Eat organic, non-GMO foods. Look for foods with the verified non-GMO seal on the package.

✔ Eat pumpkin seeds for zinc deficiency (often associated with psoriasis).

✔ Drink 8 ounces of water every two waking hours.

✔ Chew your food to liquid to assist in the breakdown of proteins.

✔ Increase your fiber intake to move your bowels every day.

✔ Supplement your diet with the following:

Supplement	*Dosage*
Betaine HCL	300 mg with every meal
Omega-3 essential fatty acids (EFAs)	1 g yielding 180 mg EPA and 120 mg DHA three times daily
Folate (5-MTHF)	2,000 to 10,000 mcg twice daily
Vitamin D3	1,000 to 10,000 IU daily, depending on blood levels (see Appendix A)
Zinc glycinate chelate	20 mg twice daily (see Appendix A for precautions)
Colostrum	10,000 mg once daily
Proline-rich polypeptides	4 sprays in mouth, hold for 30 seconds and swallow, twice daily early morning and before bed for a total of 16 mg daily
Vitamin A (retinyl palmitate and beta-carotene)	2,500 IU retinyl palmitate and 2,500 IU beta-carotene (see Appendix A for precautions)
Probiotics (multistrain of *Lactobacillus acidophilus* and *Bifidobacterium* Rosell)	5 billion CFU twice daily

Consult your healthcare provider to test for the following conditions: leaky gut (see Chapter 13), gluten/wheat sensitivity (see Chapter 13), autoimmune thyroid (see Chapter 18), and candidiasis (see Chapter 19).

Clearing up general rashes

A *rash* is an outbreak on the skin characterized by discoloration and inflammation. Keeping the affected area clean and dry and exposing it to air as much as possible is usually sufficient for clearing up most rashes, but if that's not enough, try one or more of the following treatments:

- **Bentonite clay:** Apply extra-virgin, untreated bentonite clay over the affected area several times daily.

- **Apple cider vinegar:** Use an apple cider vinegar that has sediment on the bottom of the bottle. This contains raw enzymes and good, healthy bacteria. Soak a cotton ball and dab it on the rash several times daily.

- **Peppermint leaves:** Crush the leaves to make a paste and apply it to the rash several times daily. If the rash is hot and inflamed, make ice cubes out of the paste and rub the ice cubes gently over the rash.

- **Basil leaves:** Crush basil leaves, which contain camphor and thymol, well-known anti-itch compounds, and spread them over the rash.

- **Aloe vera:** Cut the leaf lengthwise with a knife, scoop out the gel, and place it on the rash several times daily. Aloe vera is well known for its anti-inflammatory properties.

- **Oatmeal:** Take an oatmeal bath (pour 1 cup of oatmeal into bathwater and soak your rash for 15 minutes; pat dry and let the oatmeal stay on your body for an hour). Alternatively, make an oatmeal poultice (add a small amount of water to ⅔ cup of oatmeal, let it turn to a paste, and apply the paste to your rash several times a day).

- **Calendula:** Dilute 5 ml calendula in a small amount of juice or water and drink it one or two times daily. Alternatively, apply it topically several times daily. Calendula contains saponins and carotenes that support healthy skin.

- **Chamomile:** Dilute 5 ml chamomile in a small amount of juice or water and drink one or two times daily. Alternatively apply the chamomile topically several times a day.

If the rash is in your mouth, take 100 mg sarsaparilla two to three times daily and/or 250 mg gotu kola three to four times daily.

If you have a certain type of rash, head to the section that provides treatment recommendations specifically for that rash type:

Rash Type	See
Dermatitis	"Dealing with dermatitis and eczema" earlier in this chapter
Diaper rash	Chapter 12
Eczema	"Dealing with dermatitis and eczema" earlier in this chapter
Herpes (genital)	Chapter 18
Herpes (oral)	"Handling herpes simplex 1" earlier in this chapter
Hives	"Honing in on hives" earlier in this chapter
Jock itch	"Ditching jock itch" earlier in this chapter
Psoriasis	"Subduing psoriasis" earlier in this chapter
Ringworm	"Reining in ringworm" later in this chapter
Seborrheic dermatitis	"Curing cradle cap: Seborrhea" earlier in this chapter

Reining in ringworm

Ringworm is a very common fungal infection (not caused by worms) that often appears in ring-shaped patterns on the arms, legs, face, and torso. The fungi feed on *keratin* — a protein in skin, hair, and nails, and the resulting rash may be very itchy and thick, dry, and scaly.

Ringworm can also affect other parts of the body, including the feet (causing athlete's foot), finger nails and toe nails (causing onychomycosis), the groin area (causing jock itch), the hands, or the scalp. If ringworm affects your fingernails and toenails, they can have a discolored or crumpled appearance. Ringworm is also contagious; it can spread through direct physical contact with affected persons or pets.

If you've contracted a case of ringworm, try the following natural cures:

- **Garlic:** Peel a clove, slice it thin, place the slices on the affected area(s), and cover with a bandage overnight.

- **Apple cider vinegar:** Using a cotton ball, apply apple cider vinegar to the ringworm three to five times daily until the ringworm disappears.

- ✔ **Tea tree oil:** Dilute tea tree oil with an equal amount of water and apply it to the affected skin several times daily for several weeks.

- ✔ **Turmeric:** Make a turmeric poultice and apply it to the affected skin several times daily for several weeks.

- ✔ **Salt and vinegar:** Make a paste of salt and vinegar and apply the paste to the affected area several times daily for one or two weeks.

- ✔ **Aloe:** Apply gel from the leaf to the ringworm several times daily.

- ✔ **Bioactive colloidal silver:** Apply colloidal silver as a liquid, gel, or ointment several times a day until the ringworm disappears.

- ✔ **Lavender oil:** Apply the oil to the affected area several times daily. Lavender oil has powerful antifungal properties.

Supplement any topical treatments by ingesting one or more of the following:

Supplement	*Dosage*
Olive leaf extract	200 mg twice daily
Grapeseed extract	100 mg twice daily
Grapefruit seed extract	100 mg twice daily
Monolaurin	200 mg twice daily
Lemongrass tea	Drink several glasses daily; place the used tea-bags on affected areas and let them dry out

If symptoms don't improve over the course of several days, turn to conventional treatments. Several over-the-counter creams — including miconazole, terbinafine, clotrimazole, ketoconazole, and tolnaftate — when applied to affected areas of the skin, have proven effective in treating ringworm. Continue treatment for an additional week after the ringworm appears to be gone.

Fungi love warm, moist surfaces such as those found in locker rooms, showers, tanning beds, swimming pools, and skin folds. Avoid sharing sporting equipment, clothing, or towels. You can also contract ringworm from an infected dog or cat, so if you have a dog or cat, have it checked and treated to avoid getting re-infected. You're at a greater risk of contracting ringworm if your immune system is weak, which is common in the very young, very old, and those who have diabetes or are obese.

Rubbing out rosacea

Rosacea is a chronic inflammatory condition characterized by facial redness most prevalent on the cheeks, nose, forehead, and around the eyes. It affects women three times more than men. Although rosacea appears on the surface of the body, its causes usually run deeper: food allergies or intolerances; leaky gut; foods that contain high levels of histamine; small-intestine bacterial overgrowth (SIBO); and alcohol, spicy foods, and hot beverages.

Start by eliminating from your diet alcohol, spicy foods, hot beverages, and foods that contain high levels of histamine (or cause your body to produce a lot of histamine): chocolate, alcoholic beverages (especially those containing sulfites), cheese, soy sauce, sauerkraut, processed meat, fish, and many processed foods. If doing so fixes the problem, you can reintroduce these foods slowly to determine which are causing the problem. Also avoid taking steroids, which worsen the condition.

Next, get tested. Team up with your healthcare provider to test for food allergies and sensitivities (see Chapter 13), leaky gut syndrome (Chapter 13), and SIBO.

If testing doesn't uncover the root cause of your rosacea and nothing you've tried has worked to cure the condition, try one or more of the following natural treatments:

- **Vascular laser:** Available through skin care centers, dermatologists, and so on.

- **Intense pulsed light (broad spectrum):** Available through skin care centers. You can purchase your own machine online for home use.

- **Sandalwood oil:** Using a cotton ball, apply liberally several times daily.

- **MSM (methylsulfonylmethane):** Take 1,000 mg three times daily.

- **Silymarin:** Take 250 mg twice daily.

- **Zinc:** 20 mg zinc glycinate chelate twice daily (see Appendix A for precautions).

- **Pancreatic enzymes:** With every meal, take 50,000 USP protease; 50,000 USP amylase; and 5,500 USP lipase.

- **B vitamins:** Purchase a formula containing the more bioavailable forms of the entire spectrum of B vitamins and follow the label instructions.

If you're diagnosed with having SIBO, follow the low-FODMAP diet, as explained in Chapter 14, and alternate the following natural treatments every two or three weeks:

- ✔ **Herbs:** Dill, wormwood *(Artemisia)*, horsetail, thyme, Pau D'Arco, stinging nettle, olive leaf, and yarrow. Look for a proprietary blend of these herbs and take 2,000 mg three times daily.

- ✔ **Oil of oregano:** Take 550 mg three times daily for two weeks. Oil of oregano may be caustic, so use with caution and decrease your dosage if necessary.

- ✔ **Berberine HCL:** Take 500 mg per meal.

Shaking off scabies

Scabies is a contagious mite infestation just below the skin's surface that makes you itch like crazy. It commonly appears as tiny bumps that first appear between the fingers, around the waist or wrists, or on the buttocks or elbows. Conventional medical treatment usually consists of potent insecticides applied to the skin. If you think you have scabies, avoid physical contact with others and don't share towels or bed linens. Wash towels and linens in hot, soapy water and machine dry on high heat. Try not to scratch, which can spread the infestation and break the skin, making you susceptible to secondary infection.

One natural cure for scabies is neem (Indian lilac). Neem doesn't kill the mites or eggs, but it disrupts the mites' reproduction cycle, preventing re-infestation as the older mites die off. You can purchase neem oils, creams, ointments, and soaps at natural health food stores and online. Apply neem oil to your entire body, head to toe, several times daily for two weeks, and wash with neem soap when you bathe.

Permethrin (Nix) is a pesticide that's gentler than some of the more powerful and potentially dangerous insecticides used to treat scabies, including lindane. Permethrin kills both mites and eggs. Follow the label instructions.

If anyone in your household is infected with scabies, everyone in the household should be treated, and then all of their clothing, bedding, and towels should be washed in hot water and detergent and machine dried on high heat.

Warding off warts

Warts are ugly, contagious, and often uncomfortable. The good news is that conventional medical treatments are usually safe and effective for removing them. Your doctor can probably burn or freeze them off at your next office visit. Using over-the-counter topical treatments, you may be able to remove the warts yourself; follow the package instructions.

Don't try to cut, pick, or burn the wart yourself. You may permanently scar yourself or cause a secondary infection, and the wart will probably reappear anyway.

To remove warts naturally, start with topical treatments. Apply raw garlic, garlic extract, or *Thuja* oil to the wart twice daily and cover with a fresh bandage for up to four weeks, until the wart disappears. Complement the topical treatments with the following dietary supplements:

Supplement	Dosage
Zinc glycinate chelate	20 mg twice daily (see Appendix A for precautions)
Vitamin A (retinyl palmitate and beta-carotene)	2,500 IU retinyl palmitate and 2,500 IU beta-carotene daily (see Appendix A for precautions)
Olive leaf extract	500 mg twice daily
Selenium	200 mcg daily

Scrubbing Away Hair and Scalp Conditions

Like any other part of your body, the skin and hair on the top of your head are susceptible to illness. In this section, I offer guidance on treating common hair and scalp maladies without harsh chemicals that could pose other health risks.

Clearing acne of the scalp

Like acne on other parts of your body, scalp acne occurs when pores become clogged with oil and dirt and then infected with bacteria. Effective treatment cleans out the pores and prevents re-infection:

✔ Use all-natural shampoo with jojoba oil and trace minerals from clay, and use oil-free conditioners that contain salicylic acid. (Read the shampoo label to make sure it is free of dyes, fragrances, and chemical additives. You want a shampoo that cleanses the hair and scalp and balances the scalp's pH.)

✔ Wash your hair daily to remove excessive dirt and oil and avoid oil styling products that contain petroleum.

✔ Eat a whole foods diet.

Demolishing dandruff

Dandruff is usually more embarrassing than it is a health risk, but it may be a symptom of something more serious, such as eczema, psoriasis, or a fungal infection. If your scalp itches, avoid the temptation to scratch, which may cause bleeding and make your scalp more susceptible to infection. Try one or more of the following treatments:

✔ Use over-the-counter shampoos containing ketoconazole, zinc pyrithione, selenium sulfide, or salicylic acid. Jason Dandruff Shampoo with sulfur and salicylic acid is a good choice for most, but it contains wheat protein, so if you're allergic to wheat or have celiac disease, cross it off your list.

Rotate shampoos monthly, alternating use of different active ingredients, because scalp conditions tend to develop resistance to certain products.

✔ For stubborn cases of dandruff, try a tar shampoo, such as Neutrogena T/Gel or its generic equivalent, once a week. After applying tar shampoo, rinse your hair with lemon juice. Tar shampoos can be irritating to certain individuals, and they may change the root color, so proceed cautiously.

✔ Mix two parts apple cider vinegar, one part warm water, and several drops of one or more of the following essential oils: lavender, lemongrass, and rosemary. Mix well and apply directly to the scalp. Allow the mixture to dry on your scalp and hair, and then shampoo and rinse. Perform this procedure once or twice weekly until the dandruff has improved.

✔ Boil several neem (Indian lilac) leaves in two cups of water. Cool and strain the solution and use it to rinse your hair two or three times a week.

✔ Mix coconut oil with lemon juice, massage it into your scalp, and leave it on for 20 minutes. Shampoo and rinse. Do this two or three times weekly.

✔ Heat a small amount of extra virgin olive oil, massage it into your scalp, and leave it in for 30 minutes. Shampoo and rinse. Do this once or twice weekly.

Combatting hair loss

Normally, you shed about 50 to 100 hairs daily. If you're losing more than that, something's wrong, and you need to find out what it is. Common causes of hair loss include medical issues, such as thyroid malfunction, autoimmune conditions (including autoimmune alopecia [hair loss]), ringworm (covered earlier in this chapter), and lupus erythematous; side effects of medications, such as cholesterol lowering drugs, Parkinson's medications, proton pump inhibitors (PPIs) for blocking stomach acid, anti-inflammatories, and beta blockers; hormonal changes in both men and women; poor diet and nutrition; and other things like pregnancy, excessive stress, certain hairstyles and hair products, and so on. Therefore, before you assume that your hair loss is strictly genetic, look into these other possible causes and be sure to check side effects and adverse reactions associated with all pharmaceuticals you're taking.

If you can't track down the specific cause for your hair loss, try adjusting your diet first. Eliminate refined processed carbohydrates and poor-quality fats. Consume high-quality protein from lean meats and oily fish. Eat healthy fats from nuts and seeds, avocados, coconuts, and olives. Consume foods rich in biotin found in nuts, brown rice, oats, and brewer's yeast. Take a high-quality B nutritional supplement daily. (Nuts and seeds contain high amounts of the B vitamins.)

The following natural cures may be helpful in preventing or reversing hair loss:

Natural Cure	Dose
Biotin	2,000 to 3,000 mcg daily
Choline (choline-stabilized orthosilicic acid)	100 mg two to three times daily
Silicon (choline-stabilized orthosilicic acid)	5 mg two to three times daily
Essential fatty acids (EPA/DHA and gamma-linolenic acid from borage oil or evening primrose oil)	3,000 to 4,000 mg EPA/DHA and 1,500 mg gamma-linolenic acid daily
Saw palmetto	200 mg twice daily
Zinc glycinate chelate	20 mg twice daily (see Appendix A for precautions)
MSM	1,000 mg three times daily

Also try a shampoo with rosemary oil to improve circulation, or buy rosemary oil and add it to your shampoo.

Nit picking: Head lice

Head lice are ugly bugs that live in your hair. Over-the-counter products for ridding your hair of lice are typically powerful and potentially dangerous insecticides. Instead of exposing yourself or your children to these products, try the following approach:

1. **Saturate the hair with olive or almond oil right down to the scalp, paying close attention to the areas around the ears and hairline.**

   Add several drops of tea tree oil or neem (Indian lilac) to the oil before applying it. These essential oils serve as gentle insecticides.

2. **Leave the oil in for about 20 minutes.**

3. **Using a lice comb, comb *all* of the hair carefully in sections, rinsing the comb in hot water as you go.**

   This step removes the dead and weakened lice and their eggs.

4. **When you're done, soak the comb in a 10 percent bleach solution or a 2 percent Lysol solution for 30 minutes, and rinse it well.**

5. **Repeat Steps 1 through 4 daily for one week.**

6. **For the next two weeks, comb through the hair to make sure all the lice are gone and re-infestation has not occurred. If you're re-infested, repeat the process.**

If one member of the household is infested, chances are good that other members are infested as well. Check everyone. To prevent the lice from spreading, wash all clothing and linens in hot water with detergent and machine dry on high heat. Vacuum the surfaces of sofas and pillows that the affected individual may have used.

If you must use an over-the-counter product to treat the lice, opt for products that contain permethrin (Nix) over those that contain lindane, especially if you're using the product on children.

Curing cradle cap: Seborrhea

Seborrheic dermatitis (called *cradle cap* in infants) is a chronic, relapsing inflammatory condition characterized by greasy, itchy, flaky patches on the face, torso, and scalp. In adults, dandruff is considered a form of seborrheic dermatitis. Symptoms commonly appear anywhere on the face, behind the ears, or around the nasal folds.

Factors that commonly contribute to seborrhea include delayed food allergies or sensitivities, a diet high in refined sugars, a weakened immune system, nutrient deficiencies, *Malassezia* yeast, excessive vitamin A consumption in children, Parkinson's disease, and stroke.

Many of the treatments described the earlier section "Dealing with dermatitis and eczema" are also helpful for treating seborrhea. In addition, antifungal shampoos, sunlight, and phototherapy (UV radiation) may help if the cause is related to fungal or yeast infection. To complement other treatments, supplement your diet with the following:

Supplement	*Dosages*
Vitamin B6 (pyridoxal 5'-phosphate)	50 mg twice daily until symptoms improve and then take once daily
Flaxseed oil	*Adults:* 1 to 2 tablespoons daily (**Note:** For infants with cradle cap, the nursing mother should consume 1 tablespoon daily)
Biotin	2 to 4 mg daily for three weeks, decreasing the dosage as symptoms improve
Folate (5-MTHF)	2,000 to 10,000 mcg daily
Riboflavin (riboflavin 5'-phosphate)	25 mg twice daily
Zinc glycinate chelate	20 mg twice daily (see Appendix A for precautions)

Chipping Away at Nail Conditions

Certain nail conditions in and of themselves require treatment; others are symptomatic of other health conditions that require treatment. In this section, I explain how to treat brittle nails and shed light on how to use certain nail conditions to track down the cause of other health issues.

Making your nails less brittle

Nails become brittle for a variety of reasons, including overexposure to the elements, repeated manipulation of the nail plate by manicures, nail biting, and improper nutrition.

To make your nails less brittle, wear gloves when working outside to protect them from the environment. When caring for cuticles, avoid using a mechanical instrument that breaks down the cuticle's natural protective barrier. Instead, soak the cuticles in water and push them back with a moist hand towel. Clean your nails and soften your cuticles by scrubbing them with the nailbrush dipped in baking soda. And avoid the temptation to pick at or bite your fingernails, which make them more susceptible to pathogens. Avoid nail glue and formaldehyde and cut down on any use of nail polish remover. Soak your fingers in Epsom salts for 30 minutes per day.

The standard American diet contributes to poor nail health. Replace junk food with quality food, including protein from lean meats, vegetable proteins, pastured eggs, wild fish, organic vegetables of all kinds, and quality essential fatty acids. A protein-rich diet supports the production of *keratin,* the major protein in nails. Supplement your diet with the following:

Supplement	Dosage
Zinc glycinate chelate	20 mg twice daily (see Appendix A for precautions)
Biotin	500 mcg twice daily, or eat more Swiss chard, eggs, and salmon
Choline (choline stabilized orthosilicic acid)	100 mg twice daily
Silicon (silicon stabilized orthosilicic acid)	5 mg twice daily

Inspecting nails to diagnose illnesses

Health conditions that affect finger nails and toenails are often symptoms of more serious conditions, including heavy metal exposure. If your nails take on an abnormal appearance, inspect them carefully for the following conditions and consult your healthcare provider for further diagnosis:

- **Beau's lines** consist of horizontal grooves on most or all of the nails that may be caused by measles/mumps, syphilis, poorly controlled diabetes (see Chapter 17), myocarditis (heart condition), hypocalcemia (low blood calcium), or zinc deficiency.

- **Nail clubbing** occurs when the fingertips enlarge and the nails curve around the fingertips, which may indicate cirrhosis of the liver, chronic obstructive pulmonary disease (COPD), inflammatory bowel disease (IBD), or celiac disease.

✔ **Onycholysis** occurs when the nail separates from the nail bed. Unless the nail separation is caused by injury to the nail, the condition is probably caused by a fungal, mold, or yeast infection.

✔ **Spoon nails** occurs when nails curve upward instead of downward typically indicating iron deficiency anemia or a liver condition in which your body absorbs excess iron from the food you eat.

✔ **Terry's nails** occur when fingernails and toenails appear white and have a ground glass appearance with no lunula (the moon-shaped area at the base of the nail). It often affects patients with liver disease, diabetes, congestive heart failure, and general poor health.

✔ **Yellow nails** may indicate a respiratory disorder, psoriasis, or fungal infection. Smoking and nail polish may also turn nails yellow over time.

✔ **Leukonycia** is characterized by white discoloration of the nail bed due to abnormal keratinization. This condition may be related to hypoalbuminemia (low protein in the blood), heavy metal toxicity, or nutritional deficiencies.

✔ **Mees lines** are single horizontal white lines that extend the complete width of the nail plate on one or all fingers. The lines are narrow and are indicative of arsenic toxicity.

✔ **Muehrcke's lines** are pairs of horizontal lines caused by edema from hypoalbuminemia (low protein in the blood).

Chapter 8

Tuning In to Ear Problems

An ear that becomes ill or fails to function properly may cause a host of symptoms, including pain, pressure, or an annoying sense of fullness in the ear; itching; hearing loss; ringing in the ears; or vertigo, characterized by dizziness or a loss of balance. If you're experiencing any of these symptoms, you've come to the right place. Here you find natural cures for everything from the common earache to *vertigo* — dizziness often caused by a health condition that affects the ear.

Doses in this chapter are for adults, not children. For guidance on how to adjust dosages for children (and adults under 150 pounds), turn to Chapter 12.

Oh, My Aching Ears! Eradicating Earaches

Earaches come in two forms: middle (*otitis media,* covered in this section) and outer (*otitis externa,* or *swimmer's ear,* covered in the next section). Both conditions are painful.

Where in the ear?

Ear problems are often categorized by the section of the ear they affect:

- ✔ **Outer ear:** The part that carries the sound to the eardrum consists of the part outside your head and the auditory canal, into which people commonly stick their pinky fingers or cotton swabs.

- ✔ **Middle ear:** The part that contains the eardrum, a large cavity, and three tiny bones called *ossicles*.

- ✔ **Inner ear:** The business end of the ear that converts vibrations from the eardrum into auditory signals that nerves carry to the brain for processing. The inner ear contains the cochlea, cochlear nerve, vestibular nerve, temporal bone, and Eustachian tube.

Middle earaches

Middle earaches are most common and are typically caused by inflammation (usually resulting from an infection or a food allergy or sensitivity) or fluid buildup (when fluid is unable to drain from the ear through the *Eustachian tube* — a tube leading from the inside of the ear to the back of the throat).

Symptoms of a middle earache are easy to spot in adults and older children — ear pressure or pain, possibly a fever, and swelling or redness of the eardrum (which a doctor can spot by using a special instrument called an *otoscope*). In children, especially those too young to talk or to describe their symptoms, irritability and loss of appetite are common symptoms for parents to look for.

The natural cure for middle earache calls for a two-pronged approach: one, reduce the inflammation, and two, improve drainage via the Eustachian tube. Follow this treatment protocol for middle ear infections:

1. **Stop smoking and avoid secondhand smoke.**

2. **Eliminate sugar, dairy, wheat, and *all* processed foods from your diet.**

   Infants should be transitioned to breast-feeding or bottle-feeding with breast milk, and breastfeeding mothers should eliminate these same foods from their diets. Also avoid foods processed with molds, such as black tea, breads, and fruit juices.

3. Take the following supplements:

Supplement	Dosage
Omega-3 essential fatty acids (EFAs)	1 g yielding 180 mg EPA and 120 mg DHA three times daily
Proline-rich polypeptides	4 sprays in mouth, hold for 30 seconds and swallow, twice daily early morning and before bed, for a total of 16 mg daily
Thymus gland extract	200 mg twice daily

4. Boost your immune system with the following vitamins and nutraceuticals (taken orally):

Supplement	Dosage
Vitamin C (mineral ascorbates)	1,000 to 3,000 mg two to three times daily
Vitamin A (retinyl palmitate)	3,750 IU daily (see Appendix A for precautions)
Echinacea purpurea	300 mg twice daily

5. Drink half your body weight in ounces of water per day.

If you weigh 160 pounds, for example, drink 80 ounces of water. You can drink decaf tea as part of your water intake.

6. Improve ear drainage with one or more of the following herbal remedies (taken orally) until symptoms subside:

Remedy	Dosage
Horehound	Follow label instructions
Elderberry (syrup)	15 ml four times daily for up to five days
Elecampane (liquid form, see caution following this table)	Start with a few drops daily, increasing to a maximum of 15 drops two or three times daily
Mullein	Follow label instructions up to a maximum of 3 to 4 g daily
Wild cherry bark (as a tea or cough syrup)	*Tea:* Mix 1 teaspoon of the powdered bark in 1 cup of hot water and drink up to three times daily; *Syrup:* 1 teaspoon twice daily

Elecampane may trigger allergic reactions in people with allergies to ragweed, chrysanthemums, marigolds, daisies, sunflowers, and many other related plants. A good rule to follow with all natural products is to start slowly and monitor closely for unwanted side effects; if unwanted side effects occur, stop using the product that you suspect is causing the side effect.

7. **Improve drainage with one or both of the following techniques:**

   - For clogged Eustachian tubes, close your mouth, hold your nose, and blow gently as if you are blowing your nose. Don't blow so hard that you feel pain.

   - Apply a warm, moist washcloth or a heating pad on a low setting to your ear.

   Be careful not to burn your skin. Do not use a heating pad with a small child who can't tell you whether the pad is too hot.

8. **Apply eardrops.**

   You can find an eardrop recipe at the end of this chapter.

If you follow these steps, you should see improvement in five to seven days. If the earache does not improve or gets worse in that time, consult your natural care provider or primary care physician.

One study has shown that a daily dose of 8.4 g xylitol (two pieces of gum five times daily after meals for at least five minutes) reduces the occurrence of acute middle ear infections by 25 percent. Chewing xylitol gum has also been shown to reduce cavities. Xylitol is a natural sweetener extracted from birch trees.

Outer earaches (swimmer's ear)

An outer earache *(otitis externa)* is caused by irritation and/or inflammation of the outer ear or the ear canal. The condition is commonly called *swimmer's ear*, because it often results from water entering the ear canal, which may lead to infection. Symptoms include redness, inflammation, itching, *acute* (sudden and intense) or *chronic* (long-lasting, but not as intense), hearing loss, and (sometimes) fever.

Treatments for outer ear infections vary, depending on the cause:

- ✔ **If your symptoms occurred after swimming, diving, or bathing:** The cause is likely water trapped in the ear canal. Mix equal parts white vinegar and rubbing alcohol, and put a few drops into each affected ear to prevent infection as the water drains. If the condition persists or worsens, switch to using the eardrop recipe I offer in the later section "Making Your Own Eardrops."

If you commonly get swimmer's ear, put several drops of the vinegar-alcohol mixture into each ear after every visit to the pool or lake and after showering or bathing.

✔ **If your earache accompanies a skin condition:** Eczema or psoriasis can cause outer ear pain. See Chapter 7 for more about treating skin conditions.

✔ **If you have earwax buildup:** The buildup may be restricting the drainage of fluid from the ear. Head to the later section "Eliminating Earwax Buildup" to confirm or rule out that possibility and deal with it, if necessary.

✔ **If you felt pain after cleaning the ear with a cotton swab or putting some object into your ear:** You may have scratched or irritated your ear. Try applying eardrops, as I explain in the later section "Making Your Own Eardrops."

If the condition persists despite your best efforts, visit your healthcare provider. Your ear canal may be so inflamed that the eardrops you're using can't reach the infection to treat it. Your doctor can also determine whether something else is obstructing your ear canal and preventing drainage.

Treating a Ruptured Eardrum

Your eardrum is a thin piece of tissue that separates your outer and middle ear. A ruptured eardrum is one that has gotten a hole in it, usually from an ear infection or accidental damage from a cotton swab or other object being inserted too far into the ear canal. A very loud noise or extreme and sudden change in pressure can also burst an eardrum.

Don't put anything in your ear, not even eardrops, when you suspect that you have a ruptured eardrum. The only cure is time. To speed recovery, adopt a healthier diet and lifestyle, as directed in Chapter 2, and take supplements that boost your immune system (see Chapter 5).

Eliminating Earwax Buildup

Earwax *(cerumen)* is a permanent resident of the ear canal. It traps dirt and microbes and helps evict these invaders before they can reach and cause real damage to your middle and inner ear. Unfortunately, earwax can build up inside your ear canal and contribute to ear infections, hearing loss, and other problems.

If you suspect that you may be experiencing earwax buildup, check for the following symptoms: hearing loss; ear pain; full or plugged feeling in your ears; itching; drainage from the ear canal; frequent ear infections, especially outer ear infections; and dizziness.

Here are the two best ways to deal with earwax buildup:

✔ Head to your healthcare provider, who has the skills and tools to remove the earwax safely and thoroughly. This is the better of the two solutions.

✔ Use a Debrox earwax removal kit for at least four days. Follow the instructions in the kit, and if symptoms don't improve, see your healthcare provider.

Don't use a cotton swab to clean the ear yourself. You may be able to remove some superficial earwax on the outer part of your ear canal, but you're likely to push earwax farther inside and compound the problem. You also may damage your eardrum.

Overcoming Hearing Loss

Sooner or later, everyone experiences some degree of hearing loss. Sometimes, it occurs suddenly, perhaps as the result of a ruptured eardrum. In other cases, it happens over time — and sometimes so gradually that you may not even notice until your hearing is nearly or completely gone or someone points it out to you.

Regardless of when you notice your hearing loss, you need to put on your detective hat and start looking at possible causes. Common causes include ear infection or fluid in the inner ear (see "Oh, My Aching Ears! Eradicating Earaches"); earwax buildup or other obstructions in the ear; a ruptured eardrum; or a malformation of the ear or some part of it. Thickening of the eardrum and damage to the nerves of the inner ear caused by long-term exposure to loud sounds can also result in hearing loss, as can certain medications and illnesses, including Meniere's disease (discussed later in this chapter). Head trauma and blood sugar issues (see the sections on diabetes in Chapter 17) can also contribute to hearing loss.

Of course, the recommended course of treatment depends on the root cause of the hearing loss. First, rule out any obvious causes that are easy to address:

✔ Have your doctor check for earwax buildup or the possibility of a ruptured eardrum.

✔ Address any underlying infections or medical conditions, such as high blood pressure or poor thyroid function, that may be contributing to the problem.

✔ If you started any medication before experiencing hearing loss, ask your prescriber and your pharmacist whether the medication has hearing loss listed as a possible side effect or look the information up online.

If you can't track down and address the underlying cause of your hearing difficulties, first adopt a healthy diet. Eliminate sugar, dairy, wheat, and *all* processed foods from your diet to alleviate any blood sugar imbalances. (See Chapter 2 for more about adopting a healthy diet and Chapter 17 for more about treating conditions related to blood sugar.) The vitamins and supplements listed in Table 8-1 may help restore hearing or at least slow the progression of hearing loss.

Also try limiting calories: Set a goal of eating 30 percent fewer calories per day. Research shows that simply restricting your caloric intake improves hearing!

Table 8-1	Vitamins and Supplements for Hearing Loss	
Supplement	*Dose (Adults)*	*Best for*
Bromelain (see Appendix B for precautions)	80 to 320 mg two or three times daily	Hearing loss with tinnitus
Folate (5-MTHF)	400 mcg two times daily	Age-related hearing loss with tinnitus
Magnesium	125 mg two times daily	Noise-induced hearing loss
Vitamin A (retinyl palmitate and beta-carotene)	Adults: 3,750 IU daily	Preventing and treating hearing loss
Vitamin B12	400 mcg two times daily	Preventing and treating hearing loss
Vitamin B3 (niacin as nicotinic acid)	140 mg two times daily for 60 days	Blood circulation–related hearing loss; stop if symptoms worsen
Vitamin D3	2,000 to 10,000 IU daily to reach 80 ng/dl blood level	Preventing and treating hearing loss
Vitamin E (tocopherols and tocotrienols)	600 IU two times daily	Sudden hearing loss (30 decibels in three days or less)
Zinc glycinate chelate (see Appendix A for precautions)	20 mg two times daily	Sudden hearing loss

All the beneficial nutrients listed in Table 8-1 are generally deficient in the standard Western diet. They can supplement a healthy diet and, with the exception of zinc and bromelain, can be taken for life. Have a knowledgeable functional medicine doctor evaluate you for these and other nutrient deficiencies.

After ruling out the obvious causes of hearing loss, you may need to consult an ear, nose, and throat (ENT) doctor to check for less common issues, such as structural problems in the ear, nerve damage, and other illnesses that may have hearing loss as a symptom.

Itchy Ears

Ear itching is a tickling, irritating sensation that may be caused by excessive or insufficient earwax; food or environmental allergies or food sensitivity; swimmer's ear; eczema, seborrheic dermatitis, or psoriasis; sensitivity to shampoo or conditioner; and otomycosis (fungal ear infection). Treatments vary, depending on the cause, but here are a few natural remedies that are likely to help:

✔ Keep the ear clean and dry. If you have excessive earwax, schedule a cleaning with your healthcare provider every six months. See the earlier section "Eliminating Earwax Buildup" for details. (Avoid using cotton swabs inside your ear, because they're more likely to impact the ear wax and possibly damage the eardrum.)

✔ Place a few drops of vegetable oil, such as olive oil, into your ear every day. Doing so may help to prevent your ears from becoming too dry and irritated, a condition that may be related to insufficient earwax.

✔ Try an elimination diet, as explained in Chapter 2, to diagnose any food allergy or sensitivity that may be causing your ears to itch.

✔ If you suspect that the itching is related to water in the ear, try remedies for swimmer's ear (refer to the earlier section "Outer earaches (swimmer's ear)," earlier in this chapter.

✔ If you have a skin condition, as well as itchy ears, see Chapter 7 for guidance on treating skin conditions, including eczema, seborrheic dermatitis, or psoriasis — all of which may cause itching ears.

✔ Try using a different shampoo or soap or wearing ear plugs when you bathe to determine whether you're sensitive to a particular shampoo, conditioner, or soap. Then eliminate those products.

Ringing in the Ears (Tinnitus)

Tinnitus, characterized by an annoying high-pitched ringing or low-pitched buzzing in the ears is a common sensation, even in people who've completely lost their hearing! A majority of cases are *idiopathic,* meaning that they can't be traced to a specific cause, but tinnitus can often be attributed to a host of conditions, including high blood pressure, diabetes, temporal mandibular joint (TMJ) dysfunction, and certain prescription medications.

In most cases, tinnitus is a mildly annoying condition that most people can live with. In 1 to 2 percent of the population, however, it can interfere with sleep, quiet activities, and normal activities of daily living. The tricky part is in tracking down the cause so that you know which treatments to try. If you're stumped, here are some suggestions:

- If you're taking any prescription medications, ask your doctor and pharmacist if any of them is linked to tinnitus or hearing loss, and, if so, whether you can stop or switch medication.

- Adopt a natural cures diet and lifestyle, as explained in Chapter 2, for at least two weeks to see whether symptoms improve. (In some cases, simply eliminating refined sugar does the trick.) Also, try any or all of these nutritional supplements.

Supplement	*Dosage*
Vitamin A (retinyl palmitate and beta-carotene)	5,000 IU daily for a minimum of six months (see Appendix A for precautions)
Zinc glycinate chelate	20 mg two times daily for a minimum of six months (see Appendix A for precautions)
CoQ10	100 mg two times daily for a minimum of six months
Vitamin B12 (methylcobalamin, sublingual fast-dissolving tablet)	1,000 mcg two times daily for a minimum of six months
Melatonin (fast-dissolving tablet)	3 mg one hour before bed for a minimum of three months

- Restrict your sodium intake to 1,500 to 2,300 mg daily for two weeks to see whether high blood pressure is causing the ringing.

- If you haven't had thyroid hormone and function tests run (see Chapter 18), ask your doctor about ordering these tests.

- Try biofeedback (see Chapter 3), which is often useful in helping your brain crank down the volume of the ringing or buzzing.

As a short-term fix, if tinnitus is interfering with your sleep, try placing a source of white noise, such as a fan, near your bed. Just make sure the noise isn't so loud that it damages your hearing.

When the World Spins: Vertigo and Meniere's Disease

Vertigo is a feeling that you or your surroundings are rocking or spinning when nothing is actually moving; it is often accompanied by nausea, vomiting, and loss of balance. The cause is usually classified as *central* (related to the brain or spinal cord) or *peripheral* (related to the inner ear). Peripheral vertigo is commonly caused by calcium carbonate crystals that naturally reside in the inner ear becoming dislocated and sending mixed messages to the brain. Sudden episodes of vertigo can also be caused by a condition known as Meniere's disease. This section covers both general vertigo and Meniere's disease.

Checking out vertigo

If you experience vertigo, the first order of business is to head to the doctor for some help in tracking down in the cause. Your doctor is likely to perform the Dix-Halpike (or Nylen-Barany) maneuver to determine whether you have peripheral vertigo and, if so, to determine which ear is affected. The Dix-Halpike maneuver goes like this:

1. **The doctor has you sit up on a table; then with her standing behind you and holding your head, you lie down, letting you head hang over the edge of the table as you look at the doctor.**

2. **The doctor turns your head about 90 degrees to the left and watches your eyes for involuntary movement.**

   Such movement would indicate peripheral vertigo.

3. **You and your doctor repeat Steps 1 and 2, turning your head to the right this time.**

If the doctor determines that you have peripheral vertigo, she may proceed to do the Epley maneuver to reposition the crystals that are causing your vertigo. You can do the Epley maneuver at home, but have a spotter so that you don't fall and hurt yourself if you become disoriented. Follow these steps:

1. **Lie down, face up, on a flat surface (your bed, for example) so that your head hangs down over the edge.**

2. **Turn your head about 90 degrees in the direction of the affected ear. Hold this position for two minutes.**

   You may experience vertigo when you do this.

3. **With your head still hanging over the edge, turn your head about 180 degrees (so that you're facing the opposite direction). Hold this position for two minutes.**

4. **Turn your body 90 degrees in the direction you're facing, keeping your head turned (now you're lying on your side and looking at the floor). Hold this position for two minutes.**

5. **Sit up, turn your head to face forward, and sit still for about ten minutes.**

If symptoms return, repeat the Epley maneuver. If the Epley maneuver doesn't fix the underlying problem, try some or all of the vitamins and supplements in Table 8-2. These have shown to be effective in treating vertigo.

Table 8-2	Vitamins and Supplements for Vertigo	
Supplement	*Dose (Adults)*	*Notes*
Vitamin B6 (pyridoxal 5'-phosphate)	100 mg daily	Increases GABA, an important neurotransmitter. Insufficient amounts of GABA may contribute to vertigo and dizziness.
Vitamin B3 (niacin as nicotinic acid)	250 to 500 mg daily to start, increasing by 250 mg a week up to a maximum of 3 g; continue until a flushing effect occurs (your skin reddens and feels warm and either itches or tingles)	Niacin dilates the blood vessels in and around the labyrinth of membranes inside the ear that your body relies on for balance.
Lemon flavonoids	300 mg two or three times daily	Flavonoids reduce the permeability of the vascular system to reduce the amount of fluid inside the part of the ear that helps you keep your balance.
Vitamin C (mineral ascorbates)	1,000 mg daily	Vitamin C is a powerful antioxidant that has shown some promise in helping treat vertigo.
Folate (5-MTHF)	400 mcg two times daily	Folate and B12 support methylation, which improves cell function and detox.

(continued)

Table 8-2 *(continued)*

Supplement	Dose (Adults)	Notes
Vitamin B12 (methylcobalamin, sublingual fast-dissolving tablet)	400 mcg two times daily	B12 and folate support methylation, which improves cell function and detox.
Ginkgo biloba	120 mg daily	Take for at least one year.
Vinpocetine	15 mg daily	Vinpocetine increases blood flow to the brain.
Cocculus	Two 30C pellets three times daily for seven days	This is a homeopathic remedy. Stop taking if symptoms do not improve in seven days.

Bodywork, including acupuncture, acupressure, chiropractic manipulation, craniosacral therapy, and reflexology have had some success in treating vertigo, as well. See Chapter 3 for more information on these approaches.

Meniere's disease

Meniere's disease (also known as *endolymphatic hydrops*) is characterized by sudden episodes of vertigo, each lasting anywhere from about 20 minutes to 2 hours over the course of up to 24 hours. The vertigo is sometimes accompanied by nausea, vomiting, hearing loss, ringing in the ears, or increased ear pressure. It may affect one or both ears.

Although the specific cause of Meniere's disease is unknown, it seems to be related to the amount or consistency of *endolymph* — a fluid in the middle ear that plays a role in helping you maintain your balance. Drainage and diet may have something to do with the buildup of fluid or its consistency, so many of the treatments for a middle earache may also be effective in treating Meniere's disease; see "Middle earaches," earlier in this chapter, for details.

One quick and easy treatment for Meniere's disease is to eliminate or greatly restrict your daily intake of caffeine, nicotine, and alcohol for five to seven days to see whether your symptoms improve. If your primary symptom is vertigo, refer to the preceding section for a technique that may clear your symptoms in about 15 minutes.

Meniere's disease has been linked to blood sugar imbalances and thyroid and adrenal dysfunction, so consult your healthcare provider to have those conditions ruled out. Have your fasting glucose and fasting insulin levels tested. If your levels are high, switch to a diet to treat insulin resistance (see Chapters 2 and 17). Also have your thyroid and adrenal functions tested and, if necessary, treated to rule out those conditions.

Table 8-3 lists several vitamins, minerals, and supplements that may help in the treatment of Meniere's disease.

Table 8-3	Vitamins and Supplements for Meniere's Disease	
Supplement	*Dose (Adults)*	*Notes*
Flavonoids with vitamin C	300 mg lemon flavonoid complex and 500 mg vitamin C three times daily for at least six months	Flavonoids can help reduce the permeability of the vascular system to reduce the amount of endolymph.
Magnesium	125 mg two times daily for a minimum of six months	Magnesium plays a critical role in energy production and decreases sensitivity to oxidative stress.
Vitamin B1 (thiamin as benfontamine)	150 mg two times daily	Maximum improvement in two to three months. ***Note:*** May substitute another form of thiamin at 100 mg two times daily.
Vitamin B3 (niacin as nicotinic acid)	500 mg two times daily	Maximum improvement in two to three months.
Vitamin B6 (pyridoxal 5'-phosphate)	100 mg a day for at least six months	Vitamin B6 is a coenzyme involved in over 100 enzymatic reactions.

See your doctor immediately if your symptoms include severe headache, double vision or loss of vision, impaired speech, numbness, tingling, chest pain, weakness in your arms or legs, or difficulty walking. These may be signs of other serious conditions, such as heart attack or stroke.

Making Your Own Eardrops

Going right to the source with herbal infection fighters can speed up the healing process for a middle ear or outer ear infection or irritation. Numerous variations of garlic-in-olive-oil remedies are available for earaches.

The one I like best is *Children's Ear Oil* from Herbal Antibiotics. This fantastic formula combines garlic and eucalyptus for a double antibacterial, antiviral one-two punch.

To cook up your own ear oil formula, here's a recipe that's safe for adults and children:

1. **Place 4 ounces of extra virgin olive oil and 5 cloves of garlic, finely chopped, in a small saucepan on low heat.**

2. **Cover and simmer the olive oil – garlic mixture for eight to ten hours.**

3. **Strain the oil to remove the garlic.**

    Discard the garlic, save the oil.

4. **Add 20 drops of eucalyptus essential oil to the strained oil and mix well.**

5. **Store the ear oil in a tinted bottle to prevent spoilage; discard after two weeks.**

When you're ready to apply the eardrops, warm a glass eyedropper by running it under warm water for about one minute. Then use the eyedropper to place two drops of the ear oil into the affected ear every 30 minutes during the day and once or twice at night (if you happen to wake up) for up to one week. Use the drops for a minimum of two days.

Never place fluid in the ear if the eardrum has been perforated. Doing so could cause permanent damage, including hearing loss. See "Treating a Ruptured Eardrum," earlier in this chapter, for details.

Chapter 9

Ogling Eye and Vision Problems

- -

In This Chapter

▶ Improving your vision and overall eye health

▶ Keeping cataracts, glaucoma, and macular degeneration at bay

▶ Treating conjunctivitis, dry eyes, and sties

▶ Reducing and recovering from eye strain

- -

*I*f you're like most people, even though vision is one the most essential of your five senses, you probably don't give your eyes or vision much thought until they fall victim to illness or you notice that you're not seeing things as clearly as you once did.

In this chapter, I encourage you to pay attention to your eyes and vision *before* you notice a problem, and I provide guidance on dietary changes and supplements that can help preserve eye and vision health throughout your lifetime. I also provide guidance on how to treat numerous eye and vision conditions, ranging from common, minor problems, such as dry eyes and conjunctivitis, to chronic conditions, including glaucoma and macular degeneration.

Doses in this chapter are for adults, not children. For guidance on how to adjust dosages for children (and adults under 150 pounds), turn to Chapter 12.

Supporting Eye and Vision Health with Diet and Lifestyle Changes

You can do a great deal to preserve your eye and vision health, and the sooner you start, the better:

✔ **Quit smoking.** Smoking makes you more susceptible to cataracts, macular degeneration, and optic nerve damage. If you smoke, try to quit.

If you can't quit, reduce how much you smoke to no more than a few cigarettes a day.

✔ **Limit alcohol consumption.** In addition to causing short-term blurred vision, excessive alcohol consumption may lead to nerve damage that degrades vision. Heavy consumption of alcohol is also associated with earlier onset of macular degeneration.

✔ **Exercise regularly.** Exercise improves circulation to the eyes as well as to other parts of your body, and it reduces the risk of vision loss that may occur as a result of high blood pressure, diabetes, and narrowing or hardening of the arteries.

✔ **Stay hydrated.** Drink at least 8 ounces of water every two hours. Proper hydration improves circulation to and lubrication of your eyes.

✔ **Consume 45 to 50 total grams of dietary fiber daily.** You can supplement the amount in your diet with fiber from psyllium husks. Fiber helps detox your entire system, including your eyes.

✔ **Eat right.** Eat a healthy diet, as explained in Chapter 2. Specifically, avoid refined sugar, processed foods, and trans fats. Focus on eating more foods that are high in antioxidants, including vitamins A (beta-carotene), C, and E (tocopherols); glutathione; and the carotenoids lutein, lycopene, and zeaxanthin, which help protect against cataracts and macular degeneration.

Lutein-rich foods include yellow and orange fruits and vegetables such as carrots, mangoes, sweet potatoes, tomatoes, squash; and green, leafy vegetables, such as kale, collard greens, and bok choy. You can find lycopene in tomatoes, watermelon, grapefruit, and red peppers. Zeaxanthin-rich foods include orange bell peppers, oranges, and cantaloupe. Egg yolks are also high in both lutein and zeaxanthin.

✔ **Wear a hat and sunglasses.** Long-term exposure to sunlight damages your eyes, so when you're outside during the day, wear sunglasses with ultraviolet (UV) protection and a brimmed hat to shade your eyes.

✔ **Wear safety glasses when necessary.** To prevent physical damage to the eye, wear safety glasses when you do any work that exposes your eyes to flying objects, regardless of how small those objects may be.

✔ **Look around.** Don't get into the habit of staring at a computer screen, a smart phone screen, a book, or any other object for more than about a half hour at a time. Give your eyes the opportunity to focus on objects both near and far to keep your eye muscles limber.

Although you're better off getting nutrients from the foods you eat, you may want to supplement your diet with the following nutrients that support healthy eyes and vision:

Supplement	Dosage
Vitamin A (retinyl palmitate and beta-carotene)	2,500 IU retinyl palmitate and 2,500 IU beta-carotene daily
Vitamin C (mineral ascorbates)	1,000 mg two to four times daily
Vitamin E (tocopherols)	400 IU daily
Magnesium glycinate chelate	250 mg twice daily
Alpha-lipoic acid	150 mg daily
Bilberry extract	180 mg daily
Lutein	10 mg daily
Lycopene	6 mg daily
N-acetyl cysteine	200 mg daily
Omega-3 essential fatty acids	1 g yielding 180 mg EPA and 120 mg DHA three times daily
Quercetin	100 mg daily
Selenium	100 mcg daily
Taurine	400 mg daily
Turmeric	400 mg daily
Zeaxanthin	500 mcg daily
Zinc glycinate chelate	35 mg daily

 Instead of buying and taking all these supplements individually, look for a quality product that combines several of these ingredients. Discuss options with your healthcare provider, who can recommend a quality product that's right for you.

Uncovering the Causes of Blurred Vision

Blurred vision may be caused by a variety of conditions. Short- or long-sightedness, astigmatism, cataracts, diabetic retinopathy (damage to the retina caused by high blood sugar), macular degeneration, detached retina, eye infection or inflammation (such as conjunctivitis), migraine, stroke, and injury to the eye can all cause vision problems. Therefore, to successfully treat blurred vision, you need to know what's causing it. Consult an ophthalmologist to obtain a diagnosis and recommendation for treatment.

You can address some conditions yourself. The sections of this chapter offer guidance on how to treat many of the eye conditions that may be causing blurred vision: cataracts, conjunctivitis, and eye strain. If your blurred vision is the result of a stroke or is associated with migraines, turn to Chapter 17 for more about treating those conditions. Other conditions, however, such as near- or short-sightedness, detached retina, and so on, may require other medical procedures — prescription eyeglasses, contacts, or Lasik surgery, for example — that fall outside the scope of natural cures.

Whatever the cause of your blurred vision, you may be able to improve recovery time through proper nutrition and supplements; see the preceding section.

Clearing Away the Clouds: Cataracts

A *cataract* is a lens that's cloudy instead of clear. Prevention is the best medicine, but if you've developed cataracts despite your best efforts at preventing them, you may be able to improve clarity of the lens with the following natural cures:

- **N-acetylcarnosine:** A few studies show improvement in cataracts with long-term use of N-acetylcarnosine eye drops. Don't expect dramatic improvement overnight, but this may stop progression of the disease and possibly even reverse its course. You can purchase N-acetylcarnosine eye drops online or at local pharmacies or health food stores.

- **Triphala eyewash:** Steep ½ teaspoon of triphala powder in ½ cup of boiling water. Let the triphala settle to the bottom and allow the infusion to cool to body temperature. Soak two cotton pads in the infusion, squeeze out just enough so that the pads aren't dripping wet, lie down with your head on a towel, place one pad over each eye, and blink every 3 to 5 seconds over the course of 15 to 25 minutes to allow some of the infusion to drip into the eye. Do this two to three times daily, once just before bedtime.

- **Dusty miller *(Cineraria maritima):*** Eye drops made with dusty miller extract may help clear cloudy lenses if you catch the cataracts early enough. You can purchase *Cineraria maritima* eye drops online or at health food stores. They usually contain additional ingredients, including eyebright.

- **Pascalite:** This cream-colored bentonite clay found in the Big Horn mountains of Wyoming is said to help dissolve cataracts. Apply the clay to your eyelids or use eye drops made of water that's been filtered through the clay.

Support your eye drop treatments with proper diet and supplements, as recommended in the earlier section "Supporting Eye and Vision Health with Diet and Lifestyle Changes." Proper diet and nutritional supplements increase the presence of antioxidants that help remove the toxins that contribute to the formation of cataracts.

The only sure cure for cataracts is surgery. The surgeon replaces the cloudy lens with an artificial implant. The good news is that the surgery is very safe, and after surgery you may no longer need corrective eyeglasses or contact lenses.

Dealing with Conjunctivitis (Pinkeye)

Conjunctivitis (pinkeye) is inflammation of the tissue that lines the inside of the eyelid and the white part of the eye. It may be a sign of viral or bacterial infection, allergy, or a reaction to a chemical irritant, such as chlorine.

If the inflammation is accompanied by a gunky discharge or your eyelids are crusty in the morning, you're probably dealing with a viral or bacterial infection. Clear discharge typically indicates allergy, chemical irritant, or other irritant in the eye. If your symptoms indicate viral or bacterial infection, see Chapters 5 and 6 for guidance on fighting infection in addition to following the suggestions in this section.

Protecting your eyes during the episode

Regardless of the cause, the first order of business is to make sure you don't further irritate your eyes or spread any infection to your other eye or to someone else:

- **Don't rub your eyes.** Rubbing your eyes irritates them and is likely to worsen the inflammation, and if you're dealing with an infection, you're likely to spread it to the other eye or to someone else.

- **If you wear contact lenses, remove them.** Switch to glasses until the condition clears up.

- **Avoid any potential chemical irritants.** This includes everything from chlorine in pools to shampoos, eye makeup, and face creams.

- **Wash your hands with soap and water frequently.** This is an added precaution, just in case you forget to keep your hands away from your eyes.

- **Throw away any eye cosmetics you used since experiencing symptoms.**

- **Start each day with a new washcloth and towel and don't share towels or cosmetics.**

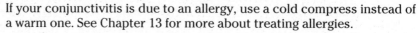

Relieving the symptoms

Compresses and eye drops applied to the eyes reduce inflammation and help the body fight any infection locally. Try one of the following treatments:

- ✔ **Warm compress:** Soak a clean washcloth in hot water, ring it out, and press it gently against your eyes for several minutes. You can use water only, or you can add one or more of the ingredients mentioned in this list, such as eyebright, to improve effectiveness. Do this several times daily, being sure to use a fresh washcloth each time.

  If your conjunctivitis is due to an allergy, use a cold compress instead of a warm one. See Chapter 13 for more about treating allergies.

- ✔ **Eyebright *(Euphrasia officinalis)*:** Brew some eyebright tea, filter it through a coffee filter, let it cool to body temperature, and use it in the form of eye drops or eyewash every four to six waking hours. To speed the healing process, drink a half cup of eyebright tea two to three times daily or take eyebright in capsule form.

- ✔ **Saltwater:** Mix 1 cup warm distilled water with ½ teaspoon sea salt, and use the solution as eye drops or eyewash every four to six waking hours.

- ✔ **Calendula or chamomile:** Brew calendula or chamomile tea, filter it through a coffee filter (if it's not already filtered), allow it to cool to body temperature, and then use in the form of eye drops or eyewash every four to six waking hours. *Note:* Don't use chamomile if you're allergic to ragweed.

- ✔ **Manuka honey:** Honey has antibacterial, antifungal, and anti-inflammatory properties. Combine ¼ teaspoon manuka honey and ¼ cup warm distilled water. Place 1 to 2 drops of the solution in each eye every couple of hours.

- ✔ **Silver:** Silver nitrate eye drops were commonly used in the past to prevent conjunctivitis and transmission of STDs to newborns. With your doctor's permission and supervision, try placing 1 to 2 drops of silver nitrate or silver hydrosol in each eye every four to six hours.

Seek medical treatment if pain or the signs of infection worsen, if you develop sensitivity to light, or if your vision becomes blurred and doesn't clear up when you blink.

Rejuvenating Dry Eyes

If your eyes sting, burn, or feel sandy, you may be suffering from a condition called *dry eyes*. Fortunately, several natural remedies can help lubricate your eyes:

- ✔ **Stay hydrated.** Drink at least 8 ounces of water every two waking hours.

- ✔ **Increase your intake of omega-3 essential fatty acids (EFAs).** Consume at least 2 g of EFAs daily, preferably from cold water fish, such as sardines, cod, herring, and salmon. Flaxseed oil is also a great source of EFAs. If you can't get your EFAs through diet alone, take a supplement. One study showed that people who consumed 450 mg EPA (eicosapentaenoic acid), 300 mg DHA (docosahexaenoic acid), and 1,000 mg flaxseed oil daily produced more tears.

- ✔ **Don't forget to blink.** If you have a tendency to stare, especially when watching TV, staring at a computer screen, or playing video games, you may need to remind yourself to blink occasionally.

- ✔ **Cover your eyes when you go outside.** If you're commonly exposed to dry, windy conditions, wear goggles to prevent your environment from drying out your eyes.

- ✔ **Humidify your indoor environment.** If the air inside your home or workplace is dry, try using a humidifier.

- ✔ **Check your medications.** Ask your doctor or pharmacist whether any of your medications may be contributing to your dry-eye condition. Antihistamines, decongestants, antidepressants, and blood pressure medications are the prime suspects.

- ✔ **Use warm compresses.** Warm compresses help clear the glands that release oils that help lubricate your eyes. Soak a clean washcloth in hot water, ring it out, and press it against your eyes for several minutes. You may use water only; use a tea with calendula, eyebright, bilberry, or chamomile (don't use chamomile if you're allergic to ragweed); or mix ½ teaspoon of sea salt with ½ cup of water.

- ✔ **Massage your eyelids.** Place a warm, moist washcloth over your eyes and gently massage your upper and lower eyelids for 5 to 10 seconds each.

- ✔ **Use eye drops or eyewashes.** Eye drops or eyewashes made from eyebright, calendula, bilberry, chamomile, or saltwater (sea salt) help soothe the eyes, keep them hydrated, and de-gunk the tear ducts and the upper and lower eyelids so that they can properly lubricate the eyes.

Although you don't want to dry yourself out by ingesting diuretics, caffeine has been shown to increase tear production. If nothing else works, try drinking a small cup (6 ounces) or two of coffee.

Giving Your Eyes a Break from Eye Strain

Eye strain occurs when your eyes get tired of being used too intently for too long. Reading, driving, texting, playing video games, or working on a computer are common activities that cause eye strain. Although you may not be able to avoid the activities that cause eye strain, you can alleviate eye strain by doing one or more of the following:

- **Get your vision checked and corrected, if necessary.** If you have to strain to see objects near or far, get the glasses, contacts, or surgery you need to correct your vision. Otherwise, you'll be straining your eyes regardless of any other measures you take.

- **Position your work at a comfortable distance.** If you're working on a computer, for example, you usually want the screen positioned at or just below eye level and about 18 to 24 inches from your face.

- **Reduce glare.** If you spend a lot of time looking at a screen, position the screen to minimize glare. This usually means placing the screen perpendicular to any sources of strong light, using window coverings to block out intense light, tilting the screen so reflected light doesn't shine in your eyes, moving lamps, and dimming overhead lighting.

- **Optimize screen brightness and contrast.** Adjust the brightness and contrast on computer screens, TVs, and other electronic devices so that you're not straining to bring a dull image into focus.

- **Keep screens clean.** Office supply stores, pharmacies, and even grocery stores carry cleaning supplies for computer screens. Distilled water and paper towels are usually sufficient; just be sure not to get the screen too wet.

- **Take frequent breaks.** Look away from what you're doing or close your eyes for five to ten seconds every so often (as long as it's safe to do so, of course). Also periodically get up and walk around or stretch in place.

To revitalize tired eyes, brew a tea or infusion, using one of the following herbs: eyebright, goldenseal, witch hazel, calendula, or chamomile (no chamomile if you're allergic to ragweed). (See Chapter 3 for more about making herbal teas and infusions.) Filter the tea through a coffee filter to remove any sediment and then refrigerate the tea or infusion. Soak cotton pads in the tea or infusion, squeeze out the excess, and place the damp pads on your eyes for five to ten minutes when your eyes feel weary. Also refer to the earlier section "Supporting Eye and Vision Health with Diet and Lifestyle Changes" for general recommendations that may also help alleviate eye strain.

Relieving the Pressure of Glaucoma

Glaucoma is a group of eye disorders that increase pressure inside the eye, which may cause damage to the optic nerve. It's the second leading cause of blindness in the U.S. Glaucoma comes in several forms:

- **Open-angle glaucoma** accounts for about 90 percent of all cases. It occurs when the channels through which fluid flows out of the eye become clogged with debris. This happens over time, and you usually don't notice symptoms until some vision loss has occurred — loss of peripheral vision or development of tunnel vision. Early detection, through regular eye exams, is crucial in slowing the progression of the illness.

- **Angle-closure glaucoma** occurs when the iris suddenly blocks the drainage channels, causing intense pain, vision problems (blurred vision or seeing halos around lights), and a noticeable hardening of the eye.

  If you notice these symptoms, seek immediate medical treatment; angle-closure glaucoma is a medical emergency.

- **Normal-tension or low-tension glaucoma** occurs when the optic nerve is damaged from something other than increased eye pressure.

- **Congenital glaucoma** is caused by incomplete development of the drainage channels in the eye. Microsurgery is usually required to repair the channels.

Treatment for glaucoma requires oral medication, medicated eye drops, or surgery to slow the flow of fluid into the eye or to improve fluid drainage out of the eye. The natural cures approach complements medical treatment through nutrition and supplements; see "Supporting Eye and Vision Health with Diet and Lifestyle Changes," earlier in this chapter, for details. If you have high blood pressure, also take steps to lower your blood pressure, as explained in Chapter 17.

Slowing Macular Degeneration's Progression

Macular degeneration (often referred to as "age-related macular degeneration, AMD, or ARMD) is a condition that results in vision loss in the center of the field of vision. (The *macula* is the center portion of the *retina* — the light-sensitive cells that line the back of the eye.) Macular degeneration comes in dry and wet forms:

- ✔ **Dry form:** This form, which makes up about 90 percent of all cases, is characterized by yellow deposits, called *drusen*, that collect on the macula, resulting in distortion or the dimming of vision in the center of the field of vision. In some cases, cells of the macula atrophy or die, causing blind spots or total loss of central vision in advanced cases.

- ✔ **Wet form:** This form is caused by abnormal blood vessels behind the macula that leak blood and fluid into the retina, making straight lines look wavy and causing blind spots or total loss of central vision in advanced cases. Although only about 10 percent of people with macular degeneration develop the wet form, it's responsible for the most serious cases of vision loss.

To prevent macular degeneration or slow its progression, adopt an eye-friendly diet and lifestyle, as explained in the earlier section "Supporting Eye and Vision Health with Diet and Lifestyle Changes." Focus on increasing consumption of a colorful diet of vegetables and fruits to boost your intake of vitamin C, antioxidants, and bioflavonoids, including diosmin, hesperidin, rutin, naringin, tangeretin, diosmetin, narirutin, neohesperidin, nobiletin, and quercetin. Bioflavonoids are especially beneficial in improving circulation to the eyes. Supplementing your diet with zinc and copper also helps.

AREDS and AREDS2

One large study conducted by the National Eye Institute of the Nation Institutes of Health (NIH), called the Age-Related Eye Disease Study (AREDS), showed that some people with intermediate to advanced dry macular degeneration decreased their risk of vision loss by taking a combination of vitamins C and E, beta-carotene, zinc, and copper. A later study, AREDS2, showed additional benefit by adding lutein and zeaxanthin to the mix. No benefit was gained with the addition of omega-3.

In another, more recent study, researchers found that high doses of omega-3 fatty acids significantly improved vision acuity in 100 percent of patients with dry AMD within four-and-a-half months of treatment. Patients were given 3.4 grams of EPA and 1.6 grams of DHA daily for six months.

Treating Sties

A *sty* is a painful abscess on the inside or outside of the eyelid typically caused by a *Staphylococcus* bacterial infection. The most effective treatment is chamomile tea eyewash. To make and apply the eyewash, follow these steps:

1. **Brew a cup of chamomile tea, using distilled water, and allow the tea to cool to room temperature (save the teabag).**

   If you're allergic to ragweed, brew green tea instead.

2. **Mix two parts tea with one part distilled water and use the solution to wash your eyes every few waking hours.**

   If you wear contact lenses, remove them before washing your eyes. You can wash your eyes using an eyedropper or eye cup, but in either case, wash your hands with soap and water first:

   • **With an eyedropper:** Hold your eye open with one hand while using an eyedropper to drip the solution into your eye as you move your eye back and forth and up and down (you may want to do this over a sink).

   • **With an eye cup:** Fill the eye cup about half way with solution, lean forward to seal your eye socket against the edge of the cup, and then raise your head so you're looking straight up. Open your eye and move it back and forth and up and down a few times. Lean forward, remove the cup, and discard the solution. Rinse the cup in warm water before washing the other eye, and wash the cup with soap and water when you're done.

3. **Apply the used (cooled) tea bags to your eyes for additional relief, if you like, but discard them after first use.**

4. **Discard unused eyewash and prepare a fresh batch daily.**

 If you get sties frequently, work on preventing infection. Keep your fingers and any foreign substances, such as makeup, away from the commonly affected areas. Clean your eyelids occasionally using a solution of baby shampoo and warm water. Dip a cotton ball in the solution, squeeze out most of the solution, and then close your eyes and gently rub the cotton ball back and forth along the line where your lower and upper eyelids meet. Use a different cotton ball for each eye to avoid spreading any infectious agents from one eye to the other.

If you have rosacea, you may be more prone to getting sties. See Chapter 7 for more about treating rosacea.

Chapter 10

Addressing Mouth and Dental Conditions

In This Chapter

▶ Improving oral health

▶ Freshening your breath naturally

▶ Curing canker sores and chapped lips

▶ Preventing tooth decay with a sugar substitute

▶ Relieving toothaches and TMJ pain

*N*early everything you consume enters your body through your mouth, so a healthy mouth is a key component to your overall health. Everything from canker sores to toothaches and gum disease is likely to affect your appetite and digestion along with your self-esteem and social interactions, which are other key components to your health and well-being. In this chapter, I offer guidance on preventing and treating several common afflictions in and around the mouth. But first, I encourage you to practice good oral hygiene, using a natural product that may be new to you.

Doses in this chapter are for adults, not children. For guidance on how to adjust dosages for children (and adults under 150 pounds), turn to Chapter 12.

Optimizing Oral Health

Maintaining healthy teeth and gums requires more than flossing, brushing, and using mouthwash. It also involves adopting a healthy diet and lifestyle, as explained in Chapter 2. Focus on eliminating or at least reducing your consumption of sugary and starchy foods, including candy, soft drinks, fruit juices, cookies, cake, and crackers. The unhealthy bacteria in your mouth are junk food junkies that thrive on this stuff and produce acid that eats away at your teeth and leads to gum disease. If you eat or drink acidy foods, such as citrus fruit, do so as part of a meal.

Eat more veggies and chew them to liquid before swallowing. Veggies, especially the green leafy variety, are higher in alkalinity and help to neutralize the acids in your mouth. As you chew, your mouth produces saliva, which further neutralizes the acids. In addition, plant-based foods, including vegetables, fruits, nuts, and seeds, contain the calcium and phosphorous your body needs to build strong teeth. (Eat sugary fruits — raisins and other dried fruit, bananas, grapes, and mangoes — in moderation, if at all.)

Drink at least 8 ounces of water every two waking hours. Water neutralizes and washes away acids and food particles while keeping your mouth hydrated. Green tea has also been shown to be effective in preventing cavities and promoting healthy gums.

To prevent cavities, follow your dentist's guidance on proper oral hygiene, which usually consists of flossing and brushing after meals. (If you can't floss and brush after a meal, at least swish some water around in your mouth to loosen the particles between your teeth and neutralize the acid.) I recommend avoiding oral hygiene products that contain fluoride and a host of other chemicals. Look for natural products that contain the ingredients listed in Table 10-1. Alternatively, use these ingredients alone or in combination to make your own oral care products.

Table 10-1	Natural Ingredients That Support Oral Care	
Ingredient	*General Information*	*How to Use It*
Baking soda	A mild abrasive that neutralizes acid	Brush your teeth with it
Peroxide	An antibacterial that cleans and disinfects	Mix one part peroxide with one or two parts water and use it as a mouthwash, but do not swallow it
Green tea	Protects teeth from erosion and abrasion (as does fluoride)	Brew green tea, let it cool, and use it as a mouthwash
Eucalyptus, menthol, or tea tree oil	Antiseptics	Add a few drops of any of these oils to your peroxide or green-tea mouthwash or your baking soda toothpaste
Xylitol	A natural sugar from birch trees that cavity-causing bacteria can't digest	Brush with it, chew xylitol gum, suck on xylitol lozenges, or dissolve it in water or green tea for use as a mouthwash

If you're a parent, you may also want to use xylitol yourself to help prevent tooth decay in your children. Several studies have shown that the children of mothers who use xylitol have up to 70 percent fewer cavities! Start your child on a low dose of xylitol and slowly increase it to 6 to 10 g daily (a teaspoon of xylitol granules is about 4 g). You can purchase xylitol sweetened gum, candy, toothpaste, and mouthwash over the counter or online. The two most common side effects of taking too much xylitol are gas and diarrhea. If either symptom occurs, back off the dosage until the symptom subsides.

Banishing Bad Breath (Halitosis)

Everyone has had a bout of bad breath, and it's usually no big deal. You floss, brush, and rinse with mouthwash, and you're good to go. However, if bad breath becomes a chronic condition, it may be a symptom of something more serious, and it's certainly something you want to attend to.

Common causes of bad breath include acid reflux (GERD); spicy foods; poor diet; improper oral hygiene, tooth decay, and gum disease; tobacco use; and a variety of health conditions such as *dysbiosis* (a bacterial imbalance in the mouth, esophagus, stomach, or intestinal tract), diabetes, liver disease, and *hypochlorydria* (inadequate gastric acid secretion).

Unless the cause of your bad breath is obvious, focus first on your diet (see Chapter 2) and take supplements to improve your digestion, as explained in Chapter 14: probiotics, betaine HCL, and digestive enzymes. In addition, take 500 to 1,000 mg of N-acetyl cysteine daily and 250 mg of milk thistle twice daily for 28 days to detox your liver.

If you can't cure your bad breath through nutrition and digestion, try the following natural cures:

- After every meal, swish water in your mouth to loosen food particles trapped between teeth and then swallow.

- Floss after you eat.

- Mix ½ teaspoon baking soda and ½ teaspoon xylitol in 1 cup of water, and use it as a mouthwash after every meal. Baking soda neutralizes odors, and xylitol starves the bacteria that often cause bad breath.

- Brew and drink fenugreek tea. To make the tea, boil 1 teaspoon of fenugreek seeds in 1 cup of water and then strain out the seeds.

- Chew on fresh parsley leaves after each meal for at least 30 seconds.

- Take a chlorophyll capsule after each meal.

✔ Mix 1 tablespoon of apple cider vinegar in 1 cup of water and drink it five minutes before eating or use it as a mouthwash and gargle after every meal.

✔ Brush with toothpaste that contains tea tree oil (available at health food stores and online).

Conquering Canker Sores

Canker sores (*aphthous ulcers*) are painful white lesions on the inside of the mouth, lips, or throat. Unlike herpes lesions (which you can read about in Chapter 7), canker sores are not contagious. Although canker sores have no known cause, several conditions are associated with their appearance, including health issues (viral infections, lupus, Crohn's disease, celiac disease); nutritional issues (poor diet, anemia, and vitamin B12 or folate deficiency); fatigue; and stress.

For immediate treatment, mix 1 teaspoon of salt, 1 teaspoon of baking soda, and 2 ounces of 3 percent hydrogen peroxide, and rinse your mouth with the mixture four times daily. Avoid acidic foods (such as citrus fruits) and spicy foods, which may aggravate the canker sore. Also avoid toothpaste that contains sodium laurel sulfate.

If any white spot in or around your mouth lasts for more than ten days, see your doctor. Something more serious may be causing the lesions, such as herpes or cancer. (Although canker sores aren't cancerous and don't cause cancer, certain types of cancer may appear as ulcers in the mouth, which may be mistakenly identified as canker sores.)

Canker sores and gluten sensitivity

Celiac disease and nonceliac gluten sensitivity are both associated with canker sores. Your doctor may test you for celiac disease, but if your test results come back negative, you may still have a nonceliac gluten sensitivity. Request to be tested for gluten sensitivity (see Chapter 13).

If you have a gluten sensitivity, adopt a healthy diet (see Chapter 2): Eliminate wheat, gluten, and sugar. Consume high-quality, nutrient-dense foods rich in antioxidants (eight servings of a variety of organic vegetables and two servings of organic fruit daily). Add good sources of essential fatty acids from wild fish and lean, grass-fed animals.

Beyond immediate relief and practicing good oral hygiene, supporting your diet with the following nutritional supplements can also reduce the incidence and severity of canker sores and heal them:

Supplement	Dosage
Proline-rich polypeptides extracted from pure colostrum	4 sprays in mouth, hold for 30 seconds and swallow, twice daily early morning and before bed, for a total of 16 mg daily
Probiotics (*Streptococcus salivarius* DDS 18)	Chew 1 billion CFU, use your tongue to spread it around your mouth, and then swallow
Vitamin B12 (methylcobalamin, sublingual fast-dissolving tablet)	5,000 mcg daily
Folate (5-MTHF)	2,000 to 10,000 mcg daily
Iron (ferrous bis-glycinate chelate)	30 mg daily
Vitamin C (mineral ascorbates)	1,000 mg two to three times daily
Vitamin A (retinyl palmitate and beta-carotene)	2,500 IU of retinyl palmitate and 2,500 IU of beta-carotene daily (see Appendix A for precautions)
Vitamin D3	2,000 to 10,000 IU daily, depending on blood levels (see Appendix A)
Whole beta glucan (from *Saccharomyces cerevisiae*)	250 to 500 mg twice daily

Rejuvenating Chapped Lips

Dry, cracked, peeling lips are often painful and always embarrassing, but they are preventable and treatable. Unfortunately, many of the over-the-counter products for treating chapped lips, including Vaseline, are petroleum products or contain ingredients — like phenol, lanolin, parabens, and artificial fragrances — that shouldn't come anywhere near your mouth.

To prevent or cure chapped lips, try these strategies:

- **Be picky about what you put on your lips.** Use lip balms that contain beeswax, shea butter, or almond oil. Alternatively, apply extra virgin organic coconut, olive, or jojoba oil to your lips several times daily. Shop for lip-friendly lipstick or use tinted lip balm that doesn't contain harsh chemicals. (Don't put anything on your lips that you wouldn't eat.)

- **Avoid licking and picking your lips, and protect them from the sun.** Use chemical-free sunscreen made with zinc oxide, organic sunflower oils, organic beeswax, vitamin E, and organic sea buckthorn. (I like Badger sunscreen products.)

> ✔ **Eat plenty of vegetables and fruits and stay hydrated.** Drink at least 8 ounces of water every two waking hours. Hydration works from the inside out to keep your lips moist. Use a humidifier at home and work (clean it regularly to prevent bacterial overgrowth).

For severely cracked lips that hurt when you smile, place a cucumber slice, fresh from the refrigerator, on your lips for several minutes a few times a day. You can also apply aloe vera gel several times daily.

Dealing with Gingivitis and Other Gum Infections

Gum infection is a broad term that covers everything from gingivitis (inflamed, sensitive gums) to periodontal disease (infection that leads to the loss of bone and tissue that hold the teeth in place). These conditions are often accompanied by bleeding gums and bad breath. The underlying cause is usually an overgrowth of harmful bacteria resulting from poor diet and poor dental hygiene, including the failure to visit the dentist twice a year for checkups and cleanings.

Gingivitis is a bacterial infection characterized by inflamed gums that tend to bleed easily with brushing or flossing and is often accompanied by bad breath. Without proper treatment, the infection may progress, leading to loss of bone and tissue that hold the teeth in place, and ultimately to tooth loss. The infection may even spread throughout the body, compromising overall health, including cardiovascular health.

If your gums bleed when you floss or brush, head to the dentist. A thorough cleaning is the first step toward restoring oral health. The next step is to follow up with appropriate self-care as explained earlier in this chapter, including adopting a healthy diet. In addition, if you use tobacco, quit or cut down as much as possible; tobacco use increases your risk of gum infection and periodontal disease. Finally, take the following supplements until your current infection clears up:

Supplement	Dosage
Probiotic (*Streptococcus salivarius* DDS 18)	1 billion CFU (chew and dissolve in mouth)
Coenzyme Q10 (Kaneka Q10)	Consume your weight in milligrams per day; you can also apply it with a cotton swab to the affected areas of your gums

Supplement	Dosage
Folic acid mouthwash	Rinse for one minute with 5 ml of the mouthwash twice daily and then spit it out
Vitamin C (mineral ascorbates)	1,000 mg twice daily
	You can also apply it topically: Place a couple grams in your dry palm and use a wet toothbrush to pick it up. Massage gently into the infected gums and don't rinse (**Note:** Don't use vitamin C as ascorbic acid, because it will erode your enamel)
Calcium (as MCHC)	550 mg twice daily
Vitamin D3	2,000 to 10,000 IU daily, depending on blood levels (see Appendix A)
Zinc glycinate chelate	20 mg daily
Multivitamin/mineral (high-quality formula containing the better form of each nutrient)	Follow label instructions
Borage seed oil	1 g three times daily

For infections with open sores, inflammation, and pain, or infections that don't respond to home remedies within a few days, see your doctor or dentist. Oral infections may spread to the bloodstream and cause life-threatening conditions.

Stopping Jaw Pain and Popping: Temporomandibular Joint (TMJ) Dysfunction

Jaw pain and popping are typically symptoms of a *temporomandibular joint dysfunction* (often referred to as TMJ or TMD). In addition to jaw pain and popping, you may experience pain in or near your ear, difficulty or discomfort chewing, facial pain, or locking of the joint that makes opening or closing your mouth difficult.

Sudden jaw pain may be an early warning sign of a heart attack or other serious cardiovascular event, so head to the emergency room ASAP.

Getting immediate relief

For immediate relief, soften your diet: Eat softer foods, including high-quality meal replacements (protein-rich smoothies), soups, and steamed veggies. Adopt a healthier diet that's lower in sugar, refined carbohydrates, unhealthy fats, and other inflammatory substances (see Chapter 2 for details). Avoid alcohol, because it promotes teeth grinding. Relax with herbal teas, including chamomile.

Taking care of the root causes

Long-term treatment for TMJ varies, depending on its cause:

- **Misalignment of the teeth and jaw, teeth grinding, and clenching of the jaw:** Dental appliances or even orthodontic surgery may be required to realign the lower jaw and teeth or help relieve the stress from night-time teeth grinding.

- **Psychological or emotional stress:** Stress-reduction techniques, such as yoga, Qigong, meditation, exercise, and biofeedback may be most helpful.

- **Magnesium or calcium deficiency:** Increasing magnesium and calcium intake through diet and supplements addresses this issue. Take 50 mg of magnesium citrate and 25 mg of calcium lactate twice daily.

- **Spinal misalignments, muscle imbalance, or arthritis:** Chiropractic, osteopathic, and naturopathic techniques may help realign bone structure and rebalance muscles.

- For muscle support, supplement your diet with the following nutrients:

Supplement	Dosage
Passionflower	100 mg twice daily
Valerian root	50 mg twice daily

- For cartilage support, supplement your diet with the following nutrients:

Supplement	Dosage
Glucosamine sulfate	1,500 mg daily
Chondroitin sulfate	1,000 mg daily
MSM	1,000 mg three times daily

Relieving a Toothache

Toothaches are triggered by any of a multitude of causes, including tooth decay, loose fillings, cracked teeth, eroded enamel, exposed roots (from gum disease), clenching or grinding of teeth, sensitivity to hot and cold foods and drinks, biting down on hard foods, and even sinus infection.

If the toothache can't be traced to a specific cause, try using a softer toothbrush and avoid brushing too hard or too long. Consider using an electric toothbrush with features that indicate how long you've been brushing and warn when you're pressing too hard. Certain toothpastes, such as Sensodyne, may help with sensitive teeth.

For short-term pain and infection-prevention, try the following natural remedies:

Remedy	Dosage
White willow bark	300 mg several times daily between meals
Boswellia extract	50 mg several times daily between meals
Turmeric	100 mg several times daily between meals
Probiotic (*Streptococcus salivarius* DDS 18)	1 billion CFU (chew and dissolve in mouth)
Whole beta glucan	250 to 500 mg two to three times daily
Hydrogen peroxide mouthwash	Mix equal parts 3 percent hydrogen peroxide and water and use it as a mouthwash several times daily; do not swallow

If the pain and discomfort fail to improve in a few days, see your dentist for evaluation and treatment.

Chapter 11

Kicking Leg and Feet Conditions to the Curb

*I*f you're like most people, your legs and feet are your primary means of transportation, and they really take a beating. In this chapter, I cover common ailments that affect feet and legs and offer guidance on how to treat them naturally to restore optimum function and, in some cases, appearance.

Doses in this chapter are for adults, not children. For guidance on how to adjust dosages for children (and adults under 150 pounds), turn to Chapter 12.

Stomping Out Athlete's Foot

Athlete's foot *(tinea pedis)* is a common and contagious fungal infection of the skin that causes redness, flaking, scaling, and itching. It often appears around the edges of the feet and between the toes and affects about 15 percent of the population. The disease is usually transmitted in moist areas where people walk barefoot, such as showers and pools. The fungus requires a warm, moist environment to flourish, such as a locker room or the inside of a shoe.

Battling athlete's foot from the outside in

The best treatment is prevention. Wear clean sandals in locker rooms and showers and around public pools. Keep your feet clean and dry. Go barefoot whenever possible or wear socks without shoes. Wear shoes or sandals that allow your feet to breathe. Don't share towels or footwear (for example, avoid renting bowling shoes).

Although symptoms of athlete's foot are only skin deep, contributing factors may run deeper. They include systemic candidiasis (yeast) infection, long-term use of antibiotics or corticosteroids, poor digestion, diets high in sugar and processed carbohydrates, a compromised immune system, and diabetes.

Focus first on treating the athlete's foot directly:

- ✔ Wash your feet daily with antifungal soap and water, and dry your feet with a clean towel. Keep your feet dry at all times.

- ✔ Apply one or more of the following antifungal oils or gels to affected areas (over-the-counter antifungal ointments and creams are also okay to use):

Oil/Gel	Application
Tea tree oil	Apply several times daily every other day for at least eight weeks
Calendula gel	Apply several times daily, alternating days with tea tree oil applications, for at least eight weeks
Oregano oil	Apply several times daily
Thuja oil	Apply two to three times daily

- ✔ Use antifungal powder in your socks and shoes. (Don't use any product that contains cornstarch, because fungus feeds on starches. Baking soda is better.)

- ✔ Let your feet breathe as much as possible. Go barefoot when relaxing for the evening or when walking around dry areas.

- ✔ When you must cover your feet, wear socks that wick away perspiration.

If the skin between your toes is red and cracked, the fungal infection may be compounded by a bacterial infection. Purchase Betadine from your local pharmacy, mix 2 capfuls with 1 quart of warm water, and soak your feet in the solution for 20 minutes. Dry your feet thoroughly and then apply the antifungal remedies listed earlier.

Betadine may trigger allergic reactions in certain individuals, resulting in intense itching, burning, and hives. Don't use Betadine if you're pregnant, and use it with caution if you have autoimmune thyroid disorder or have recently received radiation treatment for a thyroid condition. An alternative to Betadine is Chloroprep, which contains chlorhexidine and alcohol and is free of iodine.

Starving yeast/fungi from the inside out

Systemic yeast and fungal infections often appear as skin infections, so starve the fungus from the inside out. The standard American diet is high in refined sugars, highly processed carbohydrates, and unhealthy fats that create a breeding ground for opportunistic fungi. Eliminate refined sugar and yeasty breads and desserts from your diet and eat eight servings daily of a variety of vegetables and two servings daily of low-glycemic fruit — plums, strawberries, blackberries, blueberries, raspberries, cherries, kiwis, grapefruit, apples, and cantaloupes. (High-glycemic fruits include bananas, pineapples, watermelons, and mangoes.) Consume quality lean meats and healthy fats.

Support your dietary changes with the following nutritional supplements, several of which have powerful antifungal properties:

Supplement	Dosage
Probiotic (mixed multistrain of *Lactobacillus acidophilus* and *Bifidobacterium* Rosell)	5 billion CFU
Whole beta glucan (from *Saccharomyces cerevisiae*)	250 mg daily
Ground flaxseeds	1 to 2 tablespoons daily
Coconut oil	1 tablespoon three times daily (***Tip:*** Cook with it, add it to your rice or vegetables, or whip it into your coffee)
Oregano	500 mg three times daily
Garlic	500 mg twice daily
Grapefruit seed extract	200 mg three times daily

Battling Bunions

A *bunion* is a bony lump that forms at the base of the big toe when tight shoes push the big toe in toward the other toes. Bunions commonly run in families and more commonly afflict women. For immediate relief, do the following:

- ✔ Purchase from a surgical supply store a bunion pad or flexible bunion splint such as Bunion Aid. This splint can reduce pain and slow the progression of moderate to severe bunions.

- ✔ Apply an ice pack for 20 minutes at the end of the day to reduce swelling.

To strengthen your feet and toes, perform the following exercises:

- ✔ Practice picking up an article of clothing or a towel with your toes, dropping it, and then picking it up again. Perform this exercise several times daily.

- ✔ Flex and extend your toes. Press your toes against the floor and then raise your toes toward the ceiling several times daily.

For extreme pain that's not improving, see a qualified healthcare specialist. Consider surgery only as a last resort.

Of course, prevention is the best medicine. Wear quality shoes (no high heels) that have good support and plenty of room near the tip so that your toes can spread out. (Cramming your toes into a tight-fitting, pointy-toed shoe is just asking for bunions.) Custom orthotics (shoe inserts) available from trained chiropractors and podiatrists can prevent bunions from forming in the first place, if worn correctly. After a bunion has formed, the orthotics can help prevent the bunion from becoming more severe. I recommend using soft orthotics, not the hard ones, which I think do more harm than good.

Avoid wearing flip-flops, shoes, and boots (like Uggs) that have no arch support; shoes and boots that push your toes together; or high-heel shoes. If you're in the market for sandals, I recommend Birkenstock sandals, which have the three-arch support. Choose shoes that have arch support built into the foot bed. If a pair of shoes you like doesn't have the proper support, visit a local chiropractor or podiatrist to obtain custom orthotics.

Coping with Fallen Arches (Flat Feet)

Flat feet (also known as "fallen arches" or *pes planus*) is a condition in which the entire sole of the foot comes in complete or almost complete contact with the ground. This throws off your weight distribution, which may lead to problems in the hips, lower back, and the entire length of the spine. The feet roll inward, causing pronation, which places additional stress on the knees and leads to accelerated degeneration.

You can't prevent or reverse the flat footedness, but you can support the feet properly to rebalance the weight distribution and prevent the condition from causing other health problems:

- Buy comfortable, quality footwear that has built-in arch support.

- Obtain custom orthotics that support the three arches of the foot. I recommend Foot Levelers; visit `www.footlevelers.com` for more information and to locate a local chiropractor or podiatrist who can fit you for custom orthotics. Opt for the soft over the hard orthotics, the latter of which I think do more harm than good.

- Wear Birkenstock sandals or other sandals that offer good support for your arches. Avoid flip-flops.

- Roll your foot over a golf ball for five minutes at least once a day.

- Get a foot massage. Massage therapy can help rejuvenate overworked muscles in the feet.

 See a chiropractor to help correct any skeletal alignment issues that may have resulted from having flat feet.

Straightening Out a Case of Hammertoe

A *hammertoe* is a painful deformity in which the second, third, and fourth toes of the foot are permanently curled. Contributing factors include a genetic predisposition to the condition, tight footwear (high heels or shoes that are too short or narrow), bunions, arthritis, stroke, diabetes, and Charcot-Marie-Tooth disease — a genetic condition characterized by muscle weakness, decreased muscle size, high foot arches, hammertoes, and *foot drop* (difficulty lifting your foot at the ankle).

If you have hammertoes, the first order of business is to wear footwear that leaves room for your toes to stretch out. Avoid wearing high heels, which tend to push the toes against the front of the shoe. Obtain custom orthotics that support the three arches of the foot; see the preceding section for details.

To help relieve pain and straighten the toes, do the following:

- ✔ Use ice for 20 minutes several times daily to alleviate pain.

- ✔ Get regular foot massages. Chiropractors, podiatrists, and massage therapists can all provide beneficial treatments for hammertoe.

- ✔ Exercise your toes by repeatedly picking up a piece of paper or a towel off the floor with your toes, dropping it, and picking it up.

See a podiatrist sooner rather than later. Your podiatrist may be able to use splints or straps to straighten the toes over time, but such methods are more effective the earlier they're implemented.

Handling Heel Spurs

A *heel spur* is a calcium deposit on the bottom of the heel that can be extremely painful, especially after periods of rest. A standard x-ray can diagnose or rule out the presence of a heel spur. Flat feet, high-heel shoes or shoes with poor support, standing for extended periods of time, pregnancy, and obesity may apply excess pressure to the heel and, over a period of time, can contribute to the formation of a heel spur.

Heel spurs aren't the only or even the most common cause of heel pain. Plantar fasciitis is the most common cause (see "Taming Plantar Fasciitis" later in this chapter). Tendonitis, stress fractures, and other conditions may also cause heel pain. Getting an accurate diagnosis is the first step to treating whatever condition is causing the pain.

Start by treating the heel directly:

- ✔ See a podiatrist or chiropractor to get fitted for custom soft orthotics with a heel spur correction built into the foot bed; this supports the heel while suspending the heel spur to relieve pressure.

- ✔ Ice the heel for 20 minutes twice daily.

- ✔ Massage the inflamed area around the heel spur with warm massage oil or coconut oil twice daily.

- ✔ Gently massage arnica cream or ointment, such as Traumeel, into the affected heel several times daily.

- ✔ Conventional treatment with nonsteroidal anti-inflammatory (NSAID) medications, such as aspirin and ibuprofen, along with steroid injections also help.

Adopt an anti-inflammatory diet to reduce inflammation. Avoid refined sugar, processed carbohydrates, and hydrogenated vegetable oils. Consume a diet rich in vegetables, legumes, oily fish, and lean protein. Healthy fats from certain fish, flaxseed oil, and other sources are very helpful in reducing inflammation. Support your dietary changes with one or more of the following nutritional supplements:

Supplement	*Dosage*
White willow bark	300 mg twice daily between meals
Boswellia	50 mg twice daily between meals
Turmeric	100 mg twice daily between meals
Omega-3 essential fatty acids (EFAs)	1,000 mg as a combination of EPA and DHA two to three times daily
Vitamin B12 (sublingual fast-dissolving tablet)	5,000 mcg once daily

Rooting Out Ingrown Toenails

An ingrown toenail occurs when a corner of the toenail digs into the surrounding skin. To receive quick relief and ensure you're receiving proper treatment, I recommend that you see your doctor. Most people who try to self-treat suffer unnecessarily and end up having to see a doctor anyway. However, if you're a diehard do-it-yourselfer, and if you catch the ingrown nail early enough, you may be able to fix it. Here's how (follow this regimen several times daily for several weeks until the nail grows out):

1. **Soak your foot in a basin of warm water with a couple tablespoons of Epsom salts and keep the area clean with soap and water.**

2. **After soaking, roll a piece of cotton, gauze, or dental floss between your fingers to create a "wick." Try to lift the corner of the nail that's pressing into the skin, and place the wick between the nail and the skin.**

3. **Apply over-the-counter antibiotic cream to prevent infection.**

   In addition, let your toes breathe when possible and wear only white socks; dyes in colored socks may cause complications.

To speed healing, take one or more of the following nutritional supplements:

Supplement	*Dosage*
White willow bark	300 mg twice daily between meals
Boswellia	50 mg twice daily between meals
Turmeric	100 mg twice daily between meals

(continued)

(continued)

Supplement	Dosage
Omega-3 essential fatty acids (EFAs)	1 g yielding 180 mg EPA and 120 mg DHA two to three times daily
Proteolytic enzymes (trypsin and chymotrypsin)	125 mg trypsin and 40 mg chymotrypsin two to three times daily between meals

If symptoms worsen or fail to improve in a week, see your doctor. Minor surgery can repair an ingrown toenail in a jiffy, but don't try it yourself.

To prevent ingrown toenails, wear shoes with wiggle room for your toes and, when you trim your toenails, cut them straight across instead of trying to follow the contour of your toe.

Taming Plantar Fasciitis

Plantar fasciitis is an inflammation of the thick connective tissue on the bottom of the foot (plantar fascia) that helps maintain the arches of the foot. The inflammation is due to tearing of the tissue and is often a precursor to a heel spur. The heels and soles of the feet become very painful, especially after a night's rest. To relieve the pain and help your foot heal, do one or more of the following:

- ✔ See a podiatrist or chiropractor to get fitted for custom soft orthotics. I recommend Foot Levelers, which are custom made to support all three arches of the foot, providing a balanced foundation. (Visit www.footlevelers.com to find a practitioner in your area.)

- ✔ Roll your sole over a foot wheel or a golf ball to massage the trigger points on the bottom of the feet. (Brookstone sells a foot wheel called the Foot Therapy Roller.)

- ✔ Soak your foot in a basin of warm water with a couple tablespoons of Epsom salts several times daily.

- ✔ Gently massage arnica cream or ointment, such as Traumeel, into the sole of your foot several times daily.

- ✔ Wear good footwear with supporting arches. Don't wear shoes with a flat foot bed. If you wear sandals, don't wear the flat type; wear sandals, such as Birkenstocks, that support all three arches.

Adopt an anti-inflammatory diet to reduce inflammation. Avoid refined sugar, processed carbohydrates, and hydrogenated vegetable oils. Consume a diet rich in vegetables, legumes, oily fish, and lean protein. Healthy fats from certain fish, flaxseed oil, and other sources are very helpful in reducing inflammation. Support your dietary changes with one or more of the following nutritional supplements:

Supplement	*Dosage*
White willow bark	300 mg twice daily between meals
Boswellia	50 mg twice daily between meals
Turmeric	100 mg twice daily between meals
Omega-3 essential fatty acids (EFAs)	1 g yielding 180 mg EPA and 120 mg DHA two to three times daily
Proteolytic enzymes (trypsin and chymotrypsin)	125 mg trypsin and 40 mg chymotrypsin two to three times daily between meals

Purging Plantar Warts

Plantar warts, caused by the human papilloma virus (HPV), are hard growths on the soles of the feet that are often painful to walk on. You may think you've developed a callus, but plantar warts differ from calluses in two ways:

- ✔ Plantar warts don't go away when you soak them in water and remove the dead skin.

- ✔ If you examine the area closely with a magnifying glass, you're likely to see dark specks that are very characteristic of a plantar wart. These are abnormal capillaries (blood vessels).

The same HPV virus may cause warts on other areas of the body, but on the soles of the feet, pressure causes hard skin to grow over the wart. Plantar warts may go away on their own, but they may also last a lifetime, so you're usually better off having them removed.

Although natural cures are certainly available to treat plantar warts — I cover these shortly — I recommend conventional medicine. Your doctor can burn the wart off with acid or freeze it with liquid nitrogen. In either case, the treatment kills the wart, and the dead skin eventually falls away. Follow-up treatment is sometimes necessary. Unfortunately, you're likely to experience a great deal of pain a few hours and for several days after treatment until the skin grows back. I don't recommend having the wart cut out, because the resulting scar tissue may be as painful as the wart itself.

If you want to try some home remedies, here they are:

- **Salicylic acid:** Apply prescription-strength salicylic acid — available over the counter in pads, bandages, and topical applications — to remove layers of the wart a little at a time and stimulate your own immune response.

- **Duct tape:** Yes, another use for duct tape! Apply duct tape to the wart for six days, remove the tape, soak the wart in warm water for 20 minutes, gently remove the dead tissue with a pumice stone or emery board, and then leave the wart exposed to open air for 12 hours. (Throw out the emery board or pumice stone so that you don't re-infect your foot or spread the infection later.)

- **Silver nitrate:** Apply silver nitrate solution directly to the wart several times daily. (You can buy silver nitrate at health food stores and online. You may even be able to purchase it at your local pharmacy.)

Seek professional treatment if the warts spread or become extremely painful or if your immune system is compromised, as is evident if you have other health issues.

Plantar warts are not highly contagious but they do thrive in warm, moist environments. Wear your own clean, dry sandals in and around public locker rooms, pools, showers, and hot tubs.

Straightening Out Your Feet: Pronation and Supination

Pronation and supination are foot alignment problems that throw your knees and hips out of alignment, which can cause all sorts of problems, including pain in the feet, knees, hips, back, shoulders, and neck:

- **Pronation:** With *pronation,* feet roll inward. Your knees may rotate inward, and your pelvis may tilt forward. Pronation is commonly associated with shin splints, plantar fasciitis, and bunions.

- **Supination:** With *supination,* feet roll outward. Your knees may rotate outward, and your pelvis may tilt back. Supination is often associated with inversion ankle sprains, heel spurs, hammertoes, and stress fractures.

Functional orthotics that support the three arch structures, known as the *plantar vault,* is the best treatment. See a podiatrist or chiropractor to get fitted for custom soft orthotics. See the earlier section "Coping with Fallen Arches

(Flat Feet)" for details. Your chiropractor may also need to adjust your spine and address other alignment problems caused by the pronation or supination.

Shoring Up Shin Splints

Shin splints is a term used to describe a condition that causes sharp pain on the part of the leg below the knee — usually the front, bony part or, less commonly, the inside of the leg. Shin splints are very common in athletes, especially runners and soccer players.

Lower leg pain isn't always due to shin splints. You may have a stress fracture. To tell the difference, press your finger along your shin. If pressure on a certain point causes pain, you're probably dealing with a stress fracture. Try flexing your foot upward. If that's painful, you're probably dealing with shin splits. Also shin splints are typically painful when you first wake up in the morning, while stress fracture pain seems to get better with a night of rest.

The first order of business is to baby your shins with RICE:

- ✔ **Rest:** Your leg won't get better without rest. If you run, stop. For exercise, swim, lift weights, ride a bike, or engage in some other physical activity.

- ✔ **Ice:** Ice the affected area for 20 minutes every couple of hours several times daily to reduce inflammation.

- ✔ **Compression:** Wrap your leg with an elastic bandage from just above the ankle to just below the knee. (If you must run, run wrapped.)

- ✔ **Elevation:** Keep the affected leg elevated as much as possible when you're sitting down.

When the pain starts to let up, gently stretch your calf muscles and Achilles tendons. The classic calf stretch (you lean forward against a wall or a tree, place one leg forward and one leg back, and lower your back leg so your heel is resting on the ground) is great. You can also stretch the opposite way: Kneel on an exercise pad with the tops of your feet against the pad, gently sit back on your heals until you feel the tension in your shins, and hold for about ten seconds. Repeat each of these stretches several times.

If you have any pronation (see the earlier section "Straightening Out Your Feet: Pronation and Supination"), consult a podiatrist or chiropractor to obtain custom orthotics. Pronation is a common cause of shin splints.

Adopt an anti-inflammatory diet to reduce inflammation. Avoid refined sugar, processed carbohydrates, and hydrogenated vegetable oils. Consume a diet rich in vegetables, legumes, oily fish, and lean protein. Healthy fats from certain fish, flaxseed oil, and other sources are very helpful in reducing inflammation. Support your dietary changes with one or more of the following nutritional supplements:

Supplement	*Dosage*
White willow bark	300 mg twice daily between meals
Boswellia	50 mg twice daily between meals
Turmeric	100 mg twice daily between meals
Omega-3 essential fatty acids (EFAs)	1 g yielding 180 mg EPA and 120 mg DHA two to three times daily
Proteolytic enzymes (trypsin and chymotrypsin)	125 mg trypsin and 40 mg chymotrypsin two to three times daily between meals

Clearing the Air: Stinky Feet

Stinky feet aren't just an embarrassment; they indicate the presence of bacteria that emit a foul-smelling odor along the lines of fermented cheese, malt vinegar, or ammonia. The cure is to keep your feet clean, dry, and ventilated:

- **Keep your feet and shoes clean.** Wash your feet with soap and water at least one or two times a day. Also wash your sneakers every so often and let them air dry completely before wearing them.

- **Wear the right socks and shoes.** Wear cotton-blend socks with your shoes (avoid socks made of polyester and nylon), and wear shoes that breathe.

- **Soak your feet in baking soda and water.** Soak your feet for 20 minutes in a tub of water with 2 tablespoons of baking soda. Repeat daily for several weeks. (Soaking in peroxide also helps.)

- **Apply rubbing alcohol.** Swab feet with isopropyl alcohol twice daily for two weeks.

- **Address the odor.** Use activated charcoal foot inserts. You can also use a deodorizing foot powder or aluminum-free underarm deodorant. Here are a couple natural cures to address the odor:

  • Make your own food powder: Combine equal parts baking soda and dried, ground sage leaves. Store in an airtight glass jar. After a hard day's work, add 1 tablespoon of the mixture to each shoe. Repeat daily.

> • Mix 1 teaspoon sodium bicarbonate with a small amount of water and apply it to your feet twice daily. Sodium bicarbonate works as a basic deodorant free of aluminum and parabens and helps balance pH to prevent infection.

Vying with Varicose Veins

Varicose veins are twisted, enlarged veins near the surface of the skin, typically on the legs and ankles, often causing pain, swelling, heaviness, and fatigue. Advanced cases may cause *cellulitis* — a bacterial infection just beneath the skin.

Elevating your legs, wearing compression stockings, and exercising can all help with the circulation issues that contribute to varicose veins. Avoid long periods of standing or sitting. When sitting, try to elevate your legs as much as possible.

A healthy diet can also help (see Chapter 2), along with the following nutritional supplements:

Supplement	*Dosage*
Diosmin and hesperidin (micronized diosmin and hesperidin from *Citrus sinensis*)	500 mg twice daily (I recommend DioVasc from XYMOGEN)
Vitamin C (mineral ascorbates)	1,000 mg twice daily
Dietary fiber	40 to 50 g daily
Horse chestnut seed extract	250 mg twice daily
Gotu kola	60 to 120 mg one or two times daily
Butcher's broom	40 mg twice daily
Arjuna	100 mg twice daily

Chapter 12

Addressing Common Kiddie Health Issues

In This Chapter

▶ Adjusting dosages for kids

▶ Alleviating the pain and discomfort of colic, diaper rash, and teething

▶ Helping your kid cope with chicken pox

▶ Alleviating growing pains

▶ Getting some solid advice on vaccinations

*P*arents don't like to see their kids suffer, but childhood illnesses often serve as important events in building a child's future defenses against more serious illnesses. In this chapter, I offer guidance on how to treat common infant and childhood illnesses, and near the end of this chapter, I explain how you can minimize the discomfort and risk of reaction to childhood vaccines. But first, I offer some general guidance on how to adjust dosages of medicines, herbs, and other supplements for children.

Adjusting Dosages for Children 12 Years Old and Under

Throughout this book, the dosages I recommend for vitamins, minerals, herbs, and other supplements are for adults only. Consult your child's pediatrician for dosages specific for your child. Table 12-1 offers a conversion chart that can help you convert adult dosages into dosages that are safe and effective for children 12 years old and under.

Table 12-1	Conversion Chart for Dosages for Children
Child's Weight (in Pounds)	*Dosage*
5 to 29	⅛ the adult dosage
30 to 59	¼ the adult dosage
60 to 89	⅓ the adult dosage
90 to 119	½ the adult dosage
120 to 150	¾ the adult dosage

Bringing Up Baby

Except for the fact that they depend on you, as a parent, for *everything*, caring for the typical baby is pretty easy. As long as your baby has regular feedings, a clean diaper, a comfortable crib, and a loving family, he's good to go. However, when your baby is feeling pain or discomfort, he lets you know about it. That's when it takes some extra effort on your part to figure out what's ailing your infant and supply the cure. In this section, I offer guidance on how to treat three of the most common baby health issues — colic, diaper rash, and teething.

Gutting it out with colic

Colic is abdominal pain and discomfort characterized by extended periods of inconsolable crying for no apparent reason. This condition typically begins in the first few weeks of life and resolves on its own by the time the baby is 3 months old.

The first step to treating colic is to track down and remove its cause. Possible causes include allergies to milk formulas; foods that the breastfeeding mother is eating, including milk products; lactose intolerance; antibiotic use contributing to *dysbiosis* (a microbial imbalance in the digestive system); and feeding too fast.

Whether or not you know what's causing your baby's colic, the following treatments and preventive measures may help:

- Breastfeed for a minimum of six months. Breastfed children are less susceptible to colic.
- Take your child to a chiropractor for diagnosis and possible adjustments; chiropractic adjustments tend to reduce colic.
- Put your baby in motion. Rocking, going for a ride in the car, or being secured in a rocking baby swing can help calm a colicky baby.

✔ Try organic chamomile or basil tea for both the infant and the breast-feeding mother. (Mint tea is also helpful if the colic is due to gas, but it can induce acid reflux, so if the colic is due to reflux, don't use mint tea.)

✔ If you use an infant formula, switch to hypoallergenic formula, such as goat, rice, or predigested cow milk formula. Nutramigen and Alimentum contain hydrolyzed (predigested) milk protein and may be better tolerated; however, if your infant has blood in his stool or is allergic to milk, then avoid any form of milk protein formula and use an elemental formula such as Elecare or Neocate. An *elemental formula* contains the amino acids required to build proteins instead of preformed proteins.

Avoid soy. Approximately 90 percent of all soy in the United States is genetically modified. Also avoid formulas that contain high-fructose corn syrup.

If you're breastfeeding, eat more steamed vegetables and avoid the following: cow milk and dairy products, and eggs; chocolate; wheat; apples, bananas, strawberries, and oranges and other citrus fruits and fruit juices; tomatoes, onions, and cruciferous vegetables, including cabbage, brussels sprouts, cauliflower, bok choy, and broccoli; and coffee and other caffeinated beverages. If you're breastfeeding, take the following probiotics to support digestion and promote a healthy microbial balance in your breastfeeding infant:

Probiotic	Dosage
Infant probiotic containing *Lactobacillus acidophilus* and *Lactobacillus reuteri*	5 billion CFU per day
Infant probiotic containing *Bifidobacterium lactis* and *Streptococcus thermopolis*	3 billion CFU per day

If you're bottle-feeding, look for a formula that contains probiotics or create your own by adding *Bifidobacterium infantis* or another high-quality probiotic blend (you can open the capsules) to the formula you use.

Clearing up diaper rash

If you've changed more than a few diapers, you've had to deal with diaper rash — a skin irritation commonly caused by contact with stool and urine. Other factors that commonly contribute to diaper rash include food allergies, formula-feeding instead of breastfeeding, and the use of antibiotics. To cure the rash, here's what you do:

✔ Change diapers more frequently; before putting on the clean diaper, apply a barrier cream to reduce skin contact with urine and feces. I recommend Triple Paste medicated ointment. A zinc-based ointment is another alternative.

✔ Use super-absorbent, dye-free disposable diapers or diapers made with microfiber cloth and hypoallergenic baby wipes.

✔ Supplement feeding with DL-methionine to reduce the amount of ammonia secreted in the urine. Treat for a minimum of one week, following these guidelines:

Age	Amount
Infants younger than 12 months	200 mg
Children 1 to 2 years old	300 to 400 mg

Some of what goes into your child's body comes out of her body in the form of waste. Make sure you provide your child with proper nutrition, so that waste isn't more of an irritant than it needs to be.

Alleviating the discomfort of teething

When a child is teething, the teeth don't actually cut through the gums. Instead, the body releases chemicals that kill some gum cells and allow the gums to separate to make room for the emerging teeth. As you may imagine, the process often causes inflamed and painful gums — and results, understandably, in an irritable child. Here are some suggestions for relieving the pain and discomfort while helping the teeth break through the gums:

✔ Give your child a BPA-free teething ring. Some teething rings have liquid inside them so that you can freeze the teething ring for additional pain relief. You can also freeze water in a baby bottle and let your child gnaw on that, or let your child play with a spoon that's been chilled in the fridge.

✔ Feed your child chilled, soft fruits, such as applesauce, yogurt, and pureed fruits.

✔ Freeze an unpeeled banana and let your baby teethe on it under close supervision.

✔ Massage your baby's gums with a clean finger.

Some over-the-counter products may also help, including teething powder or ointments, but recently, many have come under fire, so consult your pediatrician for guidance. Commercial oral anesthetic heating gels (Orajel and Anbesol) give temporary relief for 30 to 40 minutes.

Teething may elevate your baby's temperature slightly but not enough to break 100°F to 101°F (37.8°C to 38.3°C). If the temperature rises above 100°F, the infant probably has an infection, possibly a herpes infection of the mouth. See Chapter 7 for more about treating herpes.

Chicken Pox Survival Guide

Chicken pox is an ugly, uncomfortable illness that results in hundreds of itchy red blisters that cover the entire body, last for about a week, and then scab over. Fever and body aches typically accompany the rash. The good news is that chicken pox is relatively harmless; most otherwise healthy children don't have any complications from the disease. In fact, you're better off getting it when you're young, because the initial infection gives you lifetime immunity from chicken pox, and serious complications are more common if you get it as an adult. The only catch is that the virus itself only goes dormant, and it may cause shingles later in life (see Chapter 6).

You can't cure chicken pox, but you can make the person who has it more comfortable while the illness runs its course:

✔ Keep the skin clean and dry. To alleviate itchiness, dab calamine lotion, zinc oxide, or an over-the-counter antihistamine cream or ointment on the red spots and blisters several times daily.

Swab a solution of 1 cup distilled water and ½ tablespoon baking soda (sodium bicarbonate) over the red bumps and blisters.

✔ To prevent secondary infection caused by scratching, keep the itchy skin covered with loose-fitting, comfortable cotton clothing (avoid wool and any other itchy fabrics). Also keep your child's nails trimmed or have her wear gloves or socks over her hands.

✔ Crush neem (Indian lilac) leaves, mix the leaves with a small amount of distilled water, and apply the mixture to the red spots several times daily. Neem is well-known for its antiviral properties and its ability to dry blisters.

✔ Grind 2 cups of oatmeal into a fine powder, mix it with ½ gallon of distilled water, and let sit for 15 minutes. Place the mixture in a porous cloth bag and tie it shut. Set the cloth bag in warm bathwater and let your child soak in the bath for 20 minutes — under your close supervision, of course. As you dab your child's body dry, try to leave a light coating of the oatmeal on his skin.

✔ Add ½ cup of apple cider vinegar to warm bathwater and let your child soak, closely supervised, for 20 minutes.

✔ Apply vitamin E oil to the red spots and blisters.

Never give a child aspirin — especially a child who is recovering from chicken pox or the flu — because of the risk of Reye's syndrome, a potentially deadly disease that causes swelling of the liver or brain.

The good ol' days

In the good old days, a child who had chicken pox was one of the most popular kids in the neighborhood. Parents of children who hadn't yet had chicken pox *wanted* their kids to be exposed to the highly contagious varicella virus. In fact, in 1989, the American Medical Association advised parents that "all healthy children should be exposed to chicken pox at an age at which it is no more than an inconvenience." It's still that way in the UK and in most other countries around the world, but in the U.S., parents are advised to get their children vaccinated.

Although a chicken pox vaccine is available, I advise against getting your child vaccinated unless his immune system has been compromised, placing him at a higher risk of more serious complications. Mass vaccination of children against chicken pox is anticipated to contribute to future epidemics of shingles, among other unforeseen consequences.

Alleviating Growing Pains

Growing pains is the term commonly used to refer to general aches and pains that children experience, primarily in their legs and usually just before bedtime or during sleep. Pain usually occurs in the front of the thighs, the calves, and behind the knees and can usually be traced to muscle pain, not joint pain. (Joint pain is usually characterized by red, swollen, tender, or warm joints, which may be symptomatic of more serious illness.) Growing pains are not serious; they're more likely caused by overuse of muscles from running, jumping, climbing, and other physical activities.

For short-term relief, massage your child's legs. Encourage your child to take a break from any intense physical activities that may be causing the muscle strain. A moist heating pad may also provide some relief, but don't have your child sleep with an electric heating pad, because electromagnetic fields (EMFs) may be harmful to a child's DNA.

Do not give your child aspirin. Aspirin in children can cause Reye's syndrome, which causes swelling in the brain and liver.

Food allergies and sensitivities may also contribute to growing pains. Feed your child a natural foods diet, as explained in Chapter 2. If symptoms worsen, consider testing for food allergies and sensitivities and negative reactions to food additives. See Chapter 13 for details.

The following supplements may help alleviate growing pains:

Supplement	Dosage
Zinc glycinate chelate	20 mg twice daily; stop when pain subsides
Manganese bis-glycinate chelate	2 mg twice daily
Vitamin D	2,000 to 10,000 IU daily, depending on blood levels (see Appendix A)

Reducing the Risks of Childhood Vaccinations

If you're a parent, you probably struggle with the decision of whether and at what age to immunize your child against illnesses such as measles, mumps, diphtheria, tetanus, pertussis (whooping cough), and much more. People on both sides of the controversy cite plenty of scientific and medical evidence to back their positions. I encourage you to discuss with your child's pediatrician the necessity of each vaccination your child is scheduled to receive. Ask about possible side effects, what you should look out for in case your child does have a reaction, and what you should do if a reaction occurs.

Want to read up on the topic yourself? Check out both pro- and anti-childhood vaccination sites, such as the American Academy of Pediatricians website at www2.aap.org/immunization (pro) and Vaccination Choice Canada at vaccinechoicecanada.com (con).

If you're concerned about having your child vaccinated, here are some suggestions that may allay your worries about potential side effects:

✔ Don't have your child vaccinated if she is currently ill or has taken antibiotics within the past four weeks.

✔ For babies and infants, delay all vaccines as long as possible. I recommend holding off on vaccinations until your child is 2 years old. During the first two years of life, the immune system is still developing and is more prone to injury.

✔ The decision to administer vaccines at 2-, 4-, and 6-months-old is based on convenience and insurance reimbursement. By delaying vaccinations, you may have extra office visits and higher copays, but the effort and costs are well worth it.

✔ Get one shot of a single vaccine at a time and wait at least one month between vaccines. (Don't get a shot that contains more than one vaccine.) The one exception is the measles, mumps, and rubella (MMR) vaccine, which is always given as a combination vaccine. When your child gets the MMR vaccine, don't allow any other vaccines (for example, polio, chicken pox, influenza, or rotavirus) to be given at the same time.

✔ Insist on a single-dose instead of a multidose vaccine. The multidose vaccine contains preservatives that allow the bottle to be punctured numerous times. Get the single-dose, preservative-free vaccine.

✔ Pretreat your child with vitamin C powder and vitamin A drops (mycelized) prior to the MMR, chicken pox, and polio vaccinations. See Table 12-2.

✔ Don't have your child vaccinated if she has taken antibiotics within the past four weeks.

✔ Don't have your child vaccinated for chicken pox unless he's in a high-risk category for developing complications from chicken pox. See "Chicken Pox Survival Guide," earlier in this chapter, for details.

✔ If your child develops a fever as a result of the vaccine, don't use aspirin and be cautious in using other fever-reducing medications. If the fever reaches 104°F (40 °C), then administer fever-reducing meds (*not* aspirin) and contact your physician. Opt for ibuprofen over acetaminophen, which reduces available glutathione (glutathione helps the body detox many of the chemical additives in the vaccines). Don't pretreat your child with acetaminophen prior to vaccination.

You can reduce the possibility of vaccine reactions, particularly to viral vaccines (polio, chickenpox, influenza, hepatitis A, hepatitis B, and MMR) by supplementing your child's diet with vitamins A and C in the days leading up to and following the vaccination (see Table 12-2). This doesn't guarantee that a reaction won't occur, but it does reduce the risk.

Table 12-2	Protocol for Reducing Vaccination Risks		
Age/Size	*Daily for Three Days Prior to Vaccination*	*Day of Vaccination*	*Daily for Three Days after Vaccination*
Infant and toddlers up to 30 pounds	Vitamin C in divided doses: 5 mg per pound in juice	Vitamin C in divided doses: 10 mg per pound in juice	Vitamin C in divided doses: 5 mg per pound in juice

Age/Size	Daily for Three Days Prior to Vaccination	Day of Vaccination	Daily for Three Days after Vaccination
	Vitamin A: 5,000 IU (1 drop) in juice	Vitamin A: 10,000 IU (2 drops) in juice	Vitamin A: 5,000 IU (1 drop) in juice
Toddlers 31 to 50 pounds	Vitamin C in divided doses: 15 mg per pound in juice	Vitamin C in divided doses: 30 mg per pound in juice	Vitamin C in divided doses: 15 mg per pound in juice
	Vitamin A: 10,000 IU (2 drops) in juice	Vitamin A: 15,000 IU (3 drops) in juice	Vitamin A: 10,000 IU (2 drops) in juice
Children 51 to 100 pounds	Vitamin C in divided doses: 30 mg per pound in juice	Vitamin C in divided doses: 50 mg per pound in juice	Vitamin C in divided doses: 30 mg per pound in juice
	Vitamin A: 15,000 IU (3 drops) in juice	Vitamin A: 25,000 IU (5 drops) in juice	Vitamin A: 15,000 IU (3 drops) in juice
Adults 100 pounds and over	Vitamin C: 1,000 mg four times daily	Vitamin C: 1,500 mg four times daily	Vitamin C: 1,000 mg four times daily
	Vitamin A: 20,000 IU (4 drops) in juice	Vitamin A: 50,000 IU (10 drops) in juice	Vitamin A: 20,000 IU (4 drops) in juice

As you read this table, keep these notes in mind:

✔ Use powdered vitamin C in the form of mineral ascorbates for accurate dosing. If 1 teaspoon contains 4,000 mg vitamin C, then ¼ teaspoon equals 1,000 mg. Vitamin C in high doses can cause loose stools. If this becomes a problem, decrease dosage.

✔ Use vitamin A in the form of retinyl palmitate and beta-carotene. (See Appendix A for more about the better forms of vitamins and minerals.)

Chapter 13

Alleviating Allergies, Asthma, and Food Sensitivity/Intolerance

- -

In This Chapter

▶ Defining and treating asthma

▶ Treating food and seasonal allergies

▶ Telling the difference between food allergy and intolerance

▶ Testing to identify problem foods and other allergenic substances

- -

*W*hen your immune system mistakenly identifies a food item as an alien invader or overreacts to a mild irritant, you suffer the consequences. Your nose may run, your eyes may become itchy or watery, and your throat may feel sore or scratchy. Maybe you get hives. Maybe you experience swelling of the lips, face, tongue, or throat. Maybe you even have trouble breathing. Other symptoms include stomachache, eczema, diarrhea, fatigue, headache, and even depression — signs you may not even associate with allergies.

Relief comes in two forms: avoiding whatever ails you and regulating your immune system response. In this chapter, I cover specific conditions — asthma, allergies, food sensitivities, and leaky gut syndrome — that involve allergic reactions and closely related symptoms, and I point out common causes and natural remedies that are proven to work.

Doses in this chapter are for adults, not children. For guidance on how to adjust dosages for children (and adults under 150 pounds), turn to Chapter 12.

Treating Asthma and Asthma Episodes

Asthma is a condition in which the airway muscles contract, the airway lining swells, and the airways produce excess mucus, often resulting in coughing, wheezing, and shortness of breath.

Severe episodes may be life-threatening. Ask your doctor whether you should carry an emergency inhaler and perhaps an epinephrine injector to help restore breathing in the event of a severe attack.

To cure your asthma, first you need to find out whether your asthma is allergic (more common) or nonallergic (less common). *Allergic asthma* is triggered by an environmental irritant — something you breathe, eat, or drink. The first step in treating allergic asthma is to identify and avoid substances you're allergic to. *Nonallergic asthma* may be triggered by anxiety, emotional upset, cold air, physical exertion (exercise), toxic chemicals (such as tobacco smoke), a viral or bacterial infection, acid reflux, or heart disease. In this section, I provide general guidance on how to deal with both types of asthma, but for certain types of nonallergic asthma, you need to address the underlying cause; for example, if the cause is related to acid reflux, head to Chapter 14.

Avoiding your asthma triggers

If you're not sure what's causing your asthma attacks, team up with your doctor to get tested for allergies, as explained in the later section, "Getting tested for allergies." Until then, take the following steps to avoid common asthma triggers:

- ✔ Treat any nasal allergies, as explained in the later section "Treating seasonal (nasal) allergies."

- ✔ Get tested for food allergies and sensitivities (see the later section "Getting tested for allergies") and avoid any problem foods. The later sections "Treating food allergies" and "Tackling Food Intolerances and Sensitivities" have the details.

- ✔ Avoid any foods, drinks, or medicines that contain histamines or sulfites. Many wines and beers contain both.

- ✔ Breathe through your nose, not through your mouth, especially during exercising. Your nose filters out irritants before they reach your lungs. You can find plenty of instruction and videos online on how to retrain your breathing.

- ✔ Avoid breathing cold air. Breathing through your nose helps warm the air before it reaches your lungs, but also wear a scarf or mask over your nose and mouth.

Raising your asthma trigger threshold

If your immune system reacts to a substance in a way that essentially suffocates you, it's obviously overreacting. Although you may not be able to completely eliminate these immune system overreactions, you can reduce them by raising the threshold at which your immune system overreacts. Start with your diet (see Chapter 2) and drink at least 8 ounces of water every two waking hours.

In addition to dietary changes, improve your digestion: Relax and take your time eating. Chew your food to liquid, which enables your system to absorb the nutrients in the food more easily. Also support your digestion with probiotics, pancreatic enzymes, and betaine HCL. See Chapter 14 for details on how to restore and maintain healthy digestion.

Additional supplementation may help reduce the inflammation that contributes to asthma:

Supplement	*Dosage*
Magnesium glycinate chelate	125 mg twice daily
Reduced glutathione (marketed as Setria)	250 to 500 mg three times daily
N-acetyl cysteine	500 mg three times daily
MSM	1 to 8 g in two or three divided doses daily, working up slowly over the course of three to fourth months and then slowly backing down to 1 to 2 g daily
Quercetin	1,000 mg three times daily with food
	Tip: A single dose of 1,500 to 2,000 mg may help calm an asthma attack
Pycnogenol	200 mg daily
Colostrum	10,000 mg daily
Vitamin C (mineral ascorbates)	1,000 mg three times daily
Vitamin D3	2,000 to 10,000 IU daily, depending on blood levels (see Appendix A)
Omega-3 essential fatty acids (EFAs)	1 g yielding 180 mg EPA and 120 mg DHA three times daily
Alpha linolenic acid	600 mg daily
Lycopene	30 mg daily
Vitamin E (mixed tocopherols)	400 IU daily
Vitamin A (retinyl palmitate and beta-carotene)	2,500 IU retinyl palmitate and 2,500 IU beta-carotene daily (see Appendix A for precautions)
Selenium	100 mcg daily
Apple cider vinegar	Mix 1 tablespoon of organic apple cider vinegar and 1 teaspoon of honey in 1 cup of water and drink three times daily
Coconut oil	1 teaspoon of organic coconut oil one or two times daily

The following herbs may help control asthma symptoms:

Herb	Dosage/Amount
Perilla seed oil	3 g daily
Turmeric (capsule form)	1.5 g twice daily
Ginger	1 cup of ginger tea three times daily (steep 1 teaspoon ginger in 3 cups boiling water)
Oregano (spice, capsule, or essential oil)	Inhale the vapors or add a few drops to a teaspoon of olive or coconut oil and take orally
Valerian root	50 mg twice daily

Tests to Identify Allergies

An allergy is the result of the body overreacting to an irritant or to a substance it wrongly identifies as an irritant, such as certain kinds of foods, pollen, and so on. The body's reaction results in inflammation that may cause any number of symptoms. In this section, I explain the various ways to identify substances you may be allergic to.

Taking a closer look at allergy symptoms

Seasonal allergies are usually characterized by nasal congestion, sneezing, runny nose, itchy eyes, coughing, and sore throat. Symptoms of food allergies depend on whether the allergic reaction is immediate or delayed:

✔ **Immediate reaction (IgE-mediated):** Symptoms occur within minutes after exposure or eating an allergenic food. Common problem foods include milk and other dairy products, eggs, wheat, peanuts, tree nuts, sesame seeds, fish (especially shellfish), and soy. Symptoms include hives; swelling of the lips, ears, face, tongue, or throat; difficulty breathing; abdominal cramps; and diarrhea. (*IgE* stands for immunoglobulin E, an antibody that the immune system produces to attack what it perceives is a threat.)

Immediate food allergies can cause *anaphylaxis,* a life-threatening allergic reaction, even if you haven't reacted so severely in the past. If you have a food allergy, carry an epinephrine injector at all times, and replace injectors that are past their expiration date.

✔ **Delayed reaction (non-IgE–mediated, also called a food sensitivity):** In a delayed reaction allergy, symptoms occur 2 to 72 hours after eating the allergenic food, and symptom intensity varies, depending on the amount of the food you ingest and how it's prepared. Delayed food allergies can occur as a result of an overly permeable gastrointestinal tract. They are typically associated with certain conditions such as asthma, eczema, irritable bowel syndrome (IBS), rheumatoid arthritis, headaches, chronic ear infections, behaviors associated with autism, and ADD/ADHD. Non-IgE–mediated reactions are often IgG-mediated; your healthcare provider can order tests specifically for IgG-mediated reactions.

Getting tested for allergies

Allergy testing serves two purposes: It identifies any substances you may be allergic to so that you can avoid those substances, and it rules out potential allergens so that you don't have to worry about them. If you suspect an allergy is the root cause of your symptoms, I strongly encourage you to get tested. I recommend one or more of the following tests:

✔ **Elimination diet:** Eliminate common problem foods from your diet for three to four weeks and reintroduce them slowly one at a time until you find the food(s) that cause problems. (See Chapter 2 for details.) This is the only do-it-yourself test in this list, and it's perhaps the best way to identify the food that ails you.

✔ **Skin tests:** Skin tests are useful for revealing IgE-mediated allergies. Your doctor scratches or pokes tiny amounts of suspected allergens into your skin and looks for a reaction.

✔ **RASTs:** Short for *radioallergosorbent tests*, RASTs are blood tests that measure the levels of allergen-specific IgE in your blood. They're often referred to as *immunoCAP* tests.

✔ **Food challenge:** Your doctor feeds you increasing amounts of the suspected food allergen and observes you closely for a reaction. Food challenges are often used to confirm or rule out a RAST result, because RAST tests frequently turn up false positives indicating a food allergy that's not really a problem.

Conduct food challenges only under the close supervision of a doctor whose office is properly equipped to respond to a severe reaction.

✔ **Tests for non-IgE-mediated allergies:** Many healthcare providers and several labs claim to be able to test for non-IgE–mediated food allergies. Some of these tests may provide useful results, while others are likely to turn up a false positives leading to an overly restrictive diet and nutritional deficiencies. Consult your healthcare provider for guidance in choosing tests and interpreting results.

Treating Seasonal (Nasal) Allergies

Treatment for nasal allergies includes at least three components: reducing exposure to potential allergens, irrigating nasal passages, and nurturing a healthy immune system response. In this section, I explain how to include each of these components in treating nasal allergies.

As your condition improves, try to wean yourself off antihistamines, decongestants, inhalers, corticosteroid injections, nasal sprays, and anything else that inhibits your body's natural ability to purge irritants and pathogens before they gain a foothold. These medications shut down your body's own defense systems, preventing them from expelling irritants.

Reducing exposure to potential allergens

Unless you live in a bubble, you can't isolate yourself from the potential allergens swirling in the air around you, but you can reduce your exposure by taking the following precautions:

- **Don't smoke.** And, as much as possible, avoid people who do.

- **Close car and house windows when the pollen count is high.** Do the same if the outside air is thick with other irritants.

- **Machine-dry clothing instead of hanging it outside.** This suggestion is especially important when pollen counts are high.

- **Treat your pets.** To reduce pet dander, bathe your pets regularly. Between baths, spray them with olive oil and comb the oil through their fur. Wearing a mask when you bathe or comb your pets may also help.

- **Treat your bedroom.** Use a special mattress and pillow covers to keep allergens out. Also clean your bedding weekly and window coverings every few months. If you have pets, keep them out of your bedroom. Have as much carpeting as possible removed from your home, especially in bedrooms.

- **Pay particular attention to housecleaning and home maintenance.** Vacuum weekly using a vacuum cleaner with a high-efficiency particle arresting (HEPA) filter, and clean or change the filter(s) regularly as instructed. Also clean your window coverings every few months. Change the air filter on your furnace at least twice a year. If possible, use a HEPA air filter. (You can purchase a stand-alone HEPA air filter to use in any room you spend a great deal of time in, such as your bedroom.) Have your home inspected and, if necessary, treated for mold.

If you have forced-air heating, turn on the furnace fan and run it continuously before you start vacuuming and for two hours afterward to help filter any dust that gets kicked up in the process.

✔ **Limit early-morning activities, when pollen and mold counts are high.** The period from August to the first frost is generally the worst time for ragweed pollen; March to June is worst for trees and grass pollen. Also wear a mask when you dust, vacuum, mow, or perform other chores that kick up irritants.

Irrigating your nasal passages

Instead of drying out nasal passages with antihistamines, irrigate those passages. I recommend using a xylitol solution such as Xlear (2 to 3 sprays per nostril while inhaling) at least three times daily. For optimum results, lie down for 30 seconds after spraying both nostrils to give the solution time to reach the back of the nose where irritants often collect.

Create your own nasal spray with 1 cup of distilled water (*never* use tap water), ¼ teaspoon sea salt or other noniodized salt, ⅛ teaspoon baking soda, 1 teaspoon pure xylitol crystals, and 4 drops grapefruit seed extract. Place this solution in a nasal spray bottle and use it as instructed in the preceding paragraph, snort it into each nostril from a clean teaspoon, or use a neti pot or other nasal irrigation device.

Supporting a healthy immune system

To support a healthy immune system, adopt a healthy diet and lifestyle as explained in Chapter 2 and take the following supplements:

Supplement	*Dosage*
Quercetin	1,000 mg three times daily with food, beginning about six weeks prior to allergy season
Butterbur (standardized extract)	50 to 75 mg daily
Omega-3 essential fatty acids (EFAs)	1 g yielding 180 mg EPA and 120 mg DHA three times daily
Stinging nettle (leaf or dried root extract)	8 to 12 g of leaf extract or 600 to 1,200 mg of dried root extract daily
Vitamin C (mineral ascorbates)	1,000 mg three times daily
Vitamin D3	2,000 to 10,000 IU daily, depending on blood levels (see Appendix A)
Vitamin E (mixed tocopherols)	400 IU daily

Treating Food Allergies

True IgE-mediated food allergies are tough to cure. Treatment consists of avoiding the foods that ail you, which sounds simpler than it is because a lot of packaged products contain common allergenic foods, including peanut, egg, and milk. If you have a food allergy, read all labels very closely. If you're unsure whether a product contains a food you're allergic to, either avoid the product or call the manufacturer to check.

If you test positive for numerous IgE- and IgG-mediated reactions, the foods triggering the reactions are probably not the problem. The more likely cause is leaky gut syndrome; proteins from these foods are leaking from the gut into surrounding areas where they don't belong and are activating the immune system. Fix the gut, and many of your food allergies and sensitivities will disappear.

Some people outgrow their food allergies, although researchers don't really know why. A healthy diet (see Chapter 2) along with proper digestion (see Chapter 14) may help speed the process. However, never challenge yourself with a food you've been allergic to without a doctor's approval and close supervision. Even a trace amount of a food you're allergic to can cause a life-threatening reaction.

Tackling Food Intolerances and Sensitivities

Conventional medicine is well equipped to deal with IgE-mediated food allergies, but it's much less effective at diagnosing and treating food intolerances and sensitivities:

- ✔ **Food intolerance:** A food intolerance is the inability to digest a food, which causes gas, bloating, loose stools, or diarrhea. Usually a person lacks a key enzyme for digesting the food or other substance, as is the case with lactose intolerance.

- ✔ **Food sensitivity:** A food sensitivity is a "delayed food allergy" — symptoms appear several hours or even several days after eating the reactive food, making it difficult to draw a connection between the food and the illness it's causing. Food sensitivities impact almost any organ in your body and trigger symptoms very similar to those of asthma, depression, chronic fatigue syndrome, arthritis, allergies, and other common illnesses, in addition to gastrointestinal conditions.

If you have an illness that can't be attributed to any other cause, you should be tested for food intolerance and sensitivity to identify or rule out those possibilities.

Getting tested for food intolerance or sensitivity

The easiest, cheapest test for food intolerance or sensitivity is to eliminate the suspected food item *entirely* from your diet for at least 28 days and then add it back in. (The 28-day time period gives your body the time it needs to lower its concentration of any antibodies to the food item.) If your symptoms disappear, if you start to feel better without that food item in your diet, or if you feel worse when you begin consuming that item again, chances are good that you have an intolerance or sensitivity to that food item.

Although conventional medicine has tests for detecting common food intolerances, such as lactose and fructose intolerance, and reactions to food colorings, preservatives, and other additives, such as sulfites, most doctors don't test for a host of other intolerances and sensitivities, including nonceliac gluten sensitivity, that commonly trigger serious illnesses. Consult a natural medicine practitioner — a chiropractor, functional medicine doctor, or naturopath, for example — who knows about these tests and is more open to ordering them.

Treating food intolerances

If you have a food intolerance or intolerance to a preservative or additive, treatment usually involves eliminating that item from your diet or at least reducing your consumption of it. If you have lactose intolerance, you can consume lactose-free dairy products or take lactase, the enzyme for digesting lactose (one such product is Lactaid) prior to consuming any dairy products that contain lactose.

Treating celiac disease and gluten sensitivity

Treatment for celiac disease and gluten sensitivity is the same: eliminate gluten — all gluten — from your diet. If you have a gluten sensitivity, permanently eliminating gluten from your diet is best, but if you're in good shape and don't have any gluten-related ailments (eczema, brain fog, digestive upset, cardiovascular issues, and so on), you may be able to have gluten occasionally, like once a month.

A list of the usual culprits

Substances in foods that commonly cause problems include the following:

✔ Alcohol

✔ Dyes, especially Red #40, Yellow #5, and Blue #2

✔ Fructose

✔ Histamines, in fermented foods and beverages (especially beer and wine) and foods containing vinegar

✔ Lactose, in milk and other dairy products

✔ Monosodium glutamate (MSG)

✔ Nitrates, in cured meats

✔ Phenylalanine, in anything containing the artificial sweetener aspartame

✔ Sulfites, in beer, wine, dried fruit, and processed foods

✔ Tyramine, in aged or fermented foods (aged cheeses, cured meats, pickled herring, sauerkraut, soy sauce, beer, wine, and certain other alcoholic beverages), chocolate, sour cream, avocado, raspberries, yeast, and mushrooms (*Tip:* Onion, brussels sprouts, garlic, and broccoli are useful detox agents for tyramine)

Read labels carefully and avoid any foods that contain wheat, rye, khorasan, spelt, or barley. Eating real, whole foods with a focus on high-quality animal protein and fresh vegetables and fruit is the best and easiest way to avoid gluten. For details on going gluten free, check out *Living Gluten-Free For Dummies* by Danna Korn (John Wiley & Sons, Inc.).

Sealing a Leaky Gut

Leaky gut syndrome (also known as *gastrointestinal hyperpermeability*) is a condition in which the small intestine becomes more porous than normal, allowing irritants, such as toxins, undigested food particles, waste products, and microbes to leak into surrounding areas where these substances shouldn't be. A leaky gut may lead to a host of health problems, including food allergies and sensitivities, digestive upset, diarrhea, lupus, chronic fatigue syndrome, diabetes, multiple sclerosis, high blood pressure, and cardiovascular problems. Treatment focuses on restoring the health of the entire digestive system, particularly the small intestine.

If you're experiencing digestive upset, food allergy or intolerance, chronic fatigue syndrome, any autoimmune disorder, or another health condition with an unidentifiable cause, I encourage you to get tested for gastrointestinal hyperpermeability.

To restore intestinal health, start by adopting a natural cures diet and lifestyle, as I explain in Chapter 2. Reducing stress and eating a healthy diet are two very effective ways to support a healthy digestive system. Drink half your weight, in ounces, of water daily. If you weigh 160 pounds, that's 80 ounces of water.

In addition to dietary changes, improve your digestion. Relax and take your time eating. Chew your food to liquid, to make it easier for your system to break down and absorb the nutrients in the food. Support your digestion and overall intestinal health by taking probiotics, pancreatic enzymes, and betaine HCL (see Chapter 14 for details and doses). I also recommend consuming 1 g of omega-3 three times daily and 3,500 mg L-glutamine (in powder form) one to three times daily.

Chapter 14

Battling Digestive, Urinary, and Bowel Conditions

*Y*our digestive and urinary systems work 24/7 to process everything you eat and drink and eliminate waste products from your system. When these two bodily systems function as designed, you typically feel pretty good. When either system falls victim to illness, your entire being is affected. In this chapter, I address the most common maladies that can affect your stomach, bowels, gallbladder, kidney, and urinary tract.

Doses in this chapter are for adults, not children. For guidance on how to adjust dosages for children (and adults under 150 pounds), turn to Chapter 12.

Alleviating Digestive Disorders

Indigestion (also known as *dyspepsia*) is characterized by heartburn, belching, abdominal bloating, nausea, and the sensation of fullness after eating only a small amount of food. Most health conditions related to indigestion (as well as those related to ulcers and bowel dysfunction) respond well to changes in diet, eating habits, and the use of supplements to optimize digestion. In this section, I offer advice on how to cure common stomach ailments and maintain a healthy gut. I also provide additional recommendations for treating specific stomach conditions.

Conventional medicine often tries to treat acid reflux with antacids, which may help for short-term indigestion. However, long-term use of antacids, particularly proton-pump inhibitors (PPIs) — omeprazole (Prilosec), esomeprazole (Nexium), pantoprazole (Protonix), and lansoprazole (Prevacid), for example — often cause more harm than good. Stomach acid is essential in properly digesting food, killing harmful bacteria and viruses, and enabling your body to absorb nutrients. By reducing stomach acid, you block the absorption of key nutrients, including minerals and B vitamins, which are crucial for maintaining proper homocysteine levels. High levels of homocysteine are associated with dementia, stroke, depression, anxiety, estrogen-related cancers, and a host of other disorders related to low levels of B vitamins. Blocking the absorption of minerals, such as calcium, contributes to osteoporosis and other conditions.

If you're taking an acid reducer, don't stop cold turkey, which is likely to trigger a rebound effect in which your body produces even more stomach acid than normal. Talk to your healthcare provider about weaning off of it slowly and replacing it with the dietary and supplement recommendations that follow.

Changing what and how you eat

The single most important factor for curing stomach ailments and maintaining a healthy gut is diet — what, how, and how much you eat. As you read about indigestion issues, keep these points in mind:

- ✔ **What:** Follow the modified elimination diet I present in Chapter 2 for 10 to 28 days to identify and eliminate from your diet the most troublesome trigger foods. Common culprits are wheat (gluten); dairy; spicy, fried, and greasy foods and sauces; refined and processed carbohydrates; and food additives. Caffeinated products, chocolate, and alcohol are also notorious triggers. Consume a lighter diet of fruits and vegetables, wild fish, and lean meats. Dump the bad fats (trans fats and hydrogenated vegetable oils) and replace them with healthy oils found in nuts, seeds, fatty fish, flaxseed, and so forth.

- ✔ **How:** Eat in a nonstressful environment and take your time to chew your food to liquid. Don't eat on the run or while driving to your next appointment. Make eating a conscious, mindful activity.

  Go easy on consuming beverages, even water, with meals, because they dilute your stomach acid and digestive enzymes. Drink between meals.

- ✔ **How much:** Eat small meals over the course of the day. Eat your larger meals earlier in the day and smaller meals before going to bed at night.

Supplementing digestion

If adjustments to your diet and how you eat are insufficient in curing your stomach upset, try one or more of the following nutritional supplements to stimulate digestion while reducing any stomach irritation:

Supplement	Dosage
Colostrum (powder form)	10,000 mg one or two times daily
L-glutamine (powder form)	3,500 mg one to three times daily
Aloe (powdered form)	50 mg one to three times daily
Deglycerized licorice (in powder form)	500 mg one to three times daily
Digestive enzymes (protease, amylase, and lipase)	50,000 to 100,000 USP; protease 50,000 to 100,000 USP; amylase and 8,000 to 15,000 USP lipase, with meals
Probiotics (*Saccharomyces boulardii;* a proprietary blend of a multistrain containing *Lactobacillus acidophilus, Bifidobacterium longum,* and *Lactobacillus plantarum;* and *Bifidobacterium lactis* HNO 19 [HOWARU Bifido])	250 mg *Saccharomyces boulardii* twice daily; 50 billion CFU multistrain probiotic once daily; 50 billion CFU HOWARU Bifido once daily
Vitamin B12 (methylcobalamin, sublingual quick-dissolving tablet)	5,000 mcg one or two times daily
Zinc carnosine	75 mg with each meal
Alkalizing super green drinks	1 or 2 drinks daily between meals (follow label instructions to prepare)
Cabbage juice	1 or 2 glasses daily
Peppermint tea	1 cup several times daily

Make your own alkalizing super green drink, following the recipe in the nearby sidebar or choose a low-sugar organic product that's free of artificial coloring and sweeteners. My favorite is Mighty Maca super alkalizing green drink by Vida Pure.

If your indigestion persists, consider other possible causes, including food allergies and sensitivities (wheat, dairy, and sugar are the most likely culprits); *hypochlorhydria* (insufficient stomach acid); deficiency in pancreatic enzymes; vitamin B12 deficiency; adverse reaction to one or more medications; fructose intolerance (see Chapter 13); or consumption of caffeine, fruit juices, soft drinks, alcohol, nicotine, or mints. In the next sections, I cover several common stomach maladies.

Alkalizing super green drink recipe

You can find plenty of delicious super green drink recipes online, but many use high-glycemic fruits, such as bananas and mangoes, to make them delicious. Here's a recipe for a great-tasting alkalizing super green drink that's low in sugar:

- 6-inch section of cucumber (chopped)
- 3 large kale leaves (torn) or 4 cups spinach leaves
- ½ to 1 avocado

- 1 cup coconut water or green tea
- Juice of 1 lime or lemon
- 4 stems fresh mint
- 4 stems fresh parsley
- 1-inch section of ginger (grated)
- 4 to 5 ice cubes (optional)

Place all the ingredients in a blender and blend until smooth.

 A common mistake is to assume that indigestion is caused by *too much* stomach acid when it's really being caused by *too little* stomach acid — a condition called *hypochlorhydria*. If nothing else seems to help with your indigestion, try boosting your stomach acid with 300 to 600 mg betaine hydrochloride (HCL), 50 to 100 mg pepsin, 350 mg L-glutamic acid, and 20 mg gentian taken with every meal. Start at the low end and increase your uptake slowly until symptoms improve or you reach the maximum dosage. If symptoms worsen, decrease the dosage or stop taking these supplements. If symptoms don't improve, consult your doctor.

Healing the burn of acid reflux (GERD)

Gastroesophageal reflux disease (GERD, or *acid reflux* for short) is a condition in which stomach acid and, occasionally, undigested food, back up into the esophagus, causing heartburn, belching, and chest pain. Acid reflux is often the root cause of a nagging cough or even asthma-like symptoms, because the irritation in the esophagus triggers the production of mucus as the body's attempt to rid itself of the irritant. Uncontrolled, acid reflux may damage the esophagus and increase the risk of esophageal cancer.

Your doctor can perform an endoscopy to look at your esophagus and determine whether irritation exists at the place where the esophagus enters the stomach. This examination can also tell whether you have a *hiatal hernia* — a condition in which part of the stomach pushes up into the esophagus. Other tests may be required to narrow down the exact cause of your acid reflux.

In addition to the general recommendations I give earlier (see the sections "Changing what and how you eat" and "Supplementing digestion"), consider the following treatments specifically for acid reflux:

✔ Avoid foods that are known to relax the sphincter muscle between the stomach and the esophagus, making reflux worse: mints, caffeine, alcohol, and nicotine.

✔ Stop eating two or three hours before bedtime, to give your body time to digest your last meal before lying down. (When you lie down, you don't have the benefit of gravity to help keep stomach acid from creeping up into your esophagus.)

✔ Elevate your upper body when sleeping. Try propping up the head of the bed or use an extra pillow or two to prop up your head and chest. The goal is to raise your esophagus above your stomach.

✔ If your doctor determines that you have a hiatal hernia, see a chiropractor, osteopath, or naturopath, who can treat it with gentle manipulation of the stomach and esophagus.

Grappling with gastritis

Gastritis is inflammation of the stomach lining, which may be caused by *Helicobacter pylori (H. pylori)* bacterial infection; alcohol abuse; nonsteroidal anti-inflammatory drugs (NSAIDS), such as aspirin and ibuprofen; or an autoimmune condition. Chronic gastritis may lead to stomach ulcers or cancer.

First, correct your diet. If you drink alcohol, stop. If you take NSAIDs for another condition, discuss the possibility of replacing them with other treatments. Also in addition to following my recommendations for improving overall digestion (see the earlier sections "Changing what and how you eat" and "Supplementing digestion"), take the following supplements:

Supplement	*Dosage*
Vitamin C (mineral ascorbates)	1,000 mg twice daily
Iron (ferrous bis-glycinate chelate)	30 mg twice daily depending on blood levels (see Appendix A for precautions)
Glucoraphanin (capsule form)	100 mg twice daily, or consume 10 to 30 g broccoli sprouts twice daily for seven days
Vitamin K (menaquinone-7)	45 mcg twice daily, or consume foods and drinks rich in vitamin K, including green leafy vegetables and green drinks (see Appendix A for precautions)

Healing a Hiatal Hernia

A *hiatal hernia* occurs when part of the stomach bulges up through the opening of the diaphragm muscle (the hiatus) through which the esophagus passes on its way to the stomach. Most people with hiatal hernias don't even know they have the condition. For others, it causes heartburn (especially after eating and when lying down), chest pain, and upper back pain and is often a constant source of discomfort.

The first order of business is to get tested and treated, if necessary, for food allergies and sensitivities, as explained in Chapter 13. Or follow the modified elimination diet in Chapter 2 to test for sensitivities to these highly allergenic foods: wheat, corn, dairy, grocery-store eggs, soy, sugar, and peanuts. Even if testing doesn't reveal a food allergy or sensitivity, adopt a healthier diet (see Chapter 2) to improve digestion and overall health. In addition, lay off the coffee, alcohol, and spicy foods, which irritate the digestive system.

Follow the Japanese rule of *hara hachi bu* — eat until you are 80 percent full. Doing so reduces the pressure of the stomach pressing up against the diaphragm. Also, stop eating three hours before bedtime, giving your body time to digest the food before you lie down to sleep. In addition to changing what and how you eat, make an appointment with a chiropractor or osteopath, who can physically manipulate the stomach into its proper position. Keep in mind, however, that this adjustment won't last unless you adopt a healthy diet and stop eating before you're full.

Support your dietary changes with the following supplements:

Supplement	*Dosage*
L-glutamine (powder form)	3 g twice daily between meals
Aloe (powder form)	50 mg twice daily
Deglycerized licorice (powder form)	500 mg twice daily
Digestive enzymes (protease, amylase, and lipase)	50,000 to 100,000 USP protease, 50,000 to 100,000 USP amylase, and 8,000 to 15,000 USP lipase, with meals
Probiotics (multistrain containing *Lactobacillus acidophilus, Bifidobacterium longum,* and *Lactobacillus plantarum*)	5 billion CFU
Alkalizing super green drinks	1 or 2 drinks daily between meals (follow label instructions to prepare)

Make your own alkalizing super green drinks (check out the sidebar in this chapter) or choose a low-sugar organic product that's free of artificial coloring and sweeteners. My favorite is Mighty Maca super alkalizing green drink by Vida Pure.

Nipping nausea and vomiting in the bud

Nausea and vomiting are associated with a host of problems, including food poisoning, food allergies, ulcers, motion sickness, low stomach acid, overconsumption of alcohol, *gastroparesis* (poorly functioning stomach muscles), gallbladder problems (see the later section "Grappling with Gallstones and Gallbladder Problems"), pregnancy, infection, heart attack, and some forms of cancer.

 Seek immediate medical treatment if vomiting lasts for more than 24 hours for adults or 6 hours for a child under 6 years old, if you observe blood in the vomit, or if vomiting is accompanied by rapid heartbeat and a fever higher than 102°F (38.9 °C).

 If you suffer from nausea and vomiting, do the following:

- ✔ Let your body vomit and purge itself of toxins, but prevent dehydration by consuming as much fluid as possible; this is especially important for small children. Stick to clear liquids; if your nausea is making it difficult to keep the liquids down, take small, frequent sips or suck on ice chips.

- ✔ Get plenty of bed rest so that your body can heal itself. Don't take aspirin or other NSAIDs, which irritate the gastrointestinal tract.

- ✔ Avoid solid foods until the vomiting stops and ask your doctor about discontinuing oral medications.

 Several herbs alleviate nausea, including aniseed, cinnamon, clove, cumin, fennel, ginger, and mint. Ginger is particularly useful in preventing motion sickness. Brew a cup of tea using these herbs, stir in a small amount of honey, and sip it throughout the day. Lime juice also relieves nausea. Mix 1 cup of water, 10 drops of lime juice, ¼ teaspoon of baking soda, and just enough honey to take the bite out of the lime juice. Drink this concoction one or two times daily. If the nausea persists, see your doctor.

Undermining ulcers

A *gastric ulcer* is an open sore in the stomach lining that typically causes pain in the upper abdomen just below the sternum, along with bloating, nausea, and vomiting. In severe cases, heavy bleeding may occur, or the stomach lining may become perforated, allowing the contents of the stomach to leak into the abdominal cavity — a medical emergency.

Seek immediate medical attention if you notice symptoms of internal bleeding, such as bloody or black, tarry stools; headache; extreme fatigue; dizziness; or fainting. If you experience severe pain, frequent vomiting, or unexplained weight loss, call your doctor.

Two factors account for 90 percent of gastric ulcers: *H. pylori* bacterial infection (80 percent) and aspirin and other NSAIDs (10 percent). The remaining 10 percent can be chalked up to stress, diet, and lifestyle. Your healthcare provider can order breath, blood, or stool tests to confirm or rule out the presence of *H. pylori* bacteria or you can simply treat for *H. pylori* to see whether your symptoms improve.

To treat ulcers caused by *H. pylori* bacteria, drink unsweetened cranberry juice, chew several springs of parsley twice daily, and take these supplements:

Supplement	*Dosage*
Mastic gum	500 to 1,000 mg twice daily between meals
Bismuth	525 mg four times daily
Sulfurophane (from broccoli sprouts and seeds)	100 mg twice daily
Oil of oregano (liquid)	0.5 ml twice daily
Turmeric	150 mg three times daily
Ginger	2.5 ml twice daily

Whatever the cause of your ulcer, follow the recommendations I outline in the earlier sections "Changing what and how you eat" and "Supplementing digestion." Also stop drinking alcohol, stop taking NSAIDs, and eliminate refined and processed carbohydrates (including all sugars and chocolate) from your diet. If you're able to tolerate dairy, consume full-fat quality plain Greek yogurt without any added fruit.

Battling Bowel Disorders

According to Hippocrates, the Father of Modern Medicine, "All diseases begin in the gut." Yet, the modern world has launched an all-out assault on the gut with junk food, sedentary living, chemicals, pollution, and the overuse of prescription medications, especially antibiotics. The result: an unprecedented epidemic of bowel disorders and disease, including constipation, diarrhea, irritable bowel syndrome (IBS), inflammatory bowel disorder (IBD), Crohn's disease, celiac disease, ulcerative colitis, and colon cancer. It's time to start reversing this trend. In this section, I offer guidance on nurturing a healthy colon and treating common bowel disorders.

Improving general colon health

Bowel disorders often clear up with efforts to improve overall colon health:

- ✔ Drink plenty of fluids, at least 8 ounces of water every two waking hours.

- ✔ Consume 45 to 50 total grams of dietary fiber daily. You can supplement the amount in your diet with fiber from ground psyllium husks.

- ✔ Eat smaller meals more frequently instead of three large meals daily.

- ✔ Supplement your diet with 75 mg triphala daily to promote regularity.

- ✔ Get tested for food allergies and sensitivities and eliminate from your diet any foods that commonly trigger reactions, such as wheat (gluten) and dairy. (See Chapter 13 for more about tests for food allergies and sensitivities.)

- ✔ Try increasing your stomach acid, as explained in the earlier section "Supplementing digestion."

- ✔ Ensure a healthy microbial balance in your gut by taking 5 billion CFU twice daily of a multistrain probiotic containing *Lactobacillus acidophilus* Rosell and *Bifidobacterium longum* Rosell.

Soothing the colon with supplements

Inflammatory bowel diseases, including Crohn's and diverticulitis, and chronic diarrhea, often respond well to the following supplements:

Supplements	Dosage
Colostrum (powder form preferable)	10,000 mg one or two times daily
Digestive enzymes (protease, amylase, and lipase)	50,000 to 100,000 USP protease; 50,000 to 100,000 USP amylase; and 8,000 to 15,000 USP lipase with meals
Probiotics (*Saccharomyces boulardii;* a proprietary blend of a multistrain containing *Lactobacillus acidophilus, Bifidobacterium longum,* and *Lactobacillus plantarum*; and *Bifidobacterium lactis* HNO 19 [HOWARU Bifido])	250 mg *Saccharomyces boulardii* twice daily; 50 billion CFU multistrain probiotic once daily; 50 billion CFU HOWARU Bifido once daily
Vitamin D3	2,000 to 10,000 mg daily, depending on blood levels (see Appendix A)

To reduce inflammation in the colon, take the following supplements:

Supplements	Dosage
Ginger (capsule form)	500 mg several times daily (alternatively, drink several cups of ginger tea a day)
Omega-3 essential fatty acids (EFAs)	1 g yielding 180 mg EPA and 120 mg DHA three times daily
L-glutamine (powder form)	3,500 mg one to three times daily
Aloe (in powder form)	50 mg one to three times daily
Deglycerized licorice (powder form)	500 mg one to three times daily
Alkalizing super green drinks	1 or 2 drinks daily between meals (follow label instructions to prepare)

Make your own alkalizing super green drink (see the earlier sidebar "Alkalizing super green drink recipe") or choose a low-sugar organic product that's free of artificial coloring and sweeteners. My favorite is Vida Pure's Mighty Maca super alkalizing green drink.

Restoring healthy gut microflora with fecal implants

Many bowel disorders are linked to a deficiency of good microbes in the colon and an excess of bad microbes, such as *Clostridium difficile (C. diff)*, which is often linked to Crohn's disease and colitis. To restore healthy gut flora, a few doctors are now performing *fecal implants* — taking donor feces from a healthy family member and implanting it into the intestines of the person who's ill (often during a colonoscopy). Fecal implants often restore colon health when all other medical treatments have failed and without having to surgically remove all or portions of the colon.

If you have a bowel disorder that's not responding to other treatment, discuss this option with your doctor. If you can get past the yuk factor and find a suitable and willing donor, you could be well on your way to a cure.

Curing constipation

Constipation is a condition in which you're not having at least one bowel movement a day or you have difficulty passing stools. If you're constipated, follow my earlier recommendations in the sections "Improving general colon health" and "Soothing the colon with supplements" and then follow these recommendations:

✔ Drink 4 to 6 ounces of prune juice daily.

✔ Take 1 to 2 tablespoons flaxseed oil or 2 to 3 tablespoons flaxseed meal in two divided doses daily. When taking flax meal, supplement with 10 to 20 mg vitamin B6 daily.

✔ Take 200 to 600 mg magnesium citrate daily, one hour before bed. Start on the low end of the dosage range and increase your dosage slowly, if necessary. Don't exceed 600 mg per day. In high doses, magnesium citrate draws fluid into the colon to act as a laxative.

✔ Take 1 to 5 g daily of a vitamin C powder in the form of mineral ascorbates. Take as much as your bowel can tolerate without experiencing diarrhea, up to 5 g. If you have loose stools, decrease the dosage.

✔ Don't suppress the urge to poop. When you gotta go, go.

If you've exhausted your attempts at rectifying the cause of your constipation, see a qualified healthcare provider to look into other possible causes, which may include stress, suppressed emotions, structural abnormalities, neurological or endocrine disorders, or adverse side effects of certain medications. Hypothyroidism (see Chapter 18) is often overlooked as a cause.

Over-the-counter laxatives may be useful as a quick fix, but avoid using them to treat repeated bouts of constipation. Overuse of laxatives creates dependency and worsens constipation over time.

Combating Crohn's disease

Crohn's disease is an autoimmune IBD that often causes abdominal pain, diarrhea, malabsorption of nutrients, fever, and weight loss. The cause is unclear, but Crohn's disease is often associated with a combination of genetic susceptibility, underlying immune system imbalance, and an environmental trigger that sets the illness in motion. Recurrent periods of flare-ups and remission are common.

In severe cases, characterized by fever, bloody stools, dehydration, or vomiting, seek immediate medical attention. Methotrexate and corticosteroids may be required to reduce the inflammation. Your doctor is likely to order frequent colonoscopies or other imaging tests to rule out abscesses and bowel obstruction.

If your Crohn's disease is caused by an imbalance of microflora in your gut, discuss treatment options with your healthcare provider, including the possibility of a fecal implant (see "Restoring healthy gut microflora with fecal implants"). You may also be able to lessen the severity of the illness through diet and lifestyle changes. In addition to the dietary changes and supplements recommended earlier for overall colon health, follow these recommendations:

✔ Consume a low disaccharide diet known as the *Specific Carbohydrate Diet*. This diet eliminates *all* grains, dairy, potatoes, beans, foods that contain sucrose, and a number of other foods. See *Breaking the Vicious Cycle*, by Elaine Gottschall (The Kirkton Press), for details.

The worst foods for Crohn's are dairy, corn, and wheat. Eliminate these three foods from your diet.

✔ Eliminate from your diet all foods that contain yeast, including breads, beer, cider, fruit skins (especially grapes and plums), grape juice, malt beverages, MSG, pretzels, sake, and wine.

✔ Never eat fast food.

✔ If you smoke, stop, no matter what it takes.

✔ Consult an acupuncturist.

✔ Supplement your diet with one of more of the following:

- **Proline-rich polypeptides (PRPs) extracted from bovine colostrum:** 4 sprays in mouth, hold for 30 seconds and swallow, twice daily early morning and before bed for a total of 16 mg daily.

- **Vitamins and minerals:** Team up with your doctor to have your vitamin and mineral levels tested and supplement your diet with additional vitamins and minerals to address any deficiencies. Maintaining a healthy level of vitamin D is particularly important to help maintain the tight junctions in the small intestine that prevent leaky gut syndrome. Be sure to use the better form of each vitamin and mineral, as I explain in Appendix A.

- **Iron:** 30 mg as ferrous bis-glycinate chelate one to two times daily if testing reveals a deficiency.

- **5-HTP (5-dydroxytryptophan):** 100 mg in controlled-release form twice daily.

Dealing with diarrhea

Diarrhea occurs in two types: acute and chronic. *Acute diarrhea* is the body's way of eliminating a toxin — a bacteria, virus, or contaminated food. If you have acute diarrhea, be happy, because it's a sign that your immune system is working properly to detox your body. Drink plenty of fluids to replace those lost as your body flushes the toxins from your system. People don't generally die from health conditions that cause acute diarrhea; they die from dehydration, so stay hydrated.

Don't take antidiarrheal medications to treat acute diarrhea, because they prevent your body from expelling the toxins. Let your immune system serve its purpose.

Chronic diarrhea, on the other hand, is a sign of a potentially serious underlying health condition, such as salmonella infection, IBS, ulcerative colitis, celiac disease, nonceliac gluten sensitivity, or even cancer. Drink plenty of fluids to prevent dehydration and see your doctor to rule out any serious underlying health condition. Also follow the recommendations provided earlier to support overall colon health.

To combat any underlying viral, bacterial, or fungal/yeast issues that may be causing your acute diarrhea, take the following supplements:

Supplements	Dosage
Monolaurin	200 mg twice daily
L-lysine	150 mg twice daily
Bee propolis	100 mg twice daily
Cinnamon bark extract	100 mg twice daily
Grapefruit seed extract	100 mg twice daily
Grapeseed extract	100 mg twice daily
Oil of oregano	150 mg twice daily
Olive leaf extract	500 mg twice daily

Calming a case of diverticulitis

Diverticulitis occurs when sacs or pouches that sometimes form on the inner wall of the intestine, usually the large intestine (colon), become inflamed or infected. Sudden and possibly severe pain in the lower left abdomen is a common symptom.

If you experience severe abdominal pain, seek immediate medical attention. Your doctor may order a CAT scan to determine whether the colon wall is punctured, in which case antibiotics and antifungals may be required to stop the infection.

To prevent and treat diverticulitis, follow the recommendations provided earlier for supporting overall colon health and add in the following supplements:

Supplements	Dosage
Boswellia	300 mg two to three times daily
Peppermint, slippery elm, or chamomile tea	2 to 3 cups daily without milk or sweeteners

Healing hemorrhoids

Hemorrhoids are swollen, inflamed veins in the anus and rectum, which typically cause itching, burning, pain, and sometimes bleeding. They're often caused by constipation, low-fiber diet, pregnancy, childbirth, hypothyroidism, and compromised liver function. For immediate relief, try the following:

- ✔ Soak the affected area for 15 to 20 minutes in warm water three times daily. Do this in the bathtub or use a sitz bath that fits over the toilet. (Add 1 ounce of witch hazel to the bath to help reduce swelling.)

- ✔ Keep the anal area clean by showering daily and rinsing the affected area with plain warm water. (Soap may irritate the area.)

- ✔ After a bowel movement, wipe gently with a soft paper towel soaked in witch hazel, a natural astringent that soothes the itching and pain and helps to shrink the swollen tissue. Clean the area thoroughly with as little wiping as possible.

- ✔ Apply ice packs to the area for periods of 10 to 15 minutes to reduce swelling.

If you experience rectal bleeding, seek medical care. Rectal bleeding may be a symptom of a more serious condition.

For long-term relief, follow the recommendations provided earlier to support overall colon health, and focus on increasing your intake of fiber and water. In addition, eat a couple prunes or drink 4 to 6 ounces of prune juice in the morning. Support your dietary changes with the following nutritional supplements:

Supplements	Dosage
Vitamin K (menaquinone-7)	45 mcg twice daily (or consume foods and drinks rich in vitamin K, including green leafy vegetables and green drinks; see Appendix A for precautions)
Horse chestnut	250 mg three times daily
Collinsonia root	500 mg three times daily
Rutin	400 mg three times daily

Eradicating irritable bowel syndrome

IBS is a disorder that affects the large intestine, often causing abdominal pain, cramps, bloating, gas, and constipation alternating with diarrhea. IBS is often traced to small intestinal bacterial overgrowth (SIBO), emotional stress, candida yeast overgrowth (giardia), food allergies and sensitivities, and serotonin imbalance. Your healthcare provider can order tests to identify or rule out several of these possible causes. If a test result comes back positive, you have a clearer idea of how to treat your IBS.

Whether the results are positive or negative, the following dietary adjustments are likely to help:

- Consume low-glycemic meals that don't spike your blood sugar and insulin levels.

- Avoid alcohol, coffee, and cruciferous vegetables (brussels sprouts, broccoli, and cauliflower).

- Follow the modified elimination diet (see Chapter 2), with an emphasis on removing wheat, corn, dairy, coffee, chocolate, and citrus fruits. Consider adopting the low-FODMAP diet, as explained in the nearby sidebar.

- In addition to following the earlier recommendations for colon health, supplement your diet with the following:

Supplements	*Dosage*
Turmeric	1 to 2 g daily, in divided doses
Boswellia	300 mg two to three times daily
Chamomile, ginger, or peppermint tea	2 to 3 cups daily without milk or sweeteners

Adopt the low-FODMAP diet to combat IBS

The low-FODMAP diet is widely accepted and recommended as one of the most effective dietary interventions for IBS. *FODMAP* is short for *fermentable oligosaccharides, disaccharides, monosaccharides, and polyols* — molecules in certain foods that are poorly absorbed in the bowels of people with IBS. Unabsorbed molecules travel down to the large intestine, where they feed bacteria, causing the symptoms of IBS.

Developed by Dr. Sue Shepherd, the low-FODMAP diet is a two-stage process in which you strictly avoid high-FODMAP foods for six to eight weeks and then slowly reintroduce certain foods as directed by your dietician.

(continued)

(continued)

Low-FODMAP diets typically provide two lists of foods — foods to avoid (high in FODMAPs) and foods to eat (low in FODMAPs) — and the lists are very long and detailed. Here's a short list of high-FODMAP foods to avoid:

- **Oligosaccharides:** Asparagus, baked beans, beetroot, broccoli, brussels sprouts, cabbage, chickpeas, couscous, eggplant, fennel, garlic, kidney beans, leeks, lentils, okra, onions, persimmons, rye, watermelon, wheat

- **Disaccharides:** Cow, sheep, and goat milk; ricotta and cottage cheese; yogurt; ice cream

- **Monosaccharides:** Apples, pears, mangoes, peaches, honey, fructose, high-fructose corn syrup

- **Polyols:** Apples, apricots, avocadoes, blackberries, cherries, nectarines, peaches, pears, plums, prunes, green bell peppers, cauliflower, mushrooms, sorbitol, mannitol, isomalt, malitol, xylitol

Here's a short list of low-FODMAP foods to eat:

- **Fruit:** Bananas, blueberries, cantaloupe, cranberries, grapes, grapefruit, honeydew melon, lemons, limes, mandarins, oranges, raspberries, strawberries, tangelos

- **Vegetables:** Artichokes, bok choy, carrots, celery, endive, green beans, lettuce, olives, potatoes, red bell peppers, spinach, summer squash, sweet potatoes, tomatoes, turnips, yams, zucchini

- **Grains (in moderation):** Gluten-free bread or cereal, 100 percent spelt bread, rice, oats, arrowroot, millet, psyllium, quinoa, sorghum, tapioca

- **Dairy:** Lactose-free milk and oat, rice, and soy milk (check for additives); hard cheeses along with brie and camembert; lactose-free yogurt; sorbet and gelato; olive oil (as a butter substitute)

- **Sweeteners:** Sugar (sucrose in small quantities), glucose, artificial sweeteners not ending in "-ol," golden syrup (small quantities), maple syrup (small quantities), molasses, and treacle

The low-FODMAP diet is highly individualized. I recommend that you work closely with a dietician, especially during the second stage of the diet, to identify which foods to reintroduce and when.

Grappling with Gallstones and Gallbladder Problems

The gallbladder is a digestive organ in the upper right abdominal area below the liver. The gallbladder's main function is to store and concentrate bile, which is critical for the digestion and absorption of fats and fat-soluble vitamins. In approximately 20 percent of the population, gallstones, consisting of bile saturated with cholesterol, form inside the gallbladder, and in about one in every seven people, a gallstone blocks the bile duct, producing symptoms that include pain in the upper or middle abdomen that lasts at least 30 minutes, fever, loss of appetite, nausea, vomiting, yellowing of the skin or eyes, and clay-colored stools.

When a gallstone blocks the bile duct, doctors typically remove the gallbladder, which can lead to all sorts of problems, including dietary restrictions that ban some of your favorite foods. Unless you have a life-threatening blockage of your bile duct, you can usually avoid surgery by doing the following:

✔ Get tested for food allergies and intolerances (see Chapter 13) and eliminate from your diet all problem foods. Food allergies and sensitivities are a major contributory factor to the formation of gallstones.

✔ Modify your diet or adopt a vegetarian diet: Eat fiber-rich foods. Eat more vegetable protein and less (or no) red meat. Reduce your consumption of dairy and fried foods, and eliminate refined processed carbohydrates. Use olive oil and flaxseed oil for salad dressings, reduce saturated fat, and eliminate trans fatty acids (hydrogenated and partially hydrogenated vegetable oils). Consume a handful of organic nuts daily or every other day, and eat beets, artichokes, and dandelions often, because they thin the bile.

✔ Consume a small amount of caffeinated beverages daily to prevent gallstone formation. (Although light to moderate alcohol consumption has been shown to decrease gallstone formation, don't start drinking just to prevent gallstones.)

✔ If you're overweight, lose weight, but do it slowly. Rapid weight loss increases the likelihood of developing gallstones. A program designed to help you shed a few pounds per week would be beneficial in prevention.

✔ Support your nutrition with the following supplements:

Supplements	*Dosage*
Vitamin C (mineral ascorbates)	500 to 2,000 mg daily
Iron (ferrous bis-glycinate chelate)	30 mg twice daily only if deficient (see Appendix A)

You may be able to discourage the formation of gallstones by increasing the amount of acid in your stomach. See "Supplementing digestion," earlier in this chapter, for details.

Treating Kidney Stones and Urinary Tract Infections

Two of the most common problems affecting the health of your urinary tract are kidney stones and urinary tract infections (UTIs). Several natural treatments benefit both conditions. Try drinking 2 to 3 liters of water over the course of the day to dilute the urine and flush your urinary tract. Drinking one (or more) 8-ounce glass of unsweetened cranberry juice daily can also be beneficial (if it's too tart for you, dilute it with water). Also consider these supplements:

Supplements	*Dosage*
Vitamin A (retinyl palmitate and beta-carotene)	2,500 IU retinyl palmitate and 2,500 IU beta-carotene daily (see Appendix A for precautions)
Vitamin C (mineral ascorbates)	1,000 mg several times daily
D-mannose	900 mg one to three times daily

D-mannose is a simple sugar found in cranberries and pineapple. Research suggests that D-mannose interferes with adhesion of *E. coli* (the bacteria primarily responsible for causing bladder infections) to the bladder wall, thereby supporting a healthy urinary tract.

Don't drink soft drinks, alcohol, or caffeinated beverages, because these tend to dehydrate you and irritate the urinary tract.

Crushing kidney stones

Kidney stones are mineral salts that crystalize inside the kidney. Problems arise when your body tries to pass these crystal formations through the urinary tract. Although passage of the stones causes no long-term damage, the process may be very painful.

If the pain is overwhelming, seek immediate medical attention and ask your doctor for shock wave lithotripsy (SWL), which uses sound waves to break the stone into tiny pieces that can be more easily passed through the urine.

For smaller kidney stones, drink plenty of water and follow the earlier recommendations for overall urinary tract health. Take an over-the-counter pain reliever, such as ibuprofen or acetaminophen as needed.

If kidney stones are a persistent problem, make the following dietary adjustments:

✔ Switch to a vegetarian diet or decrease your consumption of saturated fats (many cheeses, pizza, grain-based desserts, dairy desserts, sausages, franks, ribs, hamburgers, and so on).

✔ Limit the amount of foods you eat that contain high amounts of oxalates, including beans, chocolate, coffee, tea, rhubarb, tomatoes, eggplant, beets, peanuts, spinach, raspberries, strawberries, oranges, kale, carrots, sweet potatoes, and plums. (Although your body produces most of the oxalates it contains, it's still advisable to cut down on these foods if you're having recurrent kidney stone issues.)

✔ Consume ¼ cup of pumpkin seeds daily.

In addition to the supplements recommended earlier for overall urinary tract health, take one or more of the following nutritional supplements:

Supplements	*Dosage*
Magnesium glycinate chelate	250 mg twice daily
Vitamin B6 (pyridoxal 5'-phosphate)	40 mg twice daily
Vitamin D3	2,000 to 10,000 mg daily, depending on blood levels (see Appendix A)

Be careful supplementing vitamin D, because large doses may increase urinary calcium excretion, potentially increasing the risk of kidney stones. 2,000 mg is considered safe, but your doctor should monitor levels of urinary calcium excretion.

If you continue to have problems with kidney stones, investigate and address other possible causes, including a diet high in refined, processed sugars, saturated fats, or sodium; potassium or magnesium deficiency; metabolic acidosis (ask your doctor to check the pH of your urine, which should be between 7.0 and 8.0); and obesity.

Overcoming urinary tract infections (UTIs)

A *urinary tract infection* (also known as a *UTI, bladder infection*, or *cystitis*) is an inflammation of the bladder, commonly accompanied by difficult and painful urination and often caused by bacterial infection. If a fever is present, the infection has probably spread to the kidneys. UTIs are much more common in women than in men.

Because UTIs are almost always the result of bacterial infection, the first step is to starve the bacteria. Eliminate from your diet refined sugar and all processed, packaged foods. Eat fresh vegetables, low-glycemic fruits, lean pastured animal products, wild fish, and little if any whole grains. Replace trans fats with healthy fats in olive oil, avocado, and organic nuts and seeds (free of cottonseed or canola oil).

Drink 8 ounces of water every waking hour and a couple 8-ounce glasses of unsweetened cranberry juice daily. ***Note for women only:*** Don't use a tampon or diaphragm during an infection.

In addition to the supplements recommended earlier for overall urinary tract health, take one or more of the following supplements:

Supplements	*Dosage*
Uva ursi (liquid)	1 teaspoon (5 ml) twice daily
Probiotics (*Saccharomyces boulardii*; proprietary blend of a multistrain probiotic containing *Lactobacillus acidophilus, Bifidobacterium longum,* and *Lactobacillus plantarum*; and *Bifidobacterium lactis* HNO 19 [HOWARU Bifido])	250 mg *Saccharomyces boulardii* twice daily; 50 billion CFU multistrain probiotic once daily; 50 billion CFU HOWARU Bifido once daily (***Note:*** If you're taking an antibiotic, take your probiotic at least four hours between doses of your antibiotic.
Oil of oregano	500 mg twice daily)

To prevent UTIs, drink unsweetened cranberry juice several times a day, take showers instead of baths, and urinate before and after sexual activity. If you're a woman, wipe from front to rear and don't douche or use feminine hygiene products.

Chapter 15

Restoring Back, Joint, and Muscle Health

In This Chapter

▶ Routing gout

▶ Alleviating arthritis

▶ Relieving back pain

▶ Soothing muscle aches and cramps

*E*veryone, at some point, suffers from muscle, joint, or back pain, because bones and muscles take a beating. In this chapter, I offer advice on how to treat the most common conditions at the root of these aches and pains.

Doses in this chapter are for adults, not children. For guidance on how to adjust dosages for children (and adults under 150 pounds), turn to Chapter 12.

Tackling Arthritis in All Its Forms

Arthritis is any painful inflammation of the joints that may damage joints, bones, muscles, cartilage, and other connective tissue. More than 100 health conditions involve arthritis, including fibromyalgia, gout, lupus, Lyme disease, osteoarthritis, and rheumatoid arthritis. In this section, I describe the three most common and troublesome arthritic afflictions — gout, osteoarthritis, and rheumatoid arthritis — and offer guidance on treating them effectively with natural cures. (For information about lupus, fibromyalgia, and other chronic conditions, see Chapter 17.)

Getting rid of gout

Gouty arthritis (commonly called simply *gout*) is an extremely painful condition resulting from the buildup of uric acid crystals in the joints, most commonly the joint of the big toe. Men are ten times more likely than women to suffer from gout, and individuals who are insulin resistant are much more prone to gout attacks.

If you suffer from gout, the first step on your road to recovery is to modify your diet:

- ✔ If you're overweight, try shedding the excess pounds. See Chapter 2 for more about adopting a healthy diet that's likely to result in weight loss.

- ✔ Eliminate refined and processed sugars and all alcohol, especially beer.

- ✔ Follow a low-glycemic meal plan, such as a Paleo- or Mediterranean-style diet, that emphasizes reducing cereal grains, refined carbohydrates, and saturated (trans) fats. The diet I recommend in Chapter 2 also does the trick.

- ✔ Eat more veggies and fruit, especially berries (cherries, blueberries, and strawberries). Drinking 4 ounces of a fresh berry or cherry juice daily is a good way to increase your berry consumption.

- ✔ Eat less meat and more wild, oily fish, such as salmon, mackerel, and sardines.

- ✔ Add 1 to 2 tablespoons of flaxseeds to your diet daily. You can sprinkle these on your cereal or a salad.

- ✔ Drink 8 ounces of water every two waking hours.

Team up with your doctor to test and monitor your blood glucose levels, uric acid, pH levels, and concentrations of other substances in your blood that may make you more prone to gout. If your blood work looks okay, consider the possibility of yeast overgrowth in the intestines. Talk to your doctor about ordering tests to check for signs of yeast overgrowth.

Support any dietary changes you make with the following supplements:

Supplement	Dosage
Folate (5-MTHF)	2,000 mcg twice daily
Vitamin C (mineral ascorbates)	1,000 mg twice daily
Quercetin	500 mg twice daily
Celery seed extract	450 mg twice daily
Nettle root	250 mg three times daily
Omega-3 essential fatty acids (EFAs)	1 g yielding 180 mg EPA and 120 mg DHA three times daily
Super green drink	8 to 12 ounces one time daily

Make your own super green drink (you can find a recipe in Chapter 14) or choose a low-sugar organic product that's free of artificial coloring and sweeteners. My favorite is Mighty Maca super alkalizing green drink by Vida Pure.

Don't take niacin if you have gout. Studies show that 1.5 grams or more of niacin daily raises serum uric acid levels.

Overcoming osteoarthritis

Osteoarthritis occurs when the smooth, rubbery cartilage that covers the ends of bones wears down, resulting in bone-on-bone contact. Osteoarthritis typically affects joints in the knees, hips, and hands, and the vertebrae that form the spinal column, causing pain and stiffness and limiting range of motion. Most people over the age of 50 have some degree of osteoarthritis.

Through the miracles of modern medicine, specifically stem cell breakthroughs, doctors are able to assist the body in forming new cartilage and restoring joints. Until that's perfected, however, conventional medicine continues to focus on pain management and, when the pain becomes unmanageable, surgery, such as knee replacement, to deal with the problem.

My patients have found significant relief through changes in diet and the use of professional-grade nutritional supplements to support joint health, as I explain in the next sections.

For immediate pain relief, apply Biofreeze Pain Reliever to affected areas. My patients love it. Talk to your healthcare provider or go to www.biofreeze.com/wheretobuy.aspx to find sellers in your area.

Making dietary changes

Certain foods trigger an inflammatory response that accelerates joint degeneration. The biggest offenders are wheat, dairy, meat, and eggs. Get tested for allergies or food sensitivities to these foods and others and eliminate any problem foods from your diet, as explained in Chapter 13.

Here are three additional suggestions for dealing with osteoarthritis through diet:

- ✔ If you're overweight, shed a few pounds. Even minor weight loss can help.

- ✔ For six weeks, eliminate from your diet all nightshade vegetables — peppers, eggplant, potatoes, and tomato. In a small subset of people with osteoarthritis, eliminating nightshade vegetables helps.

- ✔ Eat less red meat, poultry, and pork, and eat more oily fish — salmon, mackerel, sardines, trout, and herring.

Taking supplements to support joint health

Three supplements are essential for supporting joint health: glucosamine sulfate, chondroitin sulfate, and MSM (methylsulfonylmethane). I strongly recommend that you buy and use a pharmaceutical-grade product that combines these three essential ingredients. XYMOGEN's SynovX Recovery (www.xymogen.com), Metagenics ChondroCare (www.metagenics.com), and NuMedica's Joint Tri-Basic (www.numedica.com) are all excellent products.

If you choose to create your own proprietary blend of supplements for joint health or want to add to the blend you buy, consider the following:

Supplement	Dosage
Vitamin C (mineral ascorbates)	1,000 mg twice daily
Vitamin D3	2,000 to 10,000 IU daily, depending on blood levels (see Appendix A)
Vitamin E (mixed tocopherols)	400 IU daily
Niacin (niacinamide)	500 mg three to six times daily (see Appendix A for precautions)
Glucosamine sulfate	1,500 mg daily in divided doses
Chondroitin sulfate	1,200 mg daily in divided doses
MSM	1,000 mg three times daily
SAMe	200 mg twice daily
Hyaluronic acid	20 mg twice daily
Turmeric	200 mg one or two times daily between meals
Bromelain	500 mg three times daily between meals (see Appendix B for precautions)
White willow	300 mg two times daily between meals; as symptoms improve, decrease to 200 mg one to two times daily
Ginger	1 g one or two times daily
Boswellia	100 mg one or two times daily between meals

Ridding yourself of rheumatoid arthritis

Rheumatoid arthritis is an autoimmune disease in which white blood cells attack joint cartilage, causing inflammation in numerous joints (shoulders, elbows, ankles, wrists, fingers, and toes) that over time often results in joint deformities. Pain is often worst in the morning.

Prescription meds won't fix your rheumatoid arthritis; they're designed to mask the symptoms, and they don't address the underlying cause.

Getting tested

Three factors converge to cause rheumatoid arthritis: genetic susceptibility, increased intestinal permeability, and an environmental trigger — food allergy or sensitivity, heavy-metal toxicity, viral or bacterial infection, poor digestion, or a lifestyle factor (such as stress). Therefore, before treating rheumatoid arthritis, get yourself tested to identify or rule out heavy-metal toxicity, food allergies/sensitivities, and increased intestinal permeability. Talk to your doctor about getting tested for the following.:

- ✔ **Heavy-metal toxicity:** Mercury, lead, aluminum, arsenic, and cadmium may contribute to inflammatory autoimmune joint issues. If the results show higher-than-acceptable levels of certain heavy metals, your doctor is likely to order chelation therapy. In addition, remove any heavy metal contamination from your home and workplace.

- ✔ **Food allergies and sensitivities:** See Chapter 13 for details.

- ✔ **Intestinal permeability:** Many patients with rheumatoid arthritis have increased intestinal permeability with *villous atrophy* (erosion of the microscopic finger-like tentacles in the small intestine that absorb nutrients), leading to severe malabsorption of nutrients from the diet. (See Chapter 14 for more about treating digestive conditions.)

Adjusting and supplementing your diet

A healthy diet reduces the inflammation characteristic of rheumatoid arthritis:

- ✔ Eliminate from your diet inflammatory foods — wheat, dairy, and sugar. Packaged, processed foods are often loaded with sugar and saturated fats.

  Consider a Mediterranean-style diet with emphasis on balancing blood sugar spikes. Check out *Mediterranean Diet For Dummies*, by Rachel Berman (John Wiley & Sons, Inc.).

- ✔ Consume eight servings of veggies and two servings of fruit daily. French fries, ketchup, and iceberg lettuce — the most consumed vegetables in the U.S. — don't count.

- ✔ Adopt a vegan diet — no meat, eggs, dairy, wheat, grains, corn, sugar, or alcohol — for a minimum of six to eight weeks to see whether your condition improves. Check out *Living Vegan For Dummies*, by Alexandra Jamieson (John Wiley & Sons, Inc.).

Support your diet with as many of the following supplements as possible. These supplements work synergistically, so combining them as directed improves your outcome:

Supplement	*Dosage*
Colostrum (powder form)	10,000 mg one or two times daily
Proline-rich polypeptides (extracted from bovine colostrum)	4 sprays in mouth, hold for 30 seconds and swallow, twice daily early morning and before bed for a total of 16 mg daily
Probiotics (*Saccharomyces boulardii;* proprietary blend of a multistrain probiotic containing *Lactobacillus acidophilus, Bifidobacterium longum,* and *Lactobacillus plantarum;* and *Bifidobacterium lactis* HNO 19 [HOWARU Bifido])	250 mg of *Saccharomyces boulardii* twice daily; 50 billion CFU of the proprietary multistrain probiotic once daily; 50 billion CFU of HOWARU Bifido once daily
Zinc glycinate chelate	20 mg twice daily
Omega-3 essential fatty acids (EFAs)	1 g yielding 180 mg EPA and 120 mg DHA three times daily
Omega-6 (from evening primrose oil, borage seed oil, or black currant seed oil [gamma-linolenic acid])	1 g daily
Folate (5-MTHF)	2,000 to 10,000 mcg daily
Vitamin B12 (methylcobalamin, sublingual fast-dissolving tablet)	5,000 mcg daily
Vitamin B6 (pyridoxal 5'-phosphate)	40 mg twice daily
Vitamin C (mineral ascorbates)	1,000 mg twice daily
Vitamin E (mixed tocopherols)	400 IU daily
Bromelain	500 mg three times daily
Ginger (capsule form)	1 to 2 g daily

Oh, My Aching Back! Treating Backache

Backache can range from your neck down into your legs (in the case of sciatica) and is one of the top reasons for emergency room and doctor visits. Common causes of backache include injury (typically from accidents, lifting heavy objects, or lifting the wrong way); skeletal or musculature issues (spinal misalignment, herniated or bulging spinal discs, flat feet, and strained muscles, tendons, or ligaments); other health issues (inflammatory conditions, constipation, and obesity); and things like poor posture, wearing high-heel shoes, and premenstrual syndrome.

If your back pain is severe or is associated with bowel or bladder control issues, seek immediate medical treatment. Back pain involving bowel or bladder control issues may result from infection, cancer, a ruptured thoracic aorta, or a severely herniated disc, all of which require immediate medical attention.

For severe back pain, pain relievers and muscle relaxants offer quick relief and may prevent additional damage. You can then use more natural remedies for a long-term fix. Consider surgery as a last resort and only after you've exhausted all other treatment options.

Eliminating possible causes of backache

To treat backache, start by eliminating some of the possible causes:

- ✔ **Stop doing whatever hurt your back in the first place.** Rest. Time is a wonderful healer, and resting your back gives it a chance to recuperate.
- ✔ **Get a firm, supportive mattress.** Try before you buy.
- ✔ **Opt for supportive footwear.** If you wear sandals, get Birkenstock sandals or others that support the arches in your foot, and don't wear inexpensive flip-flops. Get rid of high-heel shoes. They may look good, but they destroy your back.

Consider custom orthotics that support the three arches of the foot. (I recommend Foot Levelers; visit www.footlevelers.com for more information and to locate a local chiropractor or podiatrist who can fit you for custom orthotics.)

- ✔ **Change behaviors that can put strain on your back.** When texting, bring the device closer to your face instead of hunching over it. If you're a man, remove your wallet from your back pocket while sitting or driving, and if you're a woman, avoid carrying heavy bags or purses on your shoulders.
- ✔ **Lift things properly.** Get in the habit of lifting with your legs; bend at your knees, not at your waist.

Strengthening your back

Assuming the pain is manageable and you're not having back spasms, you can engage in some bodywork to strengthen your back, restore proper alignment, and increase flexibility.

If you're experiencing any muscle spasms, obtain massage therapy before engaging in any other body work. Otherwise, engaging in bodywork may worsen the spasms and other conditions contributing to your backache.

Here are some back-strengthening suggestions:

- ✔ See a chiropractor or osteopath to realign spinal subluxations (mis-aligned vertebrae) and twisted pelvis.

  Ask your physical therapist, chiropractor, or osteopath about *spinal decompression* — a valuable tool for treating herniated and bulging discs.

- ✔ Obtain physical therapy to treat any acute problems and find out exactly what you need to be working on. A physical therapist can teach you exercises and stretches that address the specific causes of the back pain you're experiencing.

- ✔ Take up yoga, Qigong, or Pilates, all of which strengthen and improve flexibility of your core, including your *para spinal musculature* (the small muscles that run along your neck and spine).

- ✔ Sit upright on an exercise ball while watching TV, reading, or engaging in other sedentary activities. Balancing yourself on an exercise ball engages your back and stomach muscles without any conscious effort on your part.

- ✔ Stretch to relieve tight muscles, but don't bounce or try to force it. Take it slow. Over time, you naturally become more limber.

Turning to diet to support pain-free back

Your diet can contribute to inflammatory spinal conditions, so focus on your diet. Eliminate sugar, refined processed carbohydrates, and trans fats, and eat more vegetables, fruit, oily fish, and healthy fats. Because dehydration contributes to back pain, drink at least 8 ounces of water every two waking hours. See Chapter 2 for more about consuming a healthy diet.

Support your dietary changes with the following supplements:

Supplement	Dosage
For muscle support	
Vitamin B6 (pyridoxal 5'-phosphate)	30 mg one or two times daily
Calcium lactate	50 mg one or two times daily
Magnesium citrate	100 mg one or two times daily
Passionflower	180 mg one or two times daily

Supplement	Dosage
For muscle support	
Valerian root	100 mg one or two times daily
To reduce inflammation	
White willow bark extract	300 mg two times daily between meals; decrease to 200 mg one to two times daily as symptoms improve
Boswellia extract	100 mg one or two times daily between meals
Turmeric	200 mg one or two times daily between meals
Bromelain	150 mg one or two times daily between meals (see Appendix B for precautions)
MSM	1,000 mg two to three times daily
To improve digestion (proteolytic enzymes)	
Chymotrypsin	6,000 USP two to three times daily between meals
Trypsin	6,000 USP two to three times daily between meals
For joint support	
Glucosamine sulfate	1,500 mg daily in divided doses
Chondroitin sulfate	1,000 mg daily in divided doses
Collagen	20 mg twice daily

Working Out Muscle Aches and Cramps

Muscle aches and cramps are usually the result of overuse injury, dehydration (especially in hot weather and during exercise), nutritional deficiencies, and blood sugar dysregulation. When you experience muscle aches and cramps, deal with the obvious, common causes first.

If you commonly experience muscle aches and cramps during or after engaging in physical activity, take the following precautions:

✔ Drink plenty of fluids before, during, and after rigorous physical activity, especially when you're working out indoors or in warm weather.

Water is usually fine, but you may want to replenish your electrolytes, as well. Look for a product that contains vitamins B1, B2, B3, B6, and pantothenic acid; the minerals calcium, phosphorus, magnesium, and chromium; citric acid; taurine; malic acid; and L-carnosine. And avoid products that contain artificial coloring, flavoring, refined sugar, high-fructose corn syrup, or artificial sweeteners. Remember, the best products aren't necessarily the ones that taste best.

✔ Consume plenty of vegetables high in magnesium, calcium, and potassium (see Appendix A for foods rich in these minerals), and avoid candy, soda, and refined carbohydrates, all of which cause you to lose minerals.

✔ Warm up and stretch before engaging in the activity. For example, walk about a mile and then stretch before jogging or running. Doing so warms up the muscles so that so you're stretching warm muscles instead of cold, tight muscles during the more-strenuous portion of the activity.

Supplement your diet with the following:

Supplement	Dosage
Vitamin B6 (pyridoxal 5'-phosphate)	30 mg one or two times daily
Calcium lactate	500 mg one or two times daily
Potassium	150 mg twice daily
Magnesium citrate	150 mg one or two times daily (**Note:** For nighttime cramping, take 300 mg one hour before bedtime)
MSM	1,000 mg two to three times daily
Super green drink	8 to 12 ounces one or two times daily

Make your own super green drink (you can find a recipe in Chapter 14) or choose a low-sugar organic product that's free of artificial coloring and sweeteners. My favorite is Mighty Maca super alkalizing green drink by Vida Pure.

Chronic muscle cramps may be caused by cirrhosis of the liver. If this condition is the root cause of your muscle cramps, eliminate all alcohol from your diet and support liver health with the following supplements:

Supplement	Dosage
Selenium	100 mcg twice daily
Milk thistle extract	260 mg twice daily
Alpha-lipoic acid	200 mg twice daily
N-acetyl cysteine	200 mg twice daily

Chapter 16

Putting Sleep Issues to Bed

• •

In This Chapter

▶ Falling asleep and staying asleep

▶ Preventing and coping with jet lag

▶ Alleviating snoring and sleep apnea

▶ Calming restless leg syndrome

▶ Curbing tendencies to walk in your sleep

• •

Good sleep is essential for good health, but the modern diet and many of today's lifestyles disrupt daily rhythms and undermine efforts to get the right amount of quality sleep. Insufficient or poor-quality sleep can lead to a wide range of health issues related to immune function, mood, memory, and mental function. In this chapter, I explain how to get enough quality sleep and overcome some of the most common conditions that may be preventing you from getting a good night's rest.

Doses in this chapter are for adults, not children. For guidance on how to adjust dosages for children (and adults under 150 pounds), turn to Chapter 12.

Overcoming Insomnia

Insomnia is the inability to fall asleep, stay asleep, or feel rested upon waking. If you're having trouble sleeping, the first step is to identify and address the cause. Common causes of insomnia include the obvious culprits: an uncomfortable bed, stress and anxiety, noise (such as the neighbor's barking dog or a nearby train), or having a bed partner who snores or is a restless sleeper. Other culprits include

   ✔ Caffeine (in coffee, tea, and energy drinks), nicotine, and alcohol (which may help you fall asleep but negatively affects quality of sleep and the ability to stay asleep)

✔ Medications, including certain antidepressants, stimulants (such as Ritalin), heart and blood pressure medications, corticosteroids and other allergy medications, decongestants, and weight-loss products

✔ Medical conditions, such as acid reflux, Alzheimer's disease, arthritis, asthma, bronchitis, cancer, cardiovascular conditions, depression, mania, overactive thyroid, Parkinson's disease, restless leg syndrome, sleep apnea, and stroke

✔ Going to bed hungry, or, conversely, eating too much too close to bedtime or eating foods high in trans fats

✔ Changes in environment or routine (for example, working a different shift or being away from home for whatever reason)

✔ No or poor sleep routines, such as going to bed at 10 p.m. one night and staying up to watch TV until midnight the next, or exercising too close to bedtime

Unless a specific health condition is causing you to lose sleep, you may be able to cure your insomnia by adjusting your routine, diet, and exercise regime, as I explain in this section.

Establishing a healthy sleep routine

One almost sure way to cure insomnia is to go to bed at the same time every night and wake up at the same time every morning. No staying up late on weekends and sleeping in in the morning. If you enjoy late-night TV, record the shows and watch them the next day. Here are a few additional ideas for enhancing your sleep routine:

✔ Use your bedroom exclusively for sleep and sex. Don't use it to watch TV, work at home, or pay your bills.

✔ Dim the lights at least one hour before bedtime. Light triggers your brain to think it's daytime and time to stay awake. Darkness tells your body to release melatonin, which makes you sleepy.

"Dim the lights" applies especially to TV screens, computers, cell phones, energy-efficient light bulbs, and other electronic devices that emit blue light, which disrupts the body's sleep-wake cycle. The closer the device is to your eyes, the bigger the problem.

✔ Transition to sleep mode. Do something that calms you before bedtime, such as reading, taking a warm bath, or engaging in relaxation exercises. Be careful, though, because certain activities, such as reading, may be more stimulating than calming.

Nap only if it's part of your daily routine, and limit naps to 20 to 40 minutes. Naps are like snacking; they can ruin your appetite for sleep.

Modifying your diet and eating habits

When, how, what, and how much you eat may affect your sleep. Here are some suggestions on how to adjust your eating to optimize sleep:

- Eat frequent smaller meals rather than a few large meals.

- Increase your carbohydrate intake at dinner. If you usually eat meat and veggies, add a half baked potato or brown rice.

- Avoid fried foods, especially at dinner. Opt for lean meat and veggies.

- Stop eating three hours before bedtime. If you have acid reflux, eating close to bedtime may be what's keeping you up at night, and you may not even realize it.

- If you drink alcohol, limit your consumption to one or two small drinks at dinner and then stop drinking for the rest of the evening.

- Stop or cut back on stimulants — coffee, tea, caffeinated soda, energy drinks, and chocolate. Consider not consuming stimulants after noon to allow them to work their way out of your system by bedtime.

- Drink at least 8 ounces of water every two waking hours. If you're waking up during the night to use the restroom, stop drinking anything two hours before bed.

Exercising

Regular aerobic exercise seems to improve sleep. Sleep and exercise are complementary; the more you exercise, the better you sleep; and the better you sleep, the more you feel like exercising.

Although research hasn't provided gobs of data to back up the link between exercise and sleep, here are some general recommendations based on the available data:

- Perform some sort of aerobic exercise for at least 30 to 40 minutes every other day.

- Don't exercise too close to bedtime, because it's likely to make you feel more wired than tired.

Don't expect immediate results. You may need to exercise regularly for four or five months before you start sleeping better.

Taking something to help you sleep

If you need to take something to help you sleep, try one or more of the following natural sleep aids:

Sleep Aid	Dosage
Melatonin	0.3 to 1.0 mg 90 minutes before bed (see Appendix C for precautions and additional details)
Valerian	400 to 900 mg 90 minutes before bed (valerian smells awful, but it can be very effective; see Appendix D for precautions)
L-theanine	100 mg twice daily with the last dose one hour before bed
Hops extract	50 mg one or two times daily with the last dose one hour before bed
Calcium lactate	100 mg one hour before bed
Magnesium citrate	150 mg one hour before bed
Lemon balm	150 mg one hour before bed
5-HTP	100 mg twice daily with the last dose one hour before bed
Tart cherry juice	8 ounces twice daily
Catnip tea (made with 1 to 2 teaspoons of dried catnip or 3 to 4 teaspoons of fresh catnip steeped in boiling water for at least 10 minutes)	8 ounces about 30 minutes before bed

Relaxing rituals can also help you sleep. Here are two suggestions: Brew a cup of chamomile tea. Although the science doesn't back up chamomile tea as effective in treating insomnia, the ritual of making and drinking the tea (or any warm beverage) can enhance your bedtime routine. Or take a relaxing bath before bedtime. Use lavender-scented soap or bath salts or use lavender essential oil to scent your bedroom. See Chapter 3 for more about using essential oils.

Resetting Your Internal Clock in Response to Jet Lag

Jet lag is the fatigue you feel after flying across several time zones. Exposure to light and darkness are the only true cures for jet lag, providing your brain with the information it needs to establish a healthy sleep-wake cycle. Here are a few suggestions to adjust your exposure to light and darkness and help reset the sleep schedule in your brain:

✔ **For a few days prior to your trip:** Align your exposure to light and darkness more closely with that of your destination. For example, if you're traveling west, keep the lights on a couple hours after the sun goes down, and go to bed a couple hours later than usual. Wake up two hours later, too. If light streams into your bedroom at that time, use window coverings to keep the room dark or wear a mask to block out the light. Also, because flying tends to dehydrate travelers, drink a little more than your usual 8 ounces of water every two waking hours.

✔ **Upon departure:** Set your watch to destination time.

✔ **In flight:** Try to follow the sleeping schedule you'll have when you reach your destination (take 3 to 5 mg melatonin about two hours before your "bedtime"). Continue to drink plenty of water, and avoid caffeine and alcohol.

✔ **When you reach your destination:** Spend time outdoors in the morning sun to recalibrate your internal clock. Also take 3 to 5 mg melatonin about two hours before bedtime.

Narcolepsy

Narcolepsy is a sleep disorder characterized by excessive sleepiness and the sudden onset of sleep in the midst of daily activities. Although narcolepsy has no cure, you may be able to improve alertness by getting a better night's sleep (see the earlier section "Overcoming Insomnia" for details) and eating small, light meals or snacks during the day instead of occasional large, heavy meals. Here are some other suggestions:

✔ Eliminate wheat, dairy, corn, and chocolate from your diet for at least 28 days to see whether symptoms improve. You can then reintroduce certain food categories slowly to narrow down which foods may be causing your symptoms. See Chapter 2 for guidance on following an elimination diet.

✔ Ask your doctor to check your levels of essential vitamins and minerals and then

(continued)

(continued)

supplement your diet to address any deficiencies. Low levels of the B vitamins; vitamins C, D, and E; and calcium and magnesium may contribute to narcolepsy.

✔ Try supporting dietary changes with one or more of the following supplements to increase mental alertness, boost energy, improve circulation to the brain, and more:

Supplement	Dosage
Choline (phosphotidylcholine)	300 to 400 mg three times daily
Chromium picolinate	100 mcg daily
CoQ10	100 mg twice daily
Omega-3 essential fatty acids (EFAs)	1 g yielding 180 mg EPA and 120 mg DHA three times daily
5-HTP (controlled-release form)	100 mg twice daily (see Appendix B for precautions)

Calming the Snoring Seas: Sleep Apnea

Sleep apnea is a disorder characterized by pauses in breathing that may last from seconds to minutes. Other symptoms include loud snoring punctuated by periods of silence, insomnia, dry mouth, sore throat, shortness of breath, headache, and daytime fatigue, sleepiness, and irritability. If you have sleep apnea, you may be able to resolve the problem by making the following changes:

✔ Address any nasal allergies that may be causing you to breathe through your mouth instead of your nose (see Chapters 5 and 13 for suggestions on dealing with nasal congestion).

✔ Keep your nasal passages open so you don't need to breathe through your mouth. Nasal strips can be very effective in keeping your nasal passages wide open. A hot shower before bed may also help to open your nasal passages and relax you.

✔ Take steps to get a better night's rest. See "Overcoming Insomnia," earlier in this chapter, for details. Most importantly, go to bed at the same time every night and wake up at the same time every morning.

✔ If you typically sleep on your back, try sleeping on your side. If you can't seem to stay on your side, try sleeping with a body pillow against your back. Another option is to prop up your body from the waist up or prop up the head of your bed.

✔ If you drink alcohol, stop drinking entirely, limit consumption to one or two drinks a day, or stop drinking several hours before bedtime.

✔ Ask your doctor or pharmacist whether any medications you're taking could be contributing to your sleep apnea and, if they are, explore options for taking less or switching to different medications. Sleeping pills and antihistamines are the most common contributors.

✔ If you're overweight, try shedding the excess pounds.

If you're unable to control your sleep apnea on your own, consult an acupuncturist. Certain types of acupuncture and acupressure that focus on pressure points in and around the ear have proven to be successful in treating sleep apnea.

The two most common and effective conventional medical treatments for sleep apnea could be classified as "natural cures" because they don't involve medication or invasive surgery. Oral appliances that look like mouth guards nudge the lower jaw forward to prevent snoring and keep the airway open during sleep. If that doesn't work, consider trying a *continuous positive airway pressure* (CPAP) device — a machine that blows air gently into your airway to keep it open.

Relieving Restless Leg Syndrome

Restless leg syndrome (RLS) is a neurological disorder characterized by a periodic need to move the legs or arms to relieve an unpleasant sensation in these extremities — pain, burning, itching, tingling, numbness, or a feeling that the skin is crawling. The symptoms are more severe at night and usually are preceded with a period of remaining still.

Several factors may contribute to RLS, including anemia (iron deficiency), Parkinson's disease, kidney failure, diabetes, peripheral neuropathy, antipsychotic and antidepressant medications, and pregnancy. Cold and allergy medications and sedating antihistamines may worsen the condition.

The first order of business is to identify and address the underlying cause. For example, if you're taking any medications, consult your prescribing physician to determine whether any medications you're on could be causing the RLS. Next, diagnose and treat or rule out food allergies or sensitivities (see Chapter 13). Eliminate caffeine from your diet and avoid refined sugar and processed carbohydrates (see Chapter 2 for more about adopting a healthy diet). Support your nutrition with the following supplements:

Supplement	Dosage
Iron (ferrous bis-glycinate chelate)	30 mg twice daily (**Note:** Have your doctor check iron, total iron binding capacity [TIBC], and ferritin blood levels.)
Magnesium citrate	150 mg one hour before bedtime
Folate (5-MTHF)	2,000 to 10,000 mcg daily
Vitamin E (full-spectrum formula of tocopherols)	Follow the label instructions
5-HTP (controlled-release form)	100 mg two to three times daily (consult your doctor before taking this if you're on an SSRI antidepressant)

Getting a Leg Up on Sleepwalking

Sleepwalking consists of engaging in physical activities, such as walking, talking, or driving while asleep and not remembering it later. Sleepwalking is much more common in children between 3 and 7 years old than in adults. Contributing factors include sleep deprivation, sedatives (including alcohol and sleeping pills), certain medications, stress, and fever. To reduce or eliminate sleepwalking episodes, address the various contributing factors:

- ✔ If you're depressed or anxious, treat your depression and anxiety first. See Chapter 20 for details. People with depression, anxiety, and related conditions (for example, obsessive-compulsive disorder) are many times more likely than the general population to sleepwalk.

- ✔ Get more sleep. If you're having trouble getting to sleep or staying asleep, see "Overcoming Insomnia," earlier in this chapter, for details. Otherwise, you may simply need to go to bed earlier, wake up later, or both.

- ✔ Deal with stressful events or situations in your life and adopt a less stressful lifestyle (I offer pointers in Chapter 2).

Wind down before bedtime. See "Establishing a healthy sleep routine," earlier in this chapter, for suggestions on how to de-stress before bedtime.

✔ Stop drinking alcohol or limit your consumption to a couple drinks. If your "sleepwalking" is actually your drinking to the point of blacking out and doing things that you don't recall, you definitely need to take a serious look at how much you're drinking.

✔ Ask your doctor or pharmacist whether any of your medications may be causing you to sleepwalk. (Be particularly suspicious of sedatives.) If certain medications may be contributing to the problem, look into lowering the dosage or changing to a different medication.

If you've addressed all the factors that commonly contribute to sleepwalking and are still experiencing symptoms, try hypnosis.

If you have a child who sleepwalks, take precautions to ensure her safety. If she sleeps in a bunk bed, move her to the lower level or to a different bed. Remove any glass objects from around the bed. Installing a motion detector outside her bedroom may help alert you of when she's up during the night. Consider locking doors to the outside with deadbolt locks that require a key to open from inside the house; lock the doors and remove the key prior to bedtime. You may also want to fence off stairways.

Chapter 17

Tackling Chronic Health Conditions

Chronic health conditions are those that last a long time and are difficult to shake. Fortunately, this is the area of medicine where functional medicine tends to shine. While conventional medicine battles chronic illness with powerful pharmaceutical medications that often weaken the body in the process, functional medicine works to strengthen the body so that it can more effectively rid itself of disease. In this chapter, I provide the guidance you need to equip your body to battle a host of chronic illnesses — from cancer and cardiovascular disease to osteoporosis and stroke.

Doses in this chapter are for adults, not children. For guidance on how to adjust dosages for children (and adults under 150 pounds), turn to Chapter 12.

Combatting Cancer

Cancer is uncontrolled growth of abnormal cells that may be caused by numerous factors, including genetic susceptibility, inflammatory agents in the diet and other sources, health conditions (insulin resistance, diabetes, and obesity, for example), and exposure to environmental contaminants and toxins (pollution, radiation, herbicides, pesticides, and so on). You can't control everything in the world around you, but you can control most of what you put into your body.

Start by adopting a healthy diet and lifestyle, as explained in Chapter 2, with a focus on increasing protein consumption. For people without cancer, I recommend consuming about 0.36 gram of protein per pound of body weight daily. If you have cancer, increase your daily consumption of protein to 0.45 to 0.90 gram of protein per pound. For example, if you weigh 200 pounds, then you should consume at least 200 × 0.45 = 90 grams of protein daily. Double that to get the upper limit, which would be 180 grams in this example. Also supplement a healthy diet with the following:

Supplement	Dosage
Diindolylmethane	150 mg twice daily
Vitamin A (retinyl palmitate and beta-carotene)	2,500 IU retinyl palmitate and 2,500 IU beta-carotene daily (see Appendix A for precautions)
Vitamin C (mineral ascorbates)	1,000 mg daily
Whole beta glucan	500 mg one or two times daily
Vitamin D3	2,000 to 10,000 IU daily, depending on blood levels (see Appendix A)
Vitamin E (mixed tocopherols)	400 IU daily
Vitamin B12 (methylcobalamin, sublingual fast-dissolving tablet)	1,000 to 5,000 mcg daily
Folate (5-MTHF)	1,000 to 2,000 mcg daily
Curcumin	1 to 2 g daily
Resveratrol	75 mg one or two times daily
S-acetyl glutathione	200 mg one or two times daily
Fermented wheat germ extract	5.5 g one or two times daily
Glucoraphanin (from broccoli extract) (SGS)	100 mg twice daily
Calcium glycinate chelate	150 mg daily
Magnesium glycinate chelate	125 mg twice daily
Potassium glycinate	50 mg twice daily
Selenium glycinate	100 mcg twice daily
Zinc glycinate chelate	20 mg twice daily

If you're receiving medical treatment for cancer, consult with your doctor before taking supplements. Certain supplements may interfere with chemotherapy and other medications.

In addition to diet and supplements, do what you can to reduce stress in your life. Consider centering disciplines, such as yoga, Qigong, tai chi, and mindfulness mediation. Make sure you're getting approximately eight hours of sleep per night.

Easing Chronic Fatigue Syndrome (CFS) and Fibromyalgia

Chronic fatigue syndrome (CFS) is unexplained fatigue lasting more than four months that significantly interferes with your functioning and is often associated with body aches, foggy brain, poor sleep, increased thirst, gastrointestinal issues (including irritable bowel syndrome), persistent infections (including sore throats, sinusitis, and the common cold), feeling worse the day after exercise, and multiple chemical sensitivities. Fibromyalgia is closely related to CFS but is characterized more by pain than by fatigue; many of those with fibromyalgia have tender knots in the muscles commonly referred to as *trigger points*.

To recover from CFS and fibromyalgia, you need to degunk and reenergize your body, starting with your diet. Adopt a healthy diet (see Chapter 2), replacing manufactured foods with whole foods — fresh, organic vegetables, fruits, nuts, legumes, seafood, lean meats, and healthy fats. Steer clear of dairy, grains (especially in the form of breads, baked goods, pasta, and cereals), refined sugars and other processed foods, legumes, and starches. Drink 8 ounces of pure water every two hours. Limit consumption of alcohol and caffeine. (A Paleo diet is a good option; for guidance, check out *Living Paleo For Dummies*, by Melissa Joulwan and Kellyann Petrucci [John Wiley & Sons, Inc.].)

The vast majority of CFS patients also need to be treated for yeast overgrowth. See Chapter 19 for details on treating yeast overgrowth.

If you have either CFS or fibromyalgia, apply the *sleep, hormonal support, infections, and nutritional support (SHIN)* protocol:

✔ **Sleep:** Make sure you're getting about eight hours of sleep nightly. Chapter 16 has more on dealing with sleep issues.

✔ **Hormonal support:** Get tested for and address any hormone problems and nutritional deficiencies. See Chapter 18 for more about diagnosing and treating hormone imbalances related to the adrenal and thyroid glands.

✔ **Infections:** Clean up bowel, parasitic, bacterial, fungal, and sinus infections by supplementing your diet with the following digestion and immune system support:

Supplement	Dosage
Probiotics (*Saccharomyces boulardii;* a proprietary blend of a multistrain probiotic containing *Lactobacillus acidophilus, Bifidobacterium longum,* and *Lactobacillus plantarum;* and *Bifidobacterium lactis* HNO 19 [HOWARU Bifido])	250 mg *Saccharomyces boulardii* twice daily; 50 billion CFU multistrain probiotic daily; 50 billion CFU HOWARU Bifido once daily

(continued)

(continued)

Supplement	Dosage
Monolaurin	200 mg twice daily
L-lysine	150 mg twice daily
Bee propolis	100 mg twice daily
Cinnamon bark extract	100 mg twice daily
Grapeseed extract	100 mg twice daily
Olive leaf extract	50 mg twice daily
Oregano extract	300 mg twice daily
Ginger	300 mg twice daily
Turmeric extract	200 mg twice daily
Olive extract	100 mg twice daily

✔ **Nutritional support:** Take the highest quality multivitamin/mineral formula available containing the more utilizable forms of the B vitamins and all the minerals in the form of glycinated chelates. Specifically, make sure you're supplementing your diet with the following:

Supplement	Dosage
D-ribose	5 g three times daily
Iron (ferrous bis-glycinate chelate)	30 mg up to twice daily, depending on blood levels (see Appendix A)
Vitamin B12 (methylcobalamin, sublingual fast-dissolving tablet)	5,000 to 10,000 mcg once daily
CoQ10 (Kaneka Q10)	200 to 400 mg daily
Vitamin D3	2,000 to 10,000 IU daily, depending on blood levels (see Appendix A)

To relieve the pain that accompanies CFS and fibromyalgia, take the following supplements:

Supplement	Dosage
White willow bark extract	600 mg one or two times daily between meals
Boswellia	100 mg one or two times daily between meals
Turmeric	200 mg one or two times daily between meals

You can stop all treatments after 6 to 12 months. Stay on the multivitamin/mineral, sleep support, D-ribose, and CoQ10 indefinitely.

Dealing with Cardiovascular Conditions and Stroke

Your *cardiovascular* system, consisting of your heart, veins, and arteries, circulates blood throughout your body. Over time, this system begins to show signs of wear and tear as it become subjected to *vascular insults* — injuries caused by anything from high blood pressure and fluctuating glucose levels to exposure to nicotine and alcohol. In addition, several cardiovascular conditions, including atherosclerosis, heart arrhythmia, and high blood pressure, increase the risk of stroke, so it's important to address any of these underlying conditions.

The natural cures approach to treating cardiovascular conditions and stroke is to provide the body with the nutrients it needs to prevent and recover from inflammation, oxidative stress, autoimmune dysfunction, altered gene expression, and tissue damage. In this section, I provide guidance on how to strengthen your cardiovascular system overall and then go on to address specific conditions, such as arrhythmia, atherosclerosis, heart attack, and stroke.

Improving cardiovascular health

To improve cardiovascular health, adopt a healthy diet and lifestyle, as explained in Chapter 2. Following are more specific recommendations:

- ✔ **Eat 30 percent fewer calories daily.** *Caloric restriction (CR)* reduces oxidative stress, inflammation, and autoimmune dysfunction and increases cellular energy.

  One simple way to lower your calorie intake is to eliminate wheat from your diet. Wheat stimulates the appetite; cutting wheat from your diet eliminates about 400 calories daily.

- ✔ **Fast for about 12 hours daily seven days a week.** Fast from 3 hours before bedtime until you wake up the next morning to give your digestive and cardiovascular systems a break.

- ✔ **Eat low on the glycemic index (GI).** Make most of what you eat protein and nonstarchy vegetables and fruits. Eat eight servings of low-GI vegetables and two servings of low-GI fruits daily. Avoid sugary and processed foods.

- ✔ **Eliminate trans fats.** Trans fats are mostly in the form of hydrogenated and partially hydrogenated oils used in processed foods and to fry foods in fast-food restaurants. Trans fats increase your risk of heart disease, stroke, type 2 diabetes, and other chronic conditions.

Eat monounsaturated fats (MUFAs) and select polyunsaturated fats (PUFAs), instead. MUFAs are found in nuts, avocados, and most vegetable oils, including olive, sunflower, safflower, peanut, and sesame oils. Good sources of PUFAs are walnuts, flaxseed, fatty fish (especially salmon, mackerel, tuna, sardines, and herring), algae, leafy green vegetables, and krill.

✔ **Check for and treat vitamin and mineral deficiencies.** Vitamins C, E, and B9 (folate) and the mineral selenium play key roles in cardiovascular health.

✔ **Consume 45 to 50 total grams of dietary fiber daily.** You can supplement with psyllium husks, if necessary.

✔ **Enhance your diet with heart-healthy supplements.** Antioxidants and anti-inflammatories, such as resveratrol, quercetin, red wine, green tea, dark chocolate, and flavonoids (especially diadzein and genistein from non-GMO soybeans), provide strong support for a healthy cardiovascular system.

✔ **Stay physically active.** If possible, engage in aerobic exercise for 30 minutes at least every other day, along with strength training at least three days a week.

✔ **Reduce stress.** Chronic stress increases your risk for heart disease and many other illnesses. Although you can't eliminate stress from your life, you can make reducing stress a top priority and take steps to manage stressful situations (and people) more effectively.

✔ **Get sufficient sleep.** Try to sleep approximately eight hours nightly. If you're having trouble sleeping, see Chapter 16 for suggestions.

You may be able to reduce your risk for many cardiovascular conditions, including atherosclerosis and stroke, by lowering your homocysteine levels. *Homocysteine* is an abrasive molecule that can scrape the inside lining of the arteries, increasing fatty plaque deposits. You should have your homocysteine levels checked occasionally; a healthy level is 5 to 8 micro-mol/L. To reduce homocysteine levels, follow the homocysteine-lowering protocol:

Supplement	*Dosage*
Vitamin B2 (riboflavin 5'-phosphate)	25 mg twice daily
Vitamin B6 (pyridoxine 5'-phosphate)	10 mg twice daily
Vitamin B12 (methylcobalamin, sublingual fast-dissolving tablet)	1,000 mcg daily
Folate (5-MTHF)	2,000 mcg daily
Trimethylglycine	500 mg twice daily
SAMe	200 mg twice daily

Alleviating angina

Angina is chest tightness or pain caused by insufficient blood supply to the heart. Angina can be caused by atherosclerosis (hardening or narrowing of the arteries), hypoglycemia (low blood sugar), or inflammation affecting the cardiovascular system. The first step to preventing and treating angina is to adopt a heart-healthy diet and lifestyle; see the earlier section "Improving cardiovascular health" for details.

Seek immediate medical attention for any chest tightness or pain. Angina is an early warning sign that you're at an increased risk for heart attack.

In addition to adopting a heart-healthy diet and lifestyle, increase the nitric oxide concentration in your blood. Nitric oxide is a powerful *vasodilator* (it expands the blood vessels). To increase your body's nitric oxide production, supplement your diet with the following:

Supplement	Dosage
L-arginine	2 g twice daily (see Appendix B for precautions)
Citrulline	500 mg twice daily
S-acetyl glutathione	200 mg twice daily
Aspirin	81 mg daily

Take L-arginine, citrulline, and glutathione on an empty stomach for best results.

Additional nutrients for treating angina include the following:

Supplement	Dosage
Magnesium glycinate chelate	125 mg twice daily
Acetyl-L-carnitine	350 mg twice daily
CoQ10 (Kaneka Q10)	100 to 400 mg daily
Omega-3 essential fatty acids (EFAs)	1 g yielding 180 mg EPA and 120 mg DHA four times daily
Vitamin E (mixed tocopherols)	400 IU daily
D-ribose	5 g three to four times daily (see Appendix B for precautions)
Vitamin D3	2,000 to 10,000 IU daily, depending on blood levels (see Appendix A)

Calming an erratic heartbeat: Arrhythmia

Arrhythmia is any abnormal heartbeat, including *arterial fibrillation* (fluttering), *tachycardia* (beating too fast), and *bradycardia* (beating too slow).

The first step is to get tested for food allergies and sensitivities (see Chapter 13) so that you can confirm or rule out those conditions. Eliminate caffeine, nicotine, alcohol, aspartame, and monosodium glutamate from you diet to see whether symptoms improve.

Next, adopt a healthy diet (see Chapter 2), and supplement your diet with the following nutrients, if necessary:

Supplement	Dosage
Magnesium glycinate chelate	125 mg twice daily
Potassium glycinate complex	300 mg one or two times daily, only under close medical supervision
Omega-3 essential fatty acids (EFAs)	1 g yielding 180 mg EPA and 120 mg DHA four times daily
Selenium	100 to 200 mcg daily
Copper glycinate chelate	1 to 4 mg daily
Vitamin C (mineral ascorbates)	1,000 mg twice daily
Vitamin D3	2,000 to 10,000 IU daily, depending on blood levels (see Appendix A)
D-ribose	5 g two to three times daily (see Appendix B for precautions)
CoQ10 (Kaneka Q10)	100 to 400 mg daily

Improving circulation: Atherosclerosis

Atherosclerosis is inflammation and fatty plaque buildup on the interior walls of the arteries, restricting blood flow. Atherosclerosis takes a long time to develop and doesn't start to produce symptoms until the blockage is fairly advanced. Your doctor can perform a variety of tests to determine the level of plaque buildup in your arteries. To prevent and reverse the course of inflammation and plaque buildup, start by adopting a heart-healthy diet and lifestyle; see the earlier section "Improving cardiovascular health" for details.

To determine your risk of developing atherosclerosis, your doctor may order a test to evaluate the level of lipoprotein (a) in your blood. *Lipoproteins* are molecules made of fats and proteins. Lipoprotein (a) is made in the liver and can accumulate in the endothelium, contributing to atherosclerosis, inflammation, and the formation of *foam cells* — immune cells formed in response to excess cholesterol. Lipoprotein (a) can contribute to blood clot formation. The vertical auto profile (VAP) blood test or the advanced cardiovascular test (ACT) will include this measurement, which is not performed with traditional testing.

Cook in a way that minimizes the formation of *atherogenic compounds*, which promote the formation of fatty plaque in the arteries. Store vegetable oils, butter, meat, dairy, and nuts in airtight containers. Avoid cooking at very high temperatures. For high-temp cooking, use palm or coconut oil; use olive oil for medium heat.

To help keep your blood vessels clear of plaque, make sure you're getting sufficient amounts of the following nutrients:

Supplement	*Dosage*
Omega-3 essential fatty acids (EFAs)	1 g yielding 180 mg EPA and 120 mg DHA four times daily
Vitamin E (mixed tocopherols)	400 IU daily
Trans resveratrol	200 mg twice daily
N-acetyl cysteine	1 to 2 g daily
CoQ10 (Kaneka Q10)	100 to 400 mg daily
Vitamin K2 (menaquinone-7)	45 mcg twice daily
Vitamin D3	2,000 to 10,000 IU daily, depending on blood levels (see Appendix A)
Magnesium glycinate chelate	125 mg twice daily
Whey protein	40 g daily
B vitamins (high-quality formula with the more bioavailable forms in a substantial dose)	Follow label instructions (see Appendix A)
Vitamin C (mineral ascorbates)	1,000 mg twice daily

Atherosclerosis has been linked to high levels of homocysteine in the blood. See the earlier section "Improving cardiovascular health" to find out how to lower your homocysteine levels.

TIP

Making your own exercise drink

Exercise in the morning after a 12-hour fast. Blend the following ingredients to make your own exercise drink and drink it during breaks in your exercise session to maintain healthy veins and arteries:

- 8 ounces of fresh orange juice diluted with water to 24 ounces

- 10 g of D-ribose

- 40 g whey protein

- 2 g buffered vitamin C powder

- 3,000 mg L-glutamine powder

- 2 g acetyl-L-carnitine powder

- 2,000 mg L-arginine powder

A recent study also shows that a combination of moderate red or white wine consumption five days a week and regular exercise (at least twice a week) reduces the risk of cardiovascular disease, including atherosclerosis. Moderate consumption in the study meant 0.3 to 0.4 liters (about two-and-a-half glasses) daily for men and 0.2 to 0.3 liters (one to two glasses) daily for women. However, I recommend that you drink no more than a couple ounces of wine daily.

Recovering from a heart attack

A *heart attack (myocardial infarction)* occurs when the blood supply to part of the heart muscle is totally cut off. Symptoms range from mild indigestion and heartburn to crushing tightness in the chest radiating down the arms and into the upper back and jaw, possibly accompanied by profuse sweating, ringing in the ears, and a drop in blood pressure.

WARNING!

If you're experiencing heart attack symptoms, call 911 immediately. Emergency medical attention can stop a heart attack in its tracks. Popping an aspirin may also help, but call 911 first and take aspirin only if directed to do so by medical personnel. If you're allergic to aspirin or are having a stroke due to a ruptured blood vessel, taking an aspirin is likely to do more harm than good.

For general recommendations on improving cardiovascular disease and preventing heart attacks, see the earlier section "Improving cardiovascular health." Consider supplementing your diet with the following heart attack prevention nutrients:

Supplement	*Dosage*
Omega-3 essential fatty acids (EFAs)	1 g yielding 180 mg EPA and 120 mg DHA four times daily
Vitamin E (tocopherols and tocotrienols)	400 IU daily

Supplement	Dosage
Trans resveratrol	200 mg twice daily
N-acetyl cysteine	1 to 2 g daily
CoQ10 (Kaneka Q10)	100 to 400 mg daily
Vitamin K2 (menaquinone-7)	45 mcg twice daily
Vitamin D3	2,000 to 10,000 IU daily, depending on blood levels (see Appendix A)
Magnesium glycinate chelate	125 mg twice daily
Whey protein	40 g daily
B vitamins (high-quality formula with the more bioavailable forms in a substantial dose)	Follow label instructions
Vitamin C (mineral ascorbates)	1,000 mg twice daily
L-carnitine tartrate	340 mg twice daily
D-ribose	5 g two to three times daily (see Appendix B for precautions)
Alpha-lipoic acid (controlled release)	600 mg 15 to 30 minutes before breakfast and dinner

Lowering high blood pressure (hypertension)

Blood pressure is the measure of force of the blood pushing against the walls of the blood vessels. Normal blood pressure is 120/80 mm Hg (millimeters of mercury); anything over 140/90 mm Hg is considered high. (The top number is *systolic pressure*, measured when the heart muscle is fully contracted; the bottom number is *diastolic pressure*, measured when the heart muscle is fully relaxed.) Having high blood pressure (hypertension) increases your risk of developing cardiovascular disease.

Standard blood pressure measurements can be inadequate and often misleading. I recommend getting an EndoPAT assessment, which looks at small artery elasticity, which conventional blood pressure measurements don't consider. Visit www.itamar-medical.com for details and to search for a provider near you that can conduct the assessment.

The first step in addressing high blood pressure is to adopt a healthy diet and lifestyle, as explained in the earlier section "Improving cardiovascular health." You'll be surprised at how much your blood pressure drops simply by eliminating sugar and high-glycemic foods.

Conventional medicine typically treats high blood pressure with several different classes of medications, including diuretics (which stimulate elimination of fluids), beta blockers (to block adrenaline and slow the heart-beat), calcium-channel blockers (to relax blood vessels), and angiotensin-converting-enzyme (ACE) inhibitors and other vasodilators (to expand blood vessels). Nature provides equivalents for all of these manufactured pharmaceuticals. Talk to your healthcare provider about the possibility of replacing any of your current medications with these natural alternatives or adding one or more of these to your current treatments (don't self-medicate):

Supplement	*Dosage*
Natural diuretics	
Vitamin B6 (pyridoxal 5'-phosphate)	35 mg twice daily
Taurine	250 mg twice daily
Celery	4 stalks daily
Magnesium glycinate chelate	125 mg twice daily
Protein	0.36 g per pound of body weight
CoQ10 (Kaneka Q10)	100 to 400 mg daily
Acetyl-L-carnitine	350 mg twice daily
Natural beta blocker	
Hawthorn berry	400 mg daily
Natural vasodilators	
L-arginine	2 g twice daily (see Appendix B for precautions)
Citrulline	500 mg twice daily
Omega-3 essential fatty acids (EFAs)	1 g yielding 180 mg EP and 120 mg DHA four times daily
Monounsaturated fatty acids (MUFAs)	10 ounces daily
Potassium	125 mg twice daily (see Appendix A for precautions)
Magnesium glycinate chelate	125 mg twice daily
Vitamin C (mineral ascorbates)	1,000 mg two to three times daily
Vitamin D3	2,000 to 10,000 IU daily, depending on blood levels (see Appendix A)
CoQ10 (Kaneka Q10)	100 to 400 mg daily
Natural calcium channel blockers	
Alpha-lipoic acid (controlled release)	200 mg daily
Magnesium glycinate chelate	200 mg daily
N-acetyl cysteine	500 mg daily
Vitamin C (mineral ascorbates)	1,000 mg daily
Vitamin E (tocopherols)	400 IU daily

Natural angiotensin-converting enzyme (ACE) inhibitors

Seaweed (dried wakame)	3.3 g daily
Sardines (valyl-tyrosine)	3 g daily
Bonito fish *(Sarda orientalis)*	1.5 g daily
Hydrolyzed whey protein	30 g daily
Omega-3 essential fatty acids (EFAs)	4 g daily with a ratio of 3 parts EPA to 2 parts DHA
Egg yolks	Several pastured eggs per week
Pomegranate	125 mg daily

Natural angiotensin receptor blockers (ARBs)

Potassium	250 mg daily (see Appendix A for precautions)
Trans resveratrol	200 mg daily
CoQ10 (Kaneka Q10)	100 to 400 mg daily
Gamma-linolenic acid	250 mg twice daily

Nitric oxide is a powerful vasodilator that also reduces inflammation, oxidative stress, and cardiovascular immune dysfunction. See the earlier section, "Alleviating angina," for details on increasing your body's nitric acid production.

Getting the straight story on cholesterol

If you've been diagnosed with high cholesterol, don't worry — it may not be a problem. Don't rush to go on a low-fat diet or take statin drugs, which can do more harm than good. Neither your overall cholesterol level nor your ratio of "good" HDL to "bad" LDL cholesterol necessarily affects your risk of cardio-vascular disease. A traditional lipid panel indicating your total cholesterol, HDL, LDL, and triglycerides can give you a very limited picture.

What drives the risk of cardiovascular disease is LDL particle size and the number of small, dense LDL particles. Picture the lining of your arteries as a tennis net. LDL particles the size of tennis balls won't pass through the net, but if they're the size of golf balls, they will. Small LDL particles pass through the lining of the arteries, get stuck there, and trigger the formation of fatty plaques. Small LDL particles along with a high homocysteine level, elevated lipoprotein (a), and other factors can be better assessed through a vertical auto profile (VAP) blood test rather than a traditional lipid panel.

Insist that your doctor order an *expanded lipid panel*, which reports LDL particle size and number. If the number of small LDL particles is abnormally large, take steps to reverse this unhealthy trend:

- ✔ Work toward achieving your ideal weight and body fat composition — less than 18 percent body fat for men and less than 28 percent for women.

  Body mass index (BMI) charts are readily available online to give you a ballpark idea of healthy weights based on your height.

- ✔ Adopt a Mediterranean-style diet, including plant sterols, soy foods (non-GMO), almonds, fibers, okra, and eggplant. Check out *Mediterranean Diet For Dummies,* by Rachel Berman (John Wiley & Sons, Inc.) for details.

- ✔ Team up with your healthcare provider to combine lipid-lowering medications with nutritional and nutraceutical therapies, including the following:

Supplement	*Dosage*
Curcumin	250 mg twice daily
Red yeast rice	500 mg twice daily (see note following table)
Quercetin	250 mg one to two times daily
Lycopene	4 mg twice daily
Green tea extract	250 mg twice daily
Trans resveratrol	40 mg twice daily
N-acetyl cysteine	250 mg twice daily
DGL licorice	100 mg twice daily
Berberine	200 mg twice daily
Phytosterols	800 mg twice daily
Aged garlic extract	600 mg twice daily
Omega-3 essential fatty acids (EFAs)	1 g yielding 180 mg EPA and 120 mg DHA four times daily

Niacin (B3) significantly increases HDL and HDL particle size and lowers lipoprotein (a) levels and has been shown to reduce cardiovascular disease and events by 26 percent and total mortality by 11 percent over six years. Take 1 to 4 g daily of niacin as nicotinic acid (*not* nicotinamide or hexanicotinate) while monitoring for possible undesirable side effects, which may include hyperglycemia, gout, hepatitis, flushing, elevated homocysteine, bruising, and palpitations (see Appendix A for precautions). Try one or more of the following techniques to lessen the flushing effect of niacin (tingling or itchy red skin that passes within about 30 minutes):

- ✔ Take a slower delivery form. I use a product that includes a wax coating to minimize flushing.

- ✔ Start by taking 100 mg daily and increase your dosage by 100 mg each week until you reach the maximum dosage.

- ✔ Take with food. Apple, applesauce, or apple pectin is best.

- ✔ Avoid alcohol.

- ✔ Take your niacin every day. If you start and stop, your body needs to readjust again.

- ✔ Take with baby aspirin.

- ✔ Take 200 to 500 mg quercetin daily.

Recovering from a stroke

A *stroke* is a loss of brain function due to interrupted blood flow to the brain, caused by a blocked or ruptured blood vessel. Symptoms may include weakness along one side of the body, slurred speech, vision loss, confusion, sudden intense headache (unlike anything you've ever experienced), dizziness, impaired balance, and unconsciousness. *Silent strokes* are those that go unnoticed, but over time, a series of silent strokes may cause significant brain damage.

If you have symptoms of a stroke, have someone drive you to the nearest emergency room immediately or call 911. Immediate medical treatment can prevent debilitating brain damage.

Stroke is highly preventable. Get tested to gauge your stroke risk and adjust your diet and lifestyle accordingly to lower your risk. See Chapter 2 for more about adopting a healthy diet and lifestyle with a focus on the following:

- ✔ Increasing consumption of oily fish, nuts, seeds, pastured animal products, and plenty of colorful vegetables rich in antioxidants. Dark purple organic fruits and vegetables (berries, grapes, eggplant, and cabbage) are best for preventing stroke.

- ✔ Eliminating refined sugar from your diet. Eating sugary fruit in moderation is okay, but avoid fruit juices, organic or otherwise. An 8-ounce glass of OJ contains as much sugar as a soda; you'd eat *one* orange at a sitting, *not* ten.

- ✔ Consume at least 4 g of fish oil daily and supplement with cod liver oil for additional DHA (docosahexaenoic acid), as necessary. Seventy-five percent of your brain is fat, and 25 percent of that fat is from DHA.

✔ Cut down on saturated fats from dairy and red meat, and eliminate trans fats (hydrogenated and partially hydrogenated oils) entirely. Buy only grass-fed, organic, non-GMO, pastured animal products. Never eat margarine or fried foods.

✔ Consume only non-GMO foods. Visit www.nongmoshoppingguide.com to find out what's safe and what's not. (Almost all soybean products and canola oil have been altered by genetic modification, so be very selective when purchasing those.)

✔ Take the following supplements for stroke prevention:

Supplement	Dosage
Vinpocetine	5 mg twice daily (**Note:** Don't use if you've had a stroke due to a brain hemorrhage)
DHA (cod liver oil)	2 g daily
CoQ10 (Kaneka Q10)	200 to 400 mg daily
Vitamin E (tocopherols)	400 IU daily
Alpha-lipoic acid (controlled release)	600 mg twice daily 15 minutes before meals
Phosphatidylserine	100 mg twice daily
Acetyl-L-carnitine	400 mg twice daily
Vitamin D3	2,000 to 10,000 IU daily, depending on blood levels (see Appendix A)

Delving into Diabetes and Other Blood Sugar Illnesses

Numerous chronic illnesses involve the body's inability to regulate blood glucose (sugar) levels. With *type 1 diabetes*, the pancreas produces too little or no insulin, resulting in elevated blood glucose levels. Symptoms include increased urination and thirst, blurred vision, tingling pain in the hands or feet, and weight loss despite normal or increased eating. With *type 2 diabetes (insulin resistance),* the body doesn't use insulin properly to convert sugar into energy. As a result, the pancreas produces even more insulin, and the body converts the sugar into fat instead of into energy, leading to weight gain. Without effective treatment, the overworked pancreas eventually gives out, and the person experiences symptoms identical to those of type 1 diabetes and requires insulin injections.

Metabolic syndrome is a cluster of conditions, including increased blood pressure, elevated blood sugar, excess body fat around the waist, and abnormal cholesterol levels that increase the risk of diabetes, heart disease, and stroke. Diabetes and related conditions are occurring in epidemic proportions worldwide.

The cause of type 2 diabetes and metabolic syndrome isn't solely genetic but *epigenetic,* the interplay of nature and nurture — genetics influenced by environmental factors, primarily diet. Food and other substances you ingest are more than mere sources of energy and building blocks for bodily tissues and fluids. Everything you consume "talks" to your genes, and a thousand calories of broccoli say something a whole lot different than do a thousand calories of soda. Consuming a certain amount of junk food can transform a perfectly healthy human being into someone with metabolic syndrome or type 2 diabetes.

If you're taking medication for diabetes, such as insulin, consult with your doctor before making adjustments to diet and lifestyle or taking any supplements to treat your diabetes. Your doctor needs to monitor your blood glucose levels closely and adjust your medication as these natural treatments kick in and your body requires less or no medication to regulate glucose levels. Taking more insulin than your body needs can be deadly. If your blood sugar dips too low, creating a condition called *hypoglycemia,* you may experience blurred vision, rapid heartbeat, sudden nervousness or mood change, unexplained fatigue, headache, or hunger. Eat or drink something sugary, such as a tablespoon of honey, some juice, or a piece of hard candy, and seek immediate medical attention.

Eliminating problem foods from your diet

Whether you have type 1 or type 2 diabetes or metabolic syndrome, dietary and lifestyle changes can help to level out your blood sugar levels. Adopt a healthier diet and lifestyle, as explained in Chapter 2, with a focus on eliminating the following toxins and junk:

- **Trans fats:** Eliminate all processed foods from your diet, because even if the label indicates zero trans fats, the product may contain up to 0.5 grams of trans fats in accordance with government labeling laws.

- **Sugar:** Read labels and look for ingredients that end in *-ose:* glucose, fructose, sucrose, and so on. These are all sugars.

- **Problem foods:** Eliminate wheat (gluten) and dairy (casein) products from your diet, or get tested for sensitivities, as explained in Chapter 13, and adjust your diet accordingly.

- **Artificial sweeteners:** No study has ever proven that artificial sweeteners help people lose weight. These are manufactured toxins, and some may even stimulate insulin production contributing to weight gain.

- **Food additives, monosodium glutamate (MSG), colors, and preservatives:** Many are known to be harmful. You're rolling the dice when eating this stuff.

✔ **Genetically modified organisms (GMOs):** Changing the protein structure of wheat, corn, soy, and other produce is like playing Russian roulette with foods. The human body didn't evolve over millions of years to process these foods effectively. In fact, your immune system may reject these foods, causing inflammation and other serious health conditions. Eat nature-made foods, not those developed in labs.

✔ **Hormones, antibiotics, herbicides, and pesticides:** Commercial (non-organic) produce and livestock are loaded with these toxic substances. Eat organic.

✔ **Bisphenol (BPA):** BPA leaches into your food from plastic containers and wrap, increasing the risk of diabetes and other health conditions. Drink out of glass bottles and glasses instead of plastic cups and containers. Use glass, porcelain, or stainless steel containers instead of plastic containers. Never microwave plastic containers or plastic wrap.

Your doctor should also monitor your HgbA1c levels to determine how your body has processed sugar over the past 120 days. Sugar binds to the proteins of certain tissues, causing oxidation and inflammation.

Retooling your diet is one of the best ways to address two of the other prime contributors to diabetes and related illnesses: body weight and body fat. Work toward achieving your ideal weight and body fat composition — less than 18 percent body fat for men and less than 28 percent for women. Body fat percentage is more important than weight, but it's harder to measure. You can purchase a body fat scale that measures electrical impedance to estimate your ratio of fat to muscle (electricity passes more easily through muscle than it does through fat).

Boosting your body's ability to regulate glucose level

Here are some additional suggestions for boosting your body's ability to regulate its blood glucose levels:

✔ **Start your day with a blood sugar–stabilizing smoothie.** Replace your cereal, muffin, toast, bagel, or (egad!) donut, with a healthy smoothie. See Chapter 2 for a recipe, but if you're waking up with a blood glucose level above 125 mg/dl, then leave out the fruit.

Not all breakfast smoothies are created equal. Even health food stores carry poor quality products loaded with artificial colors and flavorings, sweeteners, and inferior ingredients. You're better off blending your own smoothie using quality, organic ingredients from reputable producers.

✔ **Consume at least 50 grams of fiber daily.** Mix it up with soluble and insoluble fiber.

✔ **Minimize alcohol consumption.** Two ounces daily is healthy. Much more than that is unhealthy.

✔ **Drink oolong or unsweetened green tea.** Drink 1 cup after meals.

✔ **Exercise.** Engage in aerobic exercise 30 minutes a day five days a week and some sort of strength training three days a week. Do something physical on your nonexercise days. Take a long walk or bike ride, go swimming, or do yard work.

✔ **Reduce stress.** Your blood glucose level rises in response to stress so that you have enough energy to deal with the stress. Try to prevent stressful situations from arising and learn to deal more effectively with such situations. Honing your communication and problem-solving skills goes a long way toward reducing stress. Centering disciplines, such as Qigong and yoga, are very helpful, as well.

✔ **Take the following supplements to help your body regulate blood glucose levels:**

Supplement	*Dosage*
Alpha-lipoic acid (controlled release)	200 mg 15 to 30 minutes prior to each meal
Cinnamon	200 mg twice daily
Gymnema	200 mg twice daily
Green tea extract (EGCG)	200 mg twice daily
Chromium glycinate chelate	200 mcg twice daily
Conjugated linoleic acid (derived from pure, non-GMO safflower oil)	1.5 g twice daily
Vitamin D3	2,000 to 10,000 IU daily, depending on blood levels (see Appendix A)
Brown seaweed blend	500 mg 20 to 30 minutes before meals that contain carbohydrates
Acetyl-L-carnitine	350 mg twice daily
Multivitamin/mineral (highest quality product available with the better forms of each vitamin and mineral; see Appendix A)	Follow label instructions
Omega-3 essential fatty acids (EFAs)	1 g yielding 180 mg EPA and 120 mg DHA four times daily

Supplementing for type 1 diabetes

If you have type 1 diabetes, follow my earlier recommendations for diet and supplements to control blood sugar levels naturally. In addition, you'll need to take insulin. I also recommend the following supplements:

Supplement	Dosage
Thiamine	100 mg twice daily
Biotin	10,000 mcg twice daily after meals
Fenugreek	300 mg twice daily
Bitter gourd	150 mg twice daily

Dealing with Autoimmune Disorders

An autoimmune disorder occurs when the body's immune system attacks healthy body tissue, such as blood vessels, the thyroid gland or pancreas, joints, muscles, red blood cells, or skin. Autoimmune disorder is at the root of many illnesses, including celiac disease (Chapter 13), Hashimoto's thyroiditis (Chapter 18), type 1 diabetes (preceding section), and lupus and multiple sclerosis, which I cover in this section.

Living well with lupus

Lupus is an inflammatory disease in which the immune system attacks healthy tissues of the joints, skin, blood cells, kidney, heart, and lungs. Symptoms include fatigue, sensitivity to sunlight, rash (usually on skin exposed to the sun), swollen lymph nodes, hair loss, low-grade fever, joint and muscle pain, neuropsychiatric disorder, and accelerated atherosclerosis. Testing for lupus antibodies in the blood can confirm or rule out lupus.

As with almost all autoimmune diseases, genetic susceptibility combined with intestinal permeability and environmental stressors are implicated in the onset of lupus. You can't do anything about your genetic susceptibility, but you can treat a leaky gut and reduce or eliminate environmental stressors. Here's how:

✔ **Heal your gut.** See Chapter 13 for more about curing a leaky gut.

✔ **Adopt an anti-inflammatory diet.** See Chapter 2 for more about healthy eating. Eliminate the following from your diet:

- **Inflammatory substances:** Saturated fats, caffeine, alcohol, and fried foods, because they cause systemic inflammation

- **Artificial coloring and flavoring:** Especially tartrazine (FD&C Yellow 5)

- **Alfalfa products:** Alfalfa contains an amino acid called L-canavanine that may increase inflammation

✔ **Get tested for food allergies and insensitivities and adjust your diet accordingly.** See Chapter 13 for more about food allergies and sensitivities. Wheat/gluten and dairy/casein are the usual culprits, but there could be others.

✔ **Consume healthy fats.** Eat oily fish caught in the wild (not farm-raised), including mackerel, lake trout, herring, salmon, and sardines. Add flaxseeds to your morning smoothie and salads. These omega-3 essential fatty acids can serve as anti-inflammatories.

✔ **Detox.** Enroll yourself in a supervised detoxification program for a minimum of ten days.

In addition to adopting an anti-inflammatory diet, take the following supplements to support a healthy gut and regulate your immune system:

Supplement	*Dosage*
Colostrum	10,000 mg daily
Proline-rich polypeptides extracted from bovine colostrum	4 sprays in mouth, hold for 30 seconds and swallow, twice daily early morning and before bed for a total of 16 mg daily
Omega-3 essential fatty acids (EFAs)	1 g yielding 180 mg EPA and 120 mg DHA four times daily
Vitamin D3	2,000 to 10,000 IU daily, depending on blood levels (see Appendix A)
MSM	1,000 mg two to three times daily
Boswellia	1,500 mg two to three times daily
Indole-3-carbinol	150 mg twice daily

Managing multiple sclerosis

Multiple sclerosis (MS) is a disease in which the immune system attacks nerve fibers and *myelin,* the fatty substance that surrounds and insulates nerve fibers, interfering with communication within the brain and between the brain and body. *Sclerosis* refers to the scar tissue of the damaged myelin. Symptoms include brain fog, impaired vision and balance, brain shrinkage, and muscle weakness.

Don't stop taking any medication your doctor prescribes. Instead, work with your doctor to complement medical treatment with nutrition and other natural remedies. Find a functional medicine doctor that can help you through your journey. Visit www.functionalmedicine.org, click Find a Practitioner, and use the resulting form to conduct your search.

To treat MS, follow these guidelines:

- **Stimulate your muscles.** Any physical activity stimulates the muscles. You can also try whole body vibration, in which you stand, sit, or lie down on a machine that vibrates your entire body. If you're having trouble with *foot drop* (the front of your foot drops as you walk), you can purchase products to help with that, including WalkAide (www.walkaide.com) and Bioness (www.bioness.com).

- **Improve your sleep.** See Chapter 16 for more about increasing the quantity and quality of the sleep you're getting.

- **Reduce stress.** Try to prevent and avoid stressful situations (and people) and learn to deal more effectively with stress. Honing your communication and problem-solving skills goes a long way toward reducing stress. Centering disciplines, such as Qigong and yoga, are very helpful, as well.

- **Heal your gut.** Many chronic health conditions, including MS, are related not only to what you eat, but also to how efficiently you absorb nutrients from your food and the permeability of your digestive system (leaky gut syndrome). See Chapter 13 for more about healing your gut.

- **Get tested for food allergies and insensitivities and adjust your diet accordingly.** See Chapter 13 for more about food allergies and sensitivities. Wheat/gluten and dairy/casein are the usual culprits, but there could be others.

- **Improve your diet.** Avoid excessive sugar consumption in any form (sucrose, glucose, fructose, lactose, honey, corn syrup, and so on). Eliminate wheat/gluten from your diet regardless of test results or what your doctor says. Eat natural whole foods, including organic vegetables, fruits, meats, seafood, nuts, and seeds. (See Chapter 2 for more about adopting a healthy diet.)

- **Supplement your diet with the following:**

Supplement	Dosage
CoQ10 (Kaneka Q10) B vitamins in their better forms: B6 (pyridoxal 5′-phosphate); folate (5-MTHF); and B12 (methylcobalamin, sublingual fast-dissolving tablet)	200 to 400 mg daily; 35 mg B6 (pyridoxal 5′-phosphate) twice daily; 5 mg folate (5-MTHF) twice daily; 5,000 mcg B12 (methylcobalamin) once daily

Supplement	Dosage
Vitamin C (mineral ascorbates)	1,000 mg two to three times daily
Vitamin D3	2,000 to 10,000 IU daily, depending on blood levels (see Appendix A)
Vitamin E (tocopherols)	400 IU daily
Calcium citrate	250 mg twice daily
Magnesium glycinate chelate	350 to 400 mg twice daily
Omega-3 essential fatty acids (EFAs)	1 g four times daily with an emphasis on higher levels of DHA as found in cod liver oil
Digestive enzymes (protease, amylase, and lipase)	50,000 to 100,000 USP protease; 50,000 to 100,000 USP amylase; 8,000 to 15,000 USP lipase with meals

Mitigating Migraines

A *migraine* is a throbbing headache on one side of the head accompanied by nausea, vomiting, and extreme sensitivity to light. If you have recurrent migraines, consult your doctor, who can perform tests to diagnose or rule out glaucoma, hypertension, brain tumors, or other conditions that may be causing your migraines. Other possible causes include dramatic blood sugar fluctuations; food allergies; certain foods including chocolate, cheese, citrus fruits; caffeine and alcohol (especially red wine); monosodium glutamate; aspartame; and severe stress and sleep deprivation.

Adopt a healthy diet, as explained in Chapter 2, and avoid any food triggers: refined sugar, caffeine, alcohol (especially red wine), salt, chocolate, and the others listed previously. Better yet, team up with a functional medicine doctor to develop a personalized nutritional plan. In addition to making dietary adjustments, consider taking the following supplements, which can reduce the frequency, severity, and duration of migraines:

Supplement	Dosage
Magnesium glycinate chelate	125 mg twice daily
CoQ10 (Kaneka Q10)	100 to 400 mg daily
Folate (5-MTHF)	5 mg daily
Vitamin C (mineral ascorbates)	1,000 mg three times daily
Vitamin D3	2,000 to 10,000 IU daily, depending on blood levels (see Appendix A)

(continued)

(continued)

Supplement	Dosage
Omega-3 essential fatty acids (EFAs)	1 g yielding 180 mg EPA and 120 mg DHA four times daily
Niacin (nicotinic acid)	500 mg immediately at first sign of migraine (see note following table)
Alpha-lipoic acid (controlled release)	600 mg before meals
Butterbur	75 mg twice daily
5-HTP (controlled release)	100 mg two to three times daily
Riboflavin	200 to 400 mg daily
Feverfew	300 mg daily

Niacin is likely to cause a flushing effect — red, itchy skin — that's not dangerous and passes within 30 minutes. Refer to the earlier section "Getting the straight story on cholesterol," which includes a discussion on mitigating these effects. (See Appendix A for additional precautions.)

Strengthening Your Bones: Osteoporosis

Osteoporosis means "porous bones." It's an inflammatory condition in which bones lose density over time. Symptoms include unexplained back pain, loss of height, a stooped posture, a *dowager's hump* (curvature or bowing of the upper back), and bones that fracture easily.

As with most illnesses, preventing osteoporosis is easier than curing it. Build a strong bone bank in your childhood, adolescent, and early adult years. After the age of 35, your bone bank has more withdrawals than deposits. If you have symptoms of osteoporosis or are over the age of 35 and are concerned about your bone density, get a bone density x-ray (DEXA).

If you have osteoporosis or simply want to take steps to improve your bone density, follow these suggestions:

✔ Test for and treat any food allergies or sensitivities, with a focus on gluten sensitivity (see Chapter 13).

✔ Adopt a healthy diet and lifestyle. Eliminate sugar, soda, caffeine, salt, and alcohol, all of which raise the body's acidity and contribute to bone loss. Consume a low-glycemic, anti-inflammatory diet. (See Chapter 2 for more about diet.)

✔ If you smoke, stop.

✔ Engage in weight-bearing exercise. Your bones need resistance to develop strength.

✔ Treat hormonal imbalances (see Chapter 18).

✔ Expose your skin to sunlight several times a week without getting sunburn. Doing so raises your vitamin D level. (Contrary to popular belief, drinking milk doesn't increase bone density.)

✔ Eat unprocessed, whole foods: vegetables, fruits, nuts, seeds, wild fish, and pastured animal products.

✔ Avoid unnecessary medications, including antacids, prednisone, and many others.

✔ Try the following supplements, which can help improve bone density:

Supplement	*Dosage*
Vitamin D3	2,000 to 10,000 IU daily, depending on blood levels (see Appendix A)
Vitamin K2 (menaquinone-7)	45 mcg twice daily (see Appendix A for precautions)
Calcium and phosphorous (MCHC)	2.2 g twice daily (see Appendix A)
Choline and silicon (choline stabilized orthosilicic acid)	60 mg twice daily
Strontium	680 mg in divided doses daily for just one year in high-risk patients; then reduce dosage (*Note:* Until long-term safety data is available don't take high-dose strontium indefinitely.)

✔ Get hormone levels tested and supplement only if necessary. (See Chapter 18 for details.)

Taking the Punch out of Parkinson's Disease

Parkinson's disease is a central nervous system disorder characterized by a reduction in *dopamine,* a neurotransmitter that regulates movement and emotional response. This reduction in dopamine results in tremor (shaking), stooped-forward posture, impaired movement (as if wearing cement boots), depression, anxiety, apathy, difficulty chewing, urinary incontinence, constipation, insomnia, and loss of libido. Pharmaceutical medications, including levodopa, are used to control symptoms, but they lose their effectiveness over time and may cause undesirable side effects, such as *dyskinesia* — involuntary movement.

Don't stop taking any medications your doctor prescribes. Instead, team up with your doctor to add natural remedies to your medication regimen and strive toward decreasing the amount of medication required to control symptoms.

Instead of merely increasing dopamine levels or stimulating dopamine receptors in the brain, the natural cures approach targets the cause of the decrease in dopamine. In Parkinson's disease, you need to extinguish the fire, not just the smoke by doing the following:

- ✔ **Drink 1 to 2 cups of coffee (not decaf) daily.** Opt for organic coffee with no added sweeteners. Caffeine protects against Parkinson's.

- ✔ **Adopt an anti-inflammatory diet.** Increase consumption of sulfur-containing foods, such as cruciferous vegetables (broccoli, cauliflower, brussels sprouts, and kale), which provide the raw material for glutathione, a powerful antioxidant.

- ✔ **Avoid processed food.** Eat only organic, pesticide-free produce; fish caught in the wild; and organic, pastured livestock free of antibiotics, growth hormones, and steroids.

- ✔ **Get glutathione injections three or more times a week.** Glutathione makes brain cells more sensitive to dopamine and helps detoxify the liver and lungs. Intravenous glutathione must be administered by a qualified healthcare professional. N-acetyl cysteine and alpha-lipoic acid increase glutathione, as well, but these, too, should be administered intravenously for optimum results.

- ✔ **Supplement your diet with the following nutrients:**

Supplement	Dosage
Vitamin E (tocopherols)	400 IU daily
Vitamin C (mineral ascorbates)	1,000 mg two to three times daily
Vitamin D3	2,000 to 10,000 IU daily, depending on blood levels (see Appendix A)
N-acetyl cysteine	1 to 2 g twice daily
Alpha-lipoic acid (controlled release)	600 mg twice daily 15 minutes before meals
DHA (cod liver oil)	550 mg twice daily
CoQ10 (Kaneka Q10)	200 to 400 mg daily
Phosphatidylserine	100 mg twice daily
Vinpocetine	5 mg twice daily (see Appendix B for precautions)

- ✔ **Follow the homocysteine lowering protocol.** See the earlier section "Improving cardiovascular health" for details.

Chapter 18

Targeting Adrenal and Thyroid Conditions

....

In This Chapter

▶ De-stressing your adrenal glands

▶ Sorting out issues with an overactive thyroid

▶ Compensating for an underactive thyroid

▶ Pumping up your pituitary gland

....

*F*our glands in the human body — two adrenal glands, the pituitary gland, and the thyroid gland — are often implicated in illnesses that may cause you to feel wired or tired. In conventional medicine, when a patient complains of metabolic symptoms like sudden weight loss or gain, increased or decreased appetite, irritability or fatigue, or inability to regulate body temperature, doctors commonly focus on the thyroid gland. Unfortunately, they often overlook the adrenal and pituitary glands, which may trigger or contribute to many of these symptoms.

If you're receiving treatment for what your doctor believes is a thyroid problem, and your symptoms aren't improving, or if you and your doctor can't figure out what's making you feel so wired or tired, you've come to the right place. In this chapter, I focus on common illnesses of the adrenal, pituitary, and thyroid glands and shed light on how the adrenal and pituitary glands can affect thyroid function.

Doses in this chapter are for adults, not children. For guidance on how to adjust dosages for children (and adults under 150 pounds), turn to Chapter 12.

Addressing Adrenal Fatigue and Stress

Adrenal fatigue (also known as *hypoadrenia* or *hypoadrenalism*) is a condition in which chronic, extreme stress stimulates the adrenal glands' production of the stress hormone cortisol to the point where the adrenals burn out and levels of cortisol and the cortisol-neutralizing agent DHEA (dehydroepiandrosterone) plummet.

Fluctuations in cortisol and DHEA affect your energy levels, emotions, and resistance to disease. Symptoms of adrenal fatigue include shakiness or irritability that is relieved by eating, recurrent sore throats, infections that take a long time to heal, fatigue, and weight gain (especially around the midsection). The two most common causes of adrenal fatigue are stress and prolonged treatment with corticosteroids (synthetic cortisone) such as prednisone.

Get a salivary adrenal stress assessment to measure your response to stress. For this assessment, you gather saliva samples at four timed intervals during the course of a stressful day and then send the samples off to a lab. The resulting stress profile indicates any exaggerated hormonal stress responses to determine whether you need to modify diet and lifestyle to deal more effectively with stress. I recommend timing the first morning saliva sample with a blood draw to get an accurate assessment of your morning cortisol levels. The levels of cortisol should be highest in the early morning and then gradually taper off so that you can fall asleep at night. If your cortisol levels are below normal in the morning, you probably have adrenal fatigue.

Every time you get worked up, your cortisol level rises and you suffer the consequences. For stressed-out adrenals that have been producing too much cortisol for long periods of time, I suggest taking a mental break. Try not to take on too much. Learn how to say no. Don't sweat the small stuff. Practice mindfulness meditation, yoga, or Qigong to train your body and mind to regulate mood and calm your emotions more effectively. You can also adopt a healthy diet, as I explain in Chapter 2, and take the following adrenal-support supplements:

Supplement	Dosage
Cordyceps mycelium extract	800 mg two to three times daily
Asian ginseng root extract	400 mg two to three times daily
Rhodiola root extract	100 mg two to three times daily
Adrenal gland extract (bovine)	25 mg twice daily
Vitamin C (mineral ascorbates)	1,000 mg daily

Supplement	*Dosage*
B vitamins (comprehensive B vitamin using the more utilizable forms; see Appendix A)	Read and follow the label instructions
L-tyrosine	1 to 2 g daily
N-acetyl cysteine	400 mg twice daily
Rehmannia root	1 g twice daily
L-theanine (suntheanine)	400 mg twice daily

Doctoring Thyroid Disorders

The *thyroid gland* secretes hormones that regulate your body's heartbeat, temperature, and *metabolism,* the chemical processes that occur in the body to maintain life. If the thyroid gland secretes too much hormone (a condition called *hyperthyroidism*), your metabolism is cranked up, resulting in sudden weight loss, rapid heartbeat, nervousness, tremor, sweating, increased sensitivity to heat, more frequent bowel movements, muscle weakness, and fatigue. If the thyroid secretes too little hormone (a much more common condition called *hypothyroidism*), your metabolism slows, resulting in fatigue, weight gain, increased sensitivity to cold, constipation, muscle aches and weakness, joint pain and stiffness, slower heart rate, depression, irregular or heavier than normal menstrual periods, and impaired memory.

If you're experiencing any of these symptoms, have your thyroid hormones and function tested. (For details on what a thyroid screening looks at, head to the nearby sidebar "What's involved in a thorough thyroid screen.")

Thyroid dysfunction may be caused by dysfunction of the adrenal or pituitary gland, so issues with those glands need to be diagnosed or ruled out prior to treating thyroid dysfunction. See the earlier section "Addressing Adrenal Fatigue and Stress" and the later section "Overcoming Pituitary Gland Dysfunction" for details.

To perform a preliminary evaluation of thyroid function at home, measure your *basal body temperature* — your body temperature first thing in the morning, before you get out of bed — over the course of several days. A healthy temperature is between 97.8 and 98.7 degrees Fahrenheit. If your temperature is consistently outside that range, further testing is required to confirm or rule out thyroid dysfunction. To test for hypothyroidism, get your iodine levels checked.

What's involved in a thorough thyroid screen

A thorough thyroid screening looks at the following factors:

✔ **Thyroid stimulating hormone (TSH):** The hormone released by your pituitary gland to trigger the thyroid to secrete its hormones. The range from most labs is too liberal and needs to be narrowed to 0.2–2.0 mcU/mL.

✔ **T4:** The amount of thyroid hormone stored in the thyroid gland.

✔ **T3:** The amount of T3, the gas that fuels metabolism, outside the thyroid gland. (T4 is converted to T3 prior to being secreted by the thyroid gland.)

✔ **Reverse T3 (RT3):** The amount of RT3, a brake that slows metabolism, outside the thyroid gland.

✔ **Thyroglobulin antibodies (TgAb):** Elevated TgAb levels may indicate deficiencies or illnesses affecting the thyroid gland.

✔ **Thyroid peroxidase (TPOAb) antibodies:** Elevated TPOAb antibodies indicate *Hashimoto's thyroiditis,* an autoimmune disorder that attacks the thyroid gland and causes hypothyroidism.

✔ **TSH receptor antibodies:** The presence TSH receptor antibodies indicates Graves' disease, an autoimmune disorder that attacks the thyroid gland and causes hyperthyroidism.

For all thyroid conditions, I recommend a gluten-free diet. Every time you ingest gluten, your immune system launches an attack against not only the gluten but also the thyroid. Even if you have gluten only one time a month, you're still vulnerable because the effects of an immune response can last months. All autoimmune thyroid patients should be screened for gluten sensitivity, and anyone with gluten sensitivity should be screened for autoimmune thyroid issues. Eliminating gluten from your diet won't cure your thyroid disorder, but it will lessen the immune response and spare your thyroid gland from such attacks.

Read on for more detailed recommendations for treating hyperthyroidism and hypothyroidism.

As you read these next sections, keep this caution in mind: Don't supplement with iodine if your tests show elevated thyroid antibodies indicating an autoimmune thyroid condition, such as Graves' disease (a kind of hyperthyroidism) or Hashimoto's thyroiditis (a type of hypothyroidism and the most common cause of hypothyroidism in the U.S.). Iodine increases production of the thyroid peroxidase (TPO) enzyme that triggers the autoimmune response. Also, don't self-prescribe. Iodine dosage needs to be personalized by a knowledgeable healthcare provider.

Treating hyperthyroidism

Hyperthyroidism is an overactive thyroid. Patients with hyperthyroid absorb too much iodine, which can be seen in a thyroid scan with radioactive iodine.

Conventional treatment involves deactivating, destroying, or removing the thyroid gland and then replacing thyroid hormones with levothyroxine (Synthroid) or similar medications. A natural approach focuses on diet modifications and supplements. Ditch the standard American diet and eat a healthy diet instead (see Chapter 2 for details): Eliminate gluten and dairy. Get tested for food allergies and eliminate the offending foods (see Chapter 13). Also take the following supplements for hyperthyroidism:

Supplement	*Dosage*
Bugleweed	2 ml three times daily
Acetyl-L-carnitine	700 mg twice daily
Lemon balm	2 ml three times daily
B vitamins (comprehensive B vitamin with therapeutic levels of each nutrient in the more utilizable forms; see Appendix A)	Read and follow label instructions

Graves' disease

Graves' disease, the most common form of hyperthyroidism, is characterized by bulging eyeballs, itchy or irritated eyes, itchy skin, and other symptoms of hyperthyroidism listed earlier in this section. In addition to testing and treating for food allergies and sensitivities, take the following supplements:

Supplement	*Dosage*
Comprehensive quality multivitamin/mineral	Follow label instructions
Magnesium glycinate chelate	125 mg twice daily
Acetyl-L-carnitine	700 mg twice daily
B vitamins (comprehensive B vitamin with therapeutic levels of each nutrient in the more utilizable forms; see Appendix A)	Read and follow label instructions
Vitamin D3	2,000 to 10,000 IU daily, depending on blood levels (see Appendix A)
Omega-3 essential fatty acids (EFAs)	1 g yielding 180 mg EPA and 120 mg DHA four times daily

Because Graves' disease is an autoimmune disorder, avoid iodine supplementation and foods high in iodine, such as kelp and other seaweeds.

Toxic adenomas

Toxic adenomas are benign tumors of the thyroid, adrenal, and pituitary glands that cause excess production of thyroid hormone. Treatment requires careful monitoring by a physician, the dietary changes recommended earlier in this section, and the following supplements to optimize thyroid health and function:

Supplement	Dosage
Vitamin A	1,500 IU twice daily (see Appendix A for precautions)
Vitamin D3	2,000 to 10,000 IU daily, depending on blood levels (see Appendix A)
Vitamin E	400 IU daily
Zinc glycinate chelate	20 mg daily
Selenium	100 mcg twice daily
Rosemary	50 mg twice daily
Ashwagandha	50 mg twice daily
Iodine	Test and supplement if necessary, usually at a very low dose (about 40 mcg)
Thyroid glandular	150 mg twice daily
Adrenal glandular	50 mg twice daily
L-tyrosine	30 mg twice daily

Stimulating an underactive thyroid: Hypothyroidism

Hypothyroidism is caused by an underactive thyroid and is usually the result of an iodine deficiency. With an underactive thyroid, everything works less efficiently in your body, including digestion. Get tested for iodine deficiency and follow your doctor's orders to modify and supplement your diet.

Eating iodine-rich foods can help. These foods include seaweed (kelp, wakame, nori, and dulse, for example), oily fish, and sea salt that has a little color to it. To optimize thyroid health, eat pumpkin seeds, walnuts, and flax-seeds, and don't drink tap water that's been treated with fluoride and chlorine, because these elements displace iodine in the thyroid gland, leading to hypothyroidism.

Avoid consuming large amounts of goitrogenic vegetables and soy and don't eat these vegetables or soy within an hour of taking thyroid hormones. Goitrogenic vegetables, including bok choy, broccoli, brussels sprouts, cabbage, cauliflower, kale, kohlrabi, radishes, and rutabagas, suppress thyroid function and interfere with iodine uptake. (Contrary to what "goitrogenic" implies, these foods don't cause goiter. A goiter typically results from undiagnosed Hashimoto's thyroiditis, unrelated to iodine deficiency.)

Although the Food and Nutrition Board recommends that adults consume 150 mcg of iodine daily, you can safely take up to 12 mg and may need to take as much as 25 to 50 mg daily. Your iodine dosage really needs to be tailored to you and your condition; consult your healthcare provider to determine whether iodine supplementation is right for you and how much to take. Also, if you take calcium, take your iodine and calcium at least four hours apart.

Don't take an iodine supplement if tests show that you have elevated TPO and thyroid globulin antibodies.

To support overall thyroid health, supplement your diet with the following:

Supplement	Dosage
Vitamin A	1,500 IU twice daily (see Appendix A for precautions)
Vitamin D3	2,000 to 10,000 IU daily, depending on blood levels (see Appendix A)
Vitamin E	400 IU daily
Zinc glycinate chelate	20 mg daily
Selenium	100 mcg twice daily
Rosemary	50 mg twice daily
Ashwagandha	50 mg twice daily
Thyroid glandular	150 mg twice daily
Adrenal glandular	50 mg twice daily
L-tyrosine	30 mg twice daily
Dulse	400 mg twice daily
Irish moss	40 mg twice daily
Bladderwrack (whole plant)	15 mg twice daily

I also recommend the following supplements to support mitochondrial health (cellular energy), digestion, weight loss, and glutathione production:

Supplement	Dosage
D-ribose	5 g two to three times daily
CoQ10 (Kaneka Q10)	100 mg twice daily

(continued)

(continued)

Supplement	Dosage
Acetyl-L-carnitine	500 mg twice daily for three months and then 250 to 500 mg daily
Digestive enzymes (protease, amylase, and lipase)	50,000 to 100,000 USP protease, 50,000 to 100,000 USP amylase, and 8,000 to 15,000 USP lipase, with meals
Vitamin B12 (methylcobalamin, sublingual fast-dissolving tablets)	5,000 mcg one or two times daily
N-acetyl cysteine	400 mg twice daily

Hashimoto's thyroiditis is an autoimmune condition characterized by progressive destruction of the thyroid gland over a period of months or years. If you suspect Hashimoto's thyroiditis, ask your doctor to run a test (refer to the earlier sidebar "What's involved in a thorough thyroid screen" for details on how to test for Hashimoto's thyroiditis) and, if necessary, treat food allergies or sensitivities first, as explained in Chapter 13. Gluten sensitivity is a very common contributing factor for Hashimoto's thyroiditis, so eliminate gluten from your diet, regardless of whether you test positive for gluten sensitivity.

If you have Hashimoto's thyroiditis, avoid high doses of iodine supplements and foods that are high in iodine — kelp and other seaweeds — because iodine increases production of the thyroid peroxidase (TPO) enzyme that triggers the autoimmune response, worsening the condition. Along with the supplements listed earlier in the section "Toxic adenomas" for overall thyroid health, take a natural T4/T3 supplement, such as Nature-Throid or Armour Thyroid, to boost your thyroid hormone levels.

Overcoming Pituitary Gland Dysfunction

The pituitary gland relays orders from the captain of the ship, the *hypothalamus* (the section of the brain responsible for hormone production), to the adrenal and thyroid glands. When the pituitary gland malfunctions, it fails to communicate with the thyroid, which may contribute to hypothyroidism.

Several factors may contribute to pituitary gland dysfunction, including poor diet, inadequate sleep, stress, excess caffeine, chronic inflammation, chronic bacterial or viral infection, and pregnancy. Misuse of thyroid medications may also create a harmful feedback loop signaling the pituitary gland of the presence of excess thyroid hormone. As a result, the pituitary gland stops signaling the thyroid gland to produce hormones — a condition that may become permanent, leading to a lifetime of thyroid medication.

To support proper function of the pituitary gland, reduce stress, get plenty of quality sleep (see Chapter 16), adopt a healthy diet (see Chapter 2), treat any underlying adrenal issues (see the earlier section "Addressing Adrenal Fatigue and Stress"), and take the following supplements:

Supplement	*Dosage*
Thyroid glandular (porcine)	150 mg twice daily
Pituitary glandular (porcine)	15 mg twice daily
Sage leaf extract	5 ml twice daily
L-arginine	2 g twice daily
Gamma oryzanal	25 mg twice daily
Magnesium glycinate chelate	250 mg daily
Zinc glycinate chelate	20 mg twice daily
Manganese	2 mg daily

Don't try to fly solo. Work closely with a functional medicine practitioner to ensure that your body is getting the nutrients it needs to support pituitary gland health and function. Visit the Institute for Functional Medicine (www.functionalmedicine.org), click Find A Practitioner, and use the resulting form to track down a functional medicine practitioner near you.

Chapter 19

Addressing Sexual and Reproductive Health Conditions

• •

In This Chapter

▶ Attending to female and male sexual health issues

▶ Taking a look at infertility

▶ Treating sexually transmitted diseases (STDs)

• •

A significant portion of the human anatomy is devoted to ensuring survival of the species through reproduction. Unfortunately, the reproductive system, in both men and women, is vulnerable to a host of illnesses, including bacterial, viral, and fungal infections; various forms of inflammatory illnesses and cancer; and diseases that spread specifically through sexual contact.

In this chapter, I offer advice on treating the most common sexual and reproductive heath issues for both women and men, offer some natural cures suggestions to address infertility, and provide guidance for treating sexually transmitted diseases (STDs).

Focusing on Women's Reproductive Health

As a woman, you have the unique opportunity to conceive and bear children, but the accompanying biological complexities expose you to a host of illnesses that men don't have to deal with, such as cervical dysplasia, endometriosis, premenstrual syndrome (PMS), menopause, and vaginitis. The first steps to treating all female sex and reproductive issues are to adopt a healthy diet and lifestyle, as explained in Chapter 2; get tested for food allergies and adjust your diet accordingly (see Chapter 13); and focus on making the following dietary changes:

- ✔ **Reduce your consumption of soy products.** Unless you're going through menopause, reduce consumption of soy products to once or twice a week, and eat only organic, non-GMO, fermented soy products. If you're going through menopause, upping your intake of soy may help.

- ✔ **Eat organic whole foods free of herbicides and pesticides.** Organic whole foods are less likely to contain herbicides and pesticides that often act as *xenoestrogens,* chemicals that function as estrogen in the body.

- ✔ **Eat eight servings of vegetables daily, including at least one serving of a cruciferous vegetable and one or more servings of dark leafy green vegetables.** Cruciferous vegetables include cabbage, broccoli, brussels sprouts, cauliflower, bok choy, and kale. These vegetables clear the liver detoxification pathways that remove excess estrogen. Leafy green vegetables are higher in vitamin K.

- ✔ **Eat at least 2 tablespoons of ground flaxseeds daily.** Add a tablespoon of flaxseeds to your morning smoothie or sprinkle it on your salads. Flaxseeds are high in fiber, alpha-linolenic acid (an omega-3 essential fatty acid), and lignans, which lower the risk of breast cancer in women and prostate cancer in men, reduce the frequency and intensity of hot flashes in women, and help to regulate the menstrual cycle.

Starting in your 30s or 40s, *estrogen dominance,* a higher than normal estrogen-to-progesterone ratio, is likely to contribute to any female health issues you're experiencing. Have your hormone levels tested on a single day during days 18 to 22 of your menstrual cycle (counting from the first day of your period). If progesterone is low, supplement with bioidentical progesterone cream. Apply 20 mg twice daily directly to an inner forearm, inner thigh, or the left or right side of the back of your neck; switch areas with each application to avoid saturating one area. Don't use progesterone cream during the week of menstruation.

You also want to supplement your diet to support *estrogen methylation,* a biochemical process that removes bad estrogen from your body. Use these supplements in these dosages:

Supplement	*Dosage*
Riboflavin (riboflavin 5′-phosphate)	25 mg twice daily
Vitamin B6 (pyridoxal 5′-phosphate)	10 mg twice daily
Vitamin B12 (methylcobalamin, sublingual fast-dissolving tablet)	5,000 mcg one or two times daily
Folate (5-MTHF)	2,000 mcg daily

Supplement	Dosage
Diindolylmethane	150 mg twice daily
Trimethylglycine	500 mg twice daily
SAMe	200 mg twice daily

In addition to having your estrogen and progesterone levels evaluated, have your thyroid hormones and function tested and treated if necessary (refer to Chapter 18 for more on thyroid function).

Read on to find out about several of the most common ailments that afflict women specifically.

Treating cervical dysplasia

Cervical dysplasia consists of precancerous cell growth on the lining of the *cervix,* the opening between the vagina and the uterus. This condition is commonly associated with infection by human papillomavirus (HPV) and typically is discovered early through routine Pap smears. Only about a third of the more than 100 strains of HPV are sexually transmitted and only about a dozen (HPV 16 and HPV 18 more than others) are strongly associated with cervical cancer. Approximately 70 percent of all cases resolve within one year, and 90 percent resolve within two years without treatment. If the condition worsens or fails to improve within two years, conventional medical treatment may be necessary.

Treat cervical dysplasia with the least invasive methods first. Adopt a healthy diet and lifestyle (refer to the information earlier in this section and in Chapter 2). If you smoke, stop. Get tested and, if necessary, treated for HPV; see the later section "Human papillomavirus (HPV)" for details. You may also want to try the following local applications:

- ✔ **Escharotic treatment:** Consult a natural medicine practitioner to obtain treatment, which is performed only after a satisfactory *colposcopy,* a medical examination of the cervix using a magnifying device. Bromelain is applied to the surface of the cervix and left in place for 15 minutes with moist heat to dissolve the top layer of cells damaged by HPV. A mixture of zinc chloride and the plant *Sanguinaria* is then applied to the cervix to cause a sloughing of the abnormal tissue. This treatment is performed twice weekly for four to six weeks, with several days between treatments.

- ✔ **Vaginal suppository treatment:** *Vaginal depletion packs* (vag packs) draw infection out of the cervical cells and boost the immune system. This treatment option is suitable for mild dysplasia or to prevent HPV infection if you're in a high-risk category. You can buy vag packs online or at most health food stores.

Dealing with endometriosis

Endometriosis occurs when uterine tissue attaches itself to other organs, including fallopian tubes, ovaries, and the outer wall of the uterus. Symptoms include pelvic pain (usually worse around ovulation, menstruation, and intercourse), heavier-than-normal bleeding, nausea, vomiting, anemia, and digestive tract issues. It may cause cysts that sometime rupture, leading to agonizing pain and possibly contributing to infertility.

To treat endometriosis, start by adopting a healthy diet and lifestyle, as explained earlier in this section. Support your dietary changes with the following supplements:

Supplement	Dosage
Diindolylmethane	150 mg twice daily
Omega-3 essential fatty acids (EFAs)	1 g yielding 180 mg EPA and 120 mg DHA four times daily
Calcium D-glucarate	500 mg twice daily
Chaste berry extract *(Vitex)*	125 mg twice daily (see Appendix D for precautions)
Dandelion extract	50 mg twice daily
Ginger	30 mg twice daily
Red raspberry	25 mg twice daily, or several cups of red raspberry tea daily

Focusing on fibrocystic breasts

Fibrocystic breasts are noncancerous lumps that may be tender or painful and are most common in women who are 20 to 50 years old. Symptoms for most women occur just prior to menstruation and continue for the first several days of their menstrual cycle. Fibrocystic breasts resolve after menopause.

Breast tenderness may be caused by *hypothyroidism* (underactive thyroid), so have your thyroid function and thyroid hormone levels checked. Underactive thyroid is typically due to iodine deficiency and usually responds well to increasing consumption of iodine-rich foods. Chapter 18 has the details.

Treatment for fibrocystic breasts begins with a healthy diet, as explained earlier in this section. Eliminate caffeine, colas, and chocolate from your diet, and support your dietary changes with the following supplements:

Supplement	Dosage
Vitamin E (tocopherols)	400 IU daily
Iodine	150 mcg twice daily initially; supplement at higher doses only if tests show a deficiency
Thiamine (vitamin B1, as benfontamine)	300 mg twice daily
Diindolylmethane	150 mg twice daily
Chaste berry extract *(Vitex)*	125 mg twice daily (see Appendix D for precautions)
Omega-3 essential fatty acids (EFAs)	1 g yielding 180 mg EPA and 120 mg DHA four times daily
Red raspberry	25 mg twice daily, or several cups of red raspberry tea daily

You may also need to take thyroid hormone, but only if testing and symptoms warrant supplementation (see Chapter 18 for details).

Getting rid of uterine fibroids

Uterine fibroids are caused by the growth of noncancerous smooth muscle on the walls of the uterus. They're often detected during routine examinations and screenings and are one of the most common reasons for visits to gynecologists. Although the condition is often *asymptomatic* (without symptoms), symptoms may include heavy menstrual bleeding, painful intercourse, abdominal pain or bloating, constipation, and lower back pain.

Before agreeing to a surgical procedure to remove uterine fibroids, try curing the condition through proper nutrition. Start with a healthy diet, as explained earlier in this chapter and in Chapter 2. Support your dietary changes with the following supplements:

Supplement	Dosage
Vitamin E (tocopherols)	400 IU daily
Iodine	150 mcg twice daily (a very low dose) initially; supplement at higher doses only if tests show a deficiency
Diindolylmethane	150 mg twice daily

(continued)

(continued)

Supplement	Dosage
Chaste berry extract *(Vitex)*	125 mg twice daily (see Appendix D for precautions)
Omega-3 essential fatty acids (EFAs)	1 g yielding 180 mg EPA and 120 mg DHA four times daily
Calcium D-glucarate	500 mg twice daily
Dandelion extract	50 mg twice daily

Managing the effects of menopause

Menopause marks the end of a woman's menstrual cycle. It usually develops gradually, over the course of several years, beginning when a women enters her late-40s or sometime later and culminating in menopause when she goes 12 months without a period. The time leading up to menopause is commonly referred to as *perimenopause*, while the time after is called *post menopause*. Contrary to popular belief, menopause is not an illness and shouldn't be treated as such. It's a normal part of the aging process.

Although some women experience no symptoms, women who do have symptoms may experience irregular periods, hot flashes, vaginal dryness, night sweats, hair loss, moodiness, insomnia, reduced sex drive, fatigue, or increased susceptibility to bone loss and cardiovascular events.

Dietary changes as explained earlier in this section may be all that the body needs to execute this transition gracefully — with one exception: Instead of eating less soy, consider eating more of it. Soy foods typically eaten in Asian cultures help reduce menopausal symptoms. If you haven't been raised on soy, then consume organic, non-GMO soy only once or twice a week in the fermented form of tempeh, tofu, or miso. (Ninety percent of soy in the U.S. is genetically modified, so read labels closely and purchase products only from reputable producers.)

Steer clear of conventional *synthetic hormone replacement therapy (HRT)* — the use of synthetic hormones to make up for decreased production of estrogen and progesterone by the ovaries. Much better alternatives are available, including *bioidentical hormones* — hormones having the same molecular structure as those created by the human body.

Before implementing HRT with bioidentical hormones, have your hormone levels checked through saliva or blood and proceed with HRT only with the approval of and under the close supervision of a qualified medical practitioner. Here are some general guidelines for bioidentical HRT:

- ✔ **DHEA (dehydroepiandrosterone):** Start at a low dose (5 to 15 mg daily) and increase slowly up to 25 mg daily, if necessary.

- ✔ **Bioidentical progesterone cream:** If your estrogen-to-progesterone ratio is high, supplement with bioidentical progesterone cream, 20 mg twice daily. Apply the cream directly to an inner forearm, inner thigh, or the left or right side of the back of your neck; switch areas with each application to avoid saturating one area. Don't use progesterone cream during the week of menstruation. Postmenopausal women should apply 10 mg every day from day 10 to day 28 of each month.

In addition, take the following supplements:

Supplement	*Dosage*
Chaste berry extract *(Vitex)*	125 mg twice daily (see Appendix D for precautions)
Iodine	150 mcg twice daily initially; supplement at higher doses only if tests show a deficiency
Korean ginseng	200 mg twice daily
Wild yam	50 mg twice daily
Dong quai extract	50 mg twice daily
Black cohosh	80 mg twice daily

You may also need to take thyroid hormone or supplements to address adrenal fatigue, but only if testing and symptoms warrant supplementation (see Chapter 18 for details).

Waking up to morning sickness

Morning sickness is the term used to describe the nausea and vomiting that many women experience during the first trimester of pregnancy — regardless whether it occurs in the morning, afternoon, or any other time of the day or night. These symptoms usually dissipate after the first trimester and are not harmful to either the mother or fetus.

Morning sickness is generally nothing to worry about. However, seek immediate medical attention if you experience the following: the vomiting is severe, you pass only a small amount of dark urine, you can't keep even small amounts of liquid down, you feel dizzy or faint upon standing, your heart races, or you vomit blood. Hospitalization may be necessary to replace lost fluids and nutrients.

To prevent bouts of morning sickness, eat more protein than usual and avoid sugar, salt, fried and fatty foods, and *comfort foods* — those that are high in sodium, refined carbohydrates, and unhealthy fats. Eat small meals throughout the day instead of the traditional three large meals. Drink herbal chamomile and red raspberry tea throughout the day. The following supplements may also help reduce the frequency and intensity of morning sickness:

Supplement	*Dosage*
Multivitamin/mineral (high-quality supplement containing therapeutic levels of the B vitamins in their better forms, in powder form [see Appendix A] during first trimester; after the first trimester, switch to a quality prenatal formula)	Follow label instructions and consult your healthcare provider for specific dosages
Vitamin B6 (pyridoxal 5′-phosphate)	20 mg daily
Ginger	250 mg twice daily
Adrenal extract	130 mg two to three times daily
Vitamin K2 (menaquinone)	45 mcg one or two times daily

Calming the raging seas of PMS: Premenstrual syndrome

Premenstrual syndrome is a cluster of symptoms that may include irritability, anger, depression, bloating, sensitive breasts, headaches, fatigue, and cravings for unhealthy (salty, starchy, sugary) foods. These symptoms begin approximately one week prior to menstruation and resolve with the onset of menses. Approximately 70 to 90 percent of women experience PMS, and 30 percent of those report severe symptoms.

Aerobic exercise is the best treatment for PMS. Engage in moderate aerobic exercise for about 30 minutes daily. Support your exercise program with the dietary changes recommended earlier in this section, and focus on leveling out your blood sugar levels by doing the following:

✔ Avoid refined processed carbohydrates and dairy products. PMS has a strong connection to sugar.

✔ Eat small, frequent meals to prevent fluctuations in blood sugar levels.

✔ Avoid excess salt, caffeine, and alcohol for two weeks prior to menses.

✔ Eat less red meat and more veggies.

Get your hormone levels tested and, if your estrogen-to-progesterone ratio is high, supplement with bioidentical progesterone cream. Refer to the earlier section "Managing the effects of menopause" for details.

The following supplements may also help alleviate PMS:

Supplement	*Dosage*
Chaste berry extract *(Vitex)*	125 mg twice daily (see Appendix D for precautions)
Dong quai extract	300 to 500 mg twice daily
Vitamin B6 (pyridoxal 5'-phosphate)	25 mg one to two times daily
Magnesium glycinate chelate	250 to 500 mg daily
Vitamin E (tocopherols)	400 IU daily
Calcium citrate	600 to 1,200 mg daily
Vitamin D3	2,000 to 10,000 IU daily, depending on blood levels (see Appendix A)
5-HTP (controlled release)	100 mg two times daily
Evening primrose oil	3 to 6 g daily

PMS may also be related to *hypothyroidism* (underactive thyroid). Have your thyroid function and hormone levels tested, as explained in Chapter 18, and address any issues through nutrition and supplements. If PMS is accompanied by *candidiasis* (yeast infection), as it often is, address the infection, following the instructions I provide in the later section "Curing a yeast infection."

Overcoming sexual dysfunction

Sexual dysfunction is the inability to achieve satisfaction from sexual activity. Symptoms may include loss of libido, painful intercourse, fatigue, depression, or the inability to achieve orgasm. Successful treatment requires identifying the root cause of the disorder, which may include post-traumatic stress disorder (PTSD), anxiety, medication side effects (particularly from SSRI antidepressants), diabetes, heart disease, hypothyroidism, chronic fatigue syndrome, and neurological disorders. Menopause or having had a hysterectomy can also result in loss of libido and decreased vaginal lubrication. Team up with your doctor to identify these conditions or rule them out before seeking treatment options.

Conventional treatment for sexual dysfunction typically involves hormone replacement therapy (HRT), but I recommend HRT only if testing calls for it and only through the use of bioidentical replacement hormones, *not* synthetic versions (refer to the earlier section "Managing the effects of menopause"). DHEA at a dose of 5 to 15 mg daily may help postmenopausal women by boosting the body's sex hormone *precursors* (building blocks), but take DHEA only with medical approval and supervision. Manganese (25 to 30 mg daily) may also help.

Healthy diet and lifestyle, as explained earlier in this section and in Chapter 2, are likely to improve your sex life, as well. In addition, consider looking into relationship and sex therapies as a way to rekindle the libido and deal with other issues that may be inhibiting the pleasures of sexual activities.

Vanquishing vaginitis

Vaginitis is inflammation of the vulva and vagina, which may be associated with itching, pain, and discharge. The most common causes are bacterial or yeast infections, *trichomoniasis* (a parasite), and vaginal atrophy from lower estrogen levels due to menopause (*atrophic vaginitis*). Regardless of the cause, in this section, I provide guidance on how to support vaginal health to fight infection and alleviate any itching or pain you're experiencing. For more about treating yeast infections, see the later section "Curing a yeast infection," and for treating trichomoniasis, head to the section "Coping with Sexually Transmitted Diseases."

For *atrophic vaginitis* (vaginal inflammation due to thinning and shrinking of the tissues and decreased lubrication), try over-the-counter moisturizers or water-based lubricants. Conventional treatment involves estrogen HRT applied topically, which helps to eliminate the amount of estrogen absorbed into the bloodstream, but it still increases your risk of endometrial cancer. Try some of the remedies described in the following sections before trying HRT.

Diet

Vaginitis often responds to changes in diet. In addition to the dietary changes recommended earlier in this section and in Chapter 2, make the following adjustments:

- **Increase protein consumption.** To calculate how much protein you need to eat in grams, multiply your body weight in pounds by 0.46. If you weigh 140 pounds, for example, $140 \times 0.46 = 64.4$, so you should be eating 64.4 grams of protein daily. (If you didn't need to increase your protein consumption, you'd determine your recommended daily protein intake by multiplying your body weight by 0.36.) Sources of healthy protein include farm-fresh eggs, seafood (especially salmon, tuna, herring, and sardines), pastured livestock, nuts, seeds, and legumes.

- **Eat high-quality, full-fat, plain yogurt.** Yogurt is helpful in maintaining a healthy balance of good bacteria in your gut. Don't buy low-fat or non-fat yogurt or yogurt with fruit added. Buy plain yogurt and then doctor it up with organic nuts and berries or gluten-free granola.

✔ **Stay hydrated.** Drink 8 ounces of quality water every two waking hours.

✔ **Drink several cups of organic green tea daily.** Green tea is high in polyphenols that have potent antioxidant and antitumor properties. It's also an anti-inflammatory agent.

Probiotics

For vaginitis, especially those conditions related to bacteria or yeast infection, take probiotics orally and vaginally, in addition to supplements that support an environment in which the probiotic organisms can thrive:

✔ Orally and vaginally: Take a multistrain probiotic containing 5 billion CFU, including the following strains:

- *Lactobacillus acidophilus* Rosell-52

- *Lactobacillus rhamnosus* Rosell-11

- *Bifdobacterium longum* Rosell-175

To take a probiotic vaginally, insert the probiotic at night and cover with a pad.

✔ Eat fermented foods, such as pickled vegetables, including sauerkraut. Homemade is best.

✔ Take these supplements:

Supplement	*Dosage*
Zinc glycinate chelate	20 mg twice daily (see Appendix A for precautions)
Vitamin C (mineral ascorbates)	1,000 mg twice daily
Chaste berry extract *(Vitex)*	125 mg twice daily (see Appendix D for precautions)

Douching

Mix 3 percent hydrogen peroxide with an equal part of quality filtered water, apply with a douche, and lie on your back with your knees drawn together for at least three minutes prior to standing. Repeat daily until the infection has subsided and then douche twice a week to prevent infection.

Bathing

Draw yourself a warm bath with ½ cup Epsom salts, ⅛ cup Himalayan pink salt, 2 tablespoons tea tree oil, and ¼ cup vinegar. Bathe nightly until symptoms dissipate.

Curing a yeast infection

Yeast infection is a type of vaginitis (see the preceding section) caused by overgrowth of *Candida albicans,* which exist naturally in the body. Symptoms include itching, burning, pelvic pain, and white, milky discharge. Yeast infections often occur after treatment with antibiotics, which kill the beneficial bacteria that keep the yeast population in check. The yeast also flourishes on the standard American diet, which is high in sugar and processed carbohydrates, which are quickly converted to sugar. Other factors that contribute to yeast overgrowth are the use of birth control pills, a compromised immune system, poor hygiene, and tight clothing.

Take care of your vagina first. If you don't already do so, wipe from front to back after using the toilet. Don't use tampons, scented pads, or fancy soaps with fragrances or added chemicals. Steer clear of hot tubs, and take showers instead of baths. To reduce pain and inflammation in the labial area, apply a cold compress for a few minutes several times daily.

To rid yourself of a yeast infection, starve the yeast. Eliminate sugar, wheat, starchy foods, sugary drinks (including fruit juice), alcohol, and junk food from your diet. Stop eating foods that contain high levels of mold, including cheese, mushrooms, vinegar (and anything that contains vinegar), sour cream, alcohol (especially beer), black tea, nuts, dried fruits, and anything prepared with yeast. Stick with quality protein; fresh, nonstarchy veggies; and less-sugary fruit (no oranges). Eat foods that have antifungal properties, including garlic, onions, and coconut (coconut oil, too). In addition to dietary changes, take the following antifungal supplements:

Supplement	*Dosage*
Oregano extract	150 mg twice daily
Sodium caprylate	150 mg twice daily
Ginger	150 mg twice daily
Turmeric extract	100 mg twice daily
Olive leaf extract	500 mg twice daily

Take probiotics orally and vaginally, as explained in the preceding section "Vanquishing vaginitis."

Focusing on Male Reproductive Health Issues

Men who struggle with sex-related issues basically have two complaints — erectile dysfunction or problems urinating. And these two issues are almost always related to low testosterone or restricted blood flow. In this section, I explain how to tackle these two issues as they appear in specific conditions, including erectile dysfunction, low sperm count, low testosterone, and prostate issues.

Dealing with an enlarged prostate

Benign prostatic hypertrophy (BPH) — the fancy term for an enlarged prostate — is a noncancerous increase in the size of the prostate gland that leads to difficulty urinating. BPH may also contribute to bladder and kidney infections and damage the bladder muscles. The good news is that BPH doesn't increase your risk of cancer — that's the "benign" part.

A few, easy lifestyle changes can bring immediate relief:

✔ Don't drink anything two to three hours before bedtime.

✔ Minimize your consumption of caffeine and alcohol.

✔ Stand to urinate (to more fully empty the bladder).

✔ Team up with your doctor to evaluate your medications. Certain medications may increase urinary excretion.

In addition to the preceding changes, adopting a healthier diet (see Chapter 2) with a focus·on eliminating sugar and trans fats can also ease prostate troubles. Eat more organic produce, nuts, seeds, and oily fishes, such as salmon, mackerel, and sardines. Eliminate wheat and limit grain consumption to one small serving a day. Pumpkin seeds are a healthy prostate food, because they're very high in zinc. Drink plenty of organic green tea to assist in detoxification, and stay well-hydrated (drink plenty of water throughout the day). Also, support your dietary changes with the following nutrients:

Supplement	Dosage
Vitamin B6 (pyridoxal 5'-phosphate)	5 mg twice daily
Zinc glycinate chelate	20 mg twice daily
Saw palmetto	160 mg twice daily

(continued)

(continued)

Supplement	*Dosage*
Pumpkin seed oil	40 mg twice daily
Uva-ursi	5 mg twice daily
Oil of oregano	1,000 mg twice daily
Pygeum	100 mg twice daily
Quercetin	500 mg twice daily

Tackling erectile dysfunction

Erectile dysfunction (*ED,* also called *impotence*) is the inability to achieve or maintain an erection. Causes include certain health conditions (such as cardiovascular disease, diabetes, and hormonal changes, as well as depression and anxiety); prescription medication side effects (especially antidepressants and high blood pressure medication); and lifestyle factors (excess consumption of alcohol, poor diet, and stress).

If you're taking any medications or supplements, ask your doctor whether any of them may contribute to ED and discuss your options. Sometimes changing the dose or the time you take the medication can help. In other cases, your doctor may be able to switch you to a different medication in the same class that's less likely to contribute to ED. If you drink alcohol or smoke tobacco, try stopping those for a while to determine whether those substances are contributing to the problem.

Performance anxiety is a common and strong factor contributing to ED. I can tell you to stop worrying about it, but that's like telling you not to imagine a yellow rhinoceros. Instead, I advise you to think more about the task at hand and focus on what you and your partner are doing in the moment. Mindfulness meditation, Qigong, yoga, and other centering disciplines can help you retrain your mind to live in the moment. Anxiety, including performance anxiety, occurs only when you think too much about the future at the expense of enjoying the present moment.

Adopting a healthy diet and lifestyle (see Chapter 2) can also do wonders for your sex life. When you feel better physically, you tend to feel more physically — and psychologically — virile, and your body will be in better balance. You won't have to deal with surges and drops in blood sugar or systemic inflammation that restricts blood flow. Ditching the standard American diet is a key first step.

Also work toward boosting the level of nitric oxide (NO), a vasodilator that increases blood flow to the penis — a goal you can move toward as you implement dietary changes. Several foods promote nitric oxide production, including dark chocolate, watermelon, pomegranate, walnuts, brown rice, beets, spinach, and cranberries. Prescription medications, such as Viagra, also work by boosting production of nitric oxide, but approaching the issue naturally, through nutrition, eliminates the potential of negative side effects. The following two supplements also promote nitric oxide production (take both of them on an empty stomach):

Supplement	Dosage
L-arginine	2 g twice daily (see Appendix B for precautions)
L-citrulline	3 g daily

Other supplements that may help with erectile dysfunction include the following:

Supplement	Dosage
DHEA	25 to 50 mg daily (see Appendix C for precautions)
Maca (powder or tablets)	500 mg twice daily
Tribulus	300 mg twice daily
Horny goat weed	100 mg twice daily

Boosting your sperm count

Low sperm count is anything lower than 15 million sperm per milliliter of semen — the point at which the ability to conceive begins to decline. Factors that contribute to low sperm count include overheated or undescended testicles, sperm duct defects, certain medications, anabolic steroid use, sexually transmitted diseases (STDs), tobacco or cannabis use, excessive alcohol consumption, excessive frequency of ejaculations, environmental toxins, high stress, and obesity.

Some simple diet and lifestyle changes may help boost sperm count:

✔ Adopt a healthier diet, with a focus on eating organic foods to avoid environmental toxins. See Chapter 2 for guidance.

✔ Avoid drinking unfiltered municipal tap water, which is likely to contain chlorine and fluoride, which may lower sperm counts.

✔ Team up with your doctor to reduce or eliminate the use of pharmaceutical medications. (Don't stop taking any medications without your doctor's consent.)

- ✔ Don't use anabolic steroids; they shrink the testicles and may lead to infertility.

- ✔ If you smoke, stop, and if you drink, do so moderately — a few ounces of red wine at dinner.

- ✔ Engage in aerobic exercise for 30 to 45 minutes every day, five days a week. But don't overdo it. Excessive exercise, especially bike riding, may lower your sperm count.

- ✔ Practice mindfulness meditation, Qigong, or yoga to establish a healthier mindset.

- ✔ Strive to achieve your ideal weight. Use online body mass index (BMI) charts to set your goal.

- ✔ Avoid hot baths and hot tubs, and avoid sitting for long periods of time.

- ✔ Wear loose-fitting underwear — trade in your whitey-tighties for boxers.

- ✔ Ejaculate less frequently.

Support you dietary and lifestyle changes with the following supplements:

Supplement	Dosage
Vitamin C (mineral ascorbates)	1,000 mg one or two times daily
Zinc glycinate chelate	20 mg twice daily (see Appendix A for precautions)
Copper	4 mg of copper daily
Selenium glycinate complex	100 to 200 mcg daily
Vitamin B12 (menthylcobalamin, sublingual fast-dissolving tablet)	5,000 mcg one or two times daily
Folate (5-MTHF)	2,000 mcg daily
Tribulus	500 to 1,000 mg twice daily
Ashwagandha	400 to 800 mg twice daily
Indole-3-carbinol	150 mg twice daily

Dealing with low testosterone

Low testosterone, or *hypogonadism* (commonly referred to as *low T*), is a condition in which the testicles produce insufficient amounts of testosterone, often resulting in low sex drive, erectile dysfunction, fatigue, depression, irritability, reduced muscle mass, decreased bone density, and increased body fat.

The normal range on blood tests for testosterone is 300 to 1,200 ng/dl, but don't look exclusively at total testosterone; consider the level of *free testosterone (free T)* — the testosterone available to do the work. Many labs specify a normal range of 7.20 to 23.00 pg/ml, but ideally, free T should be below 15 pg/ml. If free T is higher, the body rapidly converts it to estrogen through the enzyme aromatase, which ramps up this conversion whenever you drink alcohol or have a higher percentage of belly fat (higher than about 22 percent). Increasing testosterone levels without addressing the conversion to estrogen increases your risk of estrogen-related cancers.

Consider the total hormonal landscape, including estrogen, testosterone, thyroid, and adrenal hormones. Boosting testosterone without considering other hormone levels and other underlying disorders may have a detrimental effect on overall health. For more about testing for and addressing adrenal and thyroid issues, see Chapter 18.

Conventional medicine typically addresses low T by supplying testosterone to the body in the form of patches, gels, or injectable pellets. However, men with prostate or breast cancer are generally advised against increasing their testosterone levels, because testosterone fuels the growth of these types of cancers. A safer option is to provide your body with the nutrients it needs to establish a healthy balance of testosterone and estrogen:

Supplement	Dosage
DHEA	25 to 50 mg daily (see Appendix C for precautions)
Diindolylmethane	150 mg one or two times daily
Vitamin D3	2,000 to 10,000 mg daily, depending on blood levels (see Appendix A)
Vitamin B6 (pyridoxal 5'-phosphate)	25 mg one to two times daily
Vitamin B12 (methylcobalamin, sublingual fast-dissolving tablet)	5,000 mcg one or two times daily
Folate (5-MTHF)	400 mcg daily
Soybean concentrate (non-GMO)	125 mg daily
Green tea extract	340 mg daily
Turmeric	160 mg daily
Lycopene	10 mg twice daily
Tribulus	500 mg twice daily
Ashwagandha	400 mg twice daily

Pumpkin seeds also tend to increase testosterone levels.

Enhancing Fertility

Infertility is the inability of a couple to make a baby over the course of 12 months, despite engaging regularly in unprotected sex. Female and male infertility are equally common, and in this section, you can find strategies for improving your chances of conceiving.

 Prior to implementing intensive and invasive medical procedures to improve fertility, a couple should, for at least 6 months, adopt a healthy diet and lifestyle (see the earlier section "Focusing on Women's Reproductive Health") for general guidance on beneficial dietary changes and Chapter 2 for more detailed information). Also be aware that sometimes the process of trying to conceive becomes so stressful that it prevents you from doing so. Chill out. You might be surprised at just how effective it is to relax and let nature take its course.

Advice for women

A number of factors contribute to infertility in women, including medical conditions (such as low progesterone, hypothyroidism, endometriosis, polycystic ovarian syndrome, and obesity); lifestyle factors (including poor diet, especially excessive sugar and unhealthy fats), excessive exercise, delaying childbearing into the 30s and 40s, and cigarette smoking); and things like high stress, excessive supplementation with beta-carotene, and environmental toxins. Address any of these contributing factors first; then try the suggestions I outline here.

 When looking at your diet, pay special attention to reducing your caffeine consumption and eliminating alcohol (even moderate alcohol consumption can be a problem) and beverages that contain brominated vegetable oil (such as Mountain Dew and several flavors of Gatorade).

To improve overall reproductive health, take the following supplements:

Supplement	Dosage
Chaste berry extract *(Vitex)*	125 mg twice daily (see Appendix D for precautions)
Iodine	150 mcg twice daily initially; supplement at higher doses only if tests show a deficiency
Vitamin B6 (pyridoxal 5'-phosphate)	35 mg daily

Chapter 19: Addressing Sexual and Reproductive Health Issues

Supplement	Dosage
Vitamin B12 (methylcobalamin, sublingual fast-dissolving tablet)	5,000 mcg one or two times daily
Folate (5-MTHF)	2,000 to 10,000 mcg daily
Omega-3 essential fatty acids (EFAs)	1 g yielding 180 mg EPA and 120 mg DHA four times daily

Supplementation with thyroid hormone may also be beneficial, but only if testing and symptoms warrant supplementation. See Chapter 18 for details.

You can also try timing your attempts to conceive so that they occur 48 hours prior to ovulation. To detect peak fertility conditions, you can purchase a test kit online or at your local pharmacy to monitor luteinizing hormone (LH) in the urine.

Advice for men

For men, infertility results from low testosterone, low sperm count, decreased sperm motility (movement), or abnormally shaped sperm. Factors that contribute to infertility include medical conditions (such as STDs that damage tissue); poor diet (especially excessive sugar and unhealthy fats); and lifestyle (excessive exercise, excessive alcohol consumption, delaying childbearing into their 30s and 40s, and cigarette smoking); and toxins such as pesticides that act as estrogen in the body and beverages that contain brominated vegetable oil (as found in Mountain Dew and several flavors of Gatorade).

To improve fertility, adopt a healthy diet and lifestyle (refer to Chapter 2) and be careful not to overdo it on exercise. Engaging in aerobic exercise for 30 to 45 minutes five times a week along with three days of strength training is sufficient.

Also, take the following supplements to support healthy sperm production and delivery and see the earlier section "Boosting your sperm count" for additional details:

Supplement	Dosage
Zinc glycinate chelate	20 mg twice daily (see Appendix A for precautions)
Copper	4 mg daily
L-arginine	2 g twice daily (see Appendix B for precautions)

(continued)

(continued)

Supplement	Dosage
L-citrulline	3 g daily
Acetyl-L-carnitine	350 mg twice daily
Vitamin E (tocopherols)	400 IU daily
Selenium	100 mcg twice daily
CoQ10 (Kaneka Q10)	100 mg twice daily
Vitamin C (mineral ascorbates)	1,000 mg twice daily
Lycopene	4 mg daily, in divided doses
Vitamin B12 (methylcobalamin, sublingual fast-dissolving tablet)	5,000 mcg one or two times daily
Omega 3 essential fatty acids (EFAs)	1 g yielding 180 mg EPA and 120 mg DHA four times daily

Coping with Sexually Transmitted Diseases

Sexually transmitted diseases (STDs) are bacterial, viral, or parasitic infections you can get from having sex with someone who has the infection. Prevention is the best medicine. Abstinence, using a condom, and having sex exclusively with one, STD-free partner are three of the best ways to prevent the spread of STDs. Despite your best efforts, however, you may contract an STD, and if you do, you've come to the right place. Here I present alternative and complementary treatments for several of the most common STDs.

For all STDs involving bacterial or viral infection, take the following supplements to boost your immune system in addition to any medications (such as antibiotics) required to clear up the infection:

Supplement	Dosage
Colostrum	10,000 mg one or two times daily
Proline-rich polypeptides extracted from bovine colostrum	4 sprays in mouth, hold for 30 seconds and swallow, twice daily early morning and before bed for a total of 16 mg daily
L-lysine	500 mg three times daily
Vitamin C (mineral ascorbates)	1,000 mg twice daily
Zinc glycinate chelate	20 mg twice daily (see Appendix A for precautions)
Whole beta glucan	500 mg twice daily for an active outbreak; 250 mg twice daily when the virus is dormant

If you're taking an antibiotic to treat an STD, take probiotics to restore the good bacteria your body needs to function properly and fight infection. You can take probiotics in the form of fermented foods or in capsule or powder form:

✔ Eat full-fat, unsweetened yogurt and fermented foods, such as kombucha, kimchi, pickles, and sauerkraut.

✔ Take a high-quality probiotic several hours from the time you take your antibiotic and for several months after discontinuing the antibiotic.

For a probiotic, I recommend taking 250 mg *Saccharomyces boulardii* twice daily along with a proprietary blend of 50 billion CFU of a multi-strain containing *Lactobacillus acidophilus, Bifidobacterium longum,* and *Lactobacillus plantarum* plus 50 billion CFU *Bifidobacterium lactis* HNO 19 (HOWARU Bifido) once daily.

Chlamydia

Chlamydia is a bacterial infection. Most women who've been infected have no symptoms, but if left untreated, it can damage a woman's reproductive organs, eyes, throat, and lungs, and ultimately cause infertility. Symptoms may include abnormal vaginal discharge and a burning sensation when urinating. In men, symptoms include a white discharge from the penis, a burning sensation when urinating, and (occasionally) pain and swelling in one or both testicles. Chlamydia is a common cause of blindness, may cause reactive arthritis in both men and women, and can permanently affect numerous joints in the body. Treatment requires antibiotics. Complement conventional antibiotic treatment with probiotics and the immune-boosting supplements recommended earlier in this section.

Genital herpes

Genital herpes is a viral infection characterized by painful blisters in the genital area, buttocks, and inner thighs. Approximately 16 percent of the population in the U.S. is infected with the herpes simplex 2 virus (HSV-2), which causes genital herpes, and more than 80 percent of those infected are unaware of their diagnosis. After the primary infection, the virus lies dormant until stress, fatigue, sunburn, or another illness reactivates it. Viral shedding can spread the disease prior to and following outbreaks.

Genital herpes has no cure, but you can prevent outbreaks by improving overall immune response. Start by adopting a healthy diet (see Chapter 2) and focus on eliminating sugar and processed carbohydrates, which lower your immunity and allow the opportunistic herpes virus to replicate.

I recommend the Herpes Simplex Series Therapy Kit from Deseret Biologicals. The homeopathic formulas in this kit are very effective in training your immune system to keep the virus in check.

Gonorrhea

Gonorrhea, commonly referred to as "the clap," is a bacterial infection. Symptoms tend to appear four to six days after infection. Women may have no symptoms or may experience vaginal discharge, pelvic pain, or vaginal bleeding between periods. Men experience a burning sensation when urinating and white, yellow, or green discharge from the penis. If left untreated, gonorrhea can lead to permanent health issues affecting the joints and heart valves. Treatment requires antibiotics. Complement conventional antibiotics with probiotics and the immune-boosting supplements mentioned earlier in this section.

HIV/AIDS

Human immunodeficiency virus (HIV) is a viral infection that begins with flu-like symptoms followed by a prolonged period with no symptoms; it ultimately makes the person more prone to infection and tumors. HIV results in AIDS, when the person's T-cell count drops below 200/cc or when an HIV-related infection or cancer develops. (T cells play a key role in defending the body against infection.)

Conventional antiretroviral medications are required to slow the progression of the disease, but you need to complement conventional treatments with nutrition and supplements to boost your body's immune system and combat the side effects of the medication.

Focus first on diet. Get tested for food allergies and sensitivities (see Chapter 13) and eliminate any problem foods from your diet. Adopt a healthy, balanced diet, as I explain in Chapter 2, to ensure that you're getting the macronutrients, micronutrients, and calories required to support overall health. Avoid wheat to ensure proper absorption of nutrients in the intestines.

Finally, support your dietary changes with the immune-boosting supplements listed earlier in this section and by taking a high-quality multivitamin/mineral with sufficient doses of the better forms of each nutrient (see Appendix A). The following supplements provide additional immune-system support:

Supplement	Dosage
Vitamin B12 (methylcobalamin, sublingual fast-dissolving tablet)	5,000 mcg once or twice daily
Folate (5-MTHF)	2,000 to 10,000 mcg daily
CoQ10 (Kaneka Q10)	Several hundred mg daily
Acetyl-L-carnitine	350 mg twice daily
Magnesium glycinate chelate	250 mg daily
N-acetyl cysteine	1 to 2 g daily
Glutamine	5 g daily
Iron	30 mg twice daily
Vitamin C (mineral ascorbates)	1,000 mg two to three times daily
Whole beta glucan	500 mg twice daily

Human papillomavirus (HPV)

Human papillomavirus (HPV) is an infection by any 1 of more than 100 types of HPVs that may cause cervical dysplasia or genital warts. A few variants of the virus, if left untreated, may cause cervical cancer. Treatment for HPV involves boosting the body's immune system, especially the so-called K (killer) cells, by taking the following supplements:

Supplement	Dosage
Shiitake mushroom extract	650 to 1,000 mg two to three times daily
Vitamin B12 (methylcobalamin, sublingual fast-dissolving tablet)	5,000 mcg one or two times daily
Folate (5-MTHF)	2,000 to 10,000 mcg daily
Vitamin A (retinyl palmitate and beta-carotene)	10,000 IU daily
Indole-3-carbinol	200 to 400 mg daily
Vitamin E (tocopherols)	400 IU daily
CoQ10 (Kaneka Q10)	100 to 200 mg daily
Vitamin C (mineral ascorbates)	1,000 to 2,000 mg daily
Green tea extract (pigallocatechin-3-gallate [EGCG])	600 mg twice daily
Coriolus versicolor	1 to 9 g daily

Folate and B12 deficiency are associated with HPV infection.

Pelvic inflammatory disease

Pelvic inflammatory disease (PID) is inflammation of the uterus, fallopian tubes, and ovaries caused by untreated STDs, having more than one sex partner, douching, or using intrauterine devices (IUDs) to prevent pregnancy. Symptoms of PID may include fever, lower pelvic pain, vaginal discharge, irregular periods, painful urination, or painful intercourse with bleeding. PID increases the risk of ectopic pregnancy (where the embryo becomes implanted somewhere other than in the uterus) and may cause infertility.

PID requires conventional treatment with broad-spectrum antibiotics. Any sex partners six months prior to diagnosis should also be treated. Complement conventional antibiotics with probiotics and the immune-boosting supplements mentioned earlier in this section.

Pubic lice

Pubic lice (commonly called "crabs") are tiny insects that infest the genital area and cause severe itching. These lice may spread to other hairy parts of the body. To eradicate pubic lice, shave the area and apply one of the following treatments to kill any remaining critters:

✔ Petroleum jelly twice daily for three to five days

✔ ½ cup of almond oil mixed with 1 tablespoon each of lavender, eucalyptus, and bergamot oils twice daily for three to five days

✔ A product with neem or tea tree oil twice daily for at least one week

After treating the area, apply calamine lotion at least twice daily to treat any itching you may have. You may itch for several days after the lice are gone, which may make you think they've returned, even if they haven't. As you apply the calamine, remain on the lookout for any survivors; you may need to re-treat yourself.

Wash your bedding and clothes in hot water and dry them in a dryer at the highest setting for at least 20 minutes. Disinfect your bathtub(s), shower(s), and toilet(s). Of course, your sex partner(s) will need to do the same.

Syphilis

Syphilis is a bacterial infection that produces four stages of symptoms:

- ✔ **Primary:** A firm, painless, non-itchy ulceration (called a *chancre*) that typically appears about 21 days after exposure but may be hidden in the vagina or rectum.

- ✔ **Secondary:** A rash that starts on the trunk of the body and then covers the entire body, sometimes even the palms of your hands and soles of the feet and is sometimes accompanied by wartlike sores in the mouth or genital area, muscle aches, fever, sore throat, and swollen lymph nodes.

- ✔ **Latent:** A period when no symptoms are present but blood testing is positive for the infection.

- ✔ **Tertiary:** The period, sometimes occurring years after exposure, in which damage to the brain, nerves, eyes, heart, blood vessels, liver, bones, and joints may occur. Fifteen to 30 percent of people with untreated syphilis develop tertiary syphilis 3 to 15 years after the initial infection.

Syphilis requires conventional treatment with antibiotics. Complement conventional antibiotics with probiotics and the immune-boosting supplements mentioned earlier in this section.

Trichomoniasis

Trichomoniasis (commonly called "trich") is a single cell parasite that's a common cause of vaginitis in women. For men, the infection can be asymptomatic in the urinary tract or it can be associated with painful, burning urination. For women, the infection can be asymptomatic or lead to vaginitis characterized by a greenish yellow frothy discharge that has a fishy odor. Several natural remedies have proven effective (used alone or in combination):

- ✔ **Garlic:** Eat garlic or take it as a supplement. Women can use garlic cloves as vaginal suppositories. Peel a clove, wrap it in gauze, dip it in vegetable oil, and insert it into the vagina. Change it every 12 hours for about five days.

- ✔ **Goldenseal:** Whether you're a man or woman, take 500 mg goldenseal daily to strengthen the body's defense against trichomoniasis. Don't take goldenseal if you're pregnant, breastfeeding, or have high blood pressure.

- **Goldenseal-and-myrrh solution:** Simmer ½ teaspoon each of myrrh and goldenseal in 1 pint of water for five minutes. Let it cool and strain through a coffee filter. For women, use the solution to douche twice daily for two weeks. (Wash and dry the douche equipment after each use to prevent reinfection.) For men, wash the penis twice daily with the solution.

- **Chickweed:** Steep fresh chickweed, strain, and add to your bath. Soak daily for at least one week.

Conventional medical treatment with metronidazole or flagyl may be required. Don't drink alcohol while taking these medications, because the combination causes nausea and vomiting. Sex partners, even if asymptomatic, should also be treated.

Chapter 20

Dealing with Mental, Emotional, and Behavioral Issues

Conventional medicine often approaches the brain as though it's floating in a beaker of chemicals instead of functioning as a key component of a complex organic system. As a result, doctors often treat brain disorders with potent prescription medications designed to restore a healthy chemical balance in the brain, regardless of what's causing the symptoms. These prescription medications are a blessing to many people who live with serious mental illnesses, such as schizophrenia and bipolar disorder, enabling them to reclaim their lives. However, the medical community is beginning to come around to the fact that brain and cognitive disorders arise due to a complex interplay of nature (genetics) and nurture (environment) and that nutrition and lifestyle play key roles in prevention and treatment.

The natural cures approach to treating brain and behavioral disorders is to focus on diet, lifestyle, therapy, and nutritional supplements to restore healthy brain function. In cases in which prescription medications are necessary, natural medicine works alongside conventional medicine to create a situation in which *less* prescription medicine, with its potential long-term side effects, is necessary to achieve the desired results.

Doses in this chapter are for adults, not children. For guidance on how to adjust dosages for children (and adults under 150 pounds), turn to Chapter 12.

Supporting a Healthy Brain

Regardless of which brain and behavior disorder you're treating, the goal is to give your body what it needs to create healthy brain cells that communicate effectively and to avoid anything that's bad for those brain cells, such as stress, alcohol, foods you're allergic or sensitive to, chemicals used in processed foods, and so on. Read on for the details of how you can use diet, supplements, and lifestyle choices to promote a healthy brain.

Team up with your doctor and therapist to forge a treatment plan that works for you. Treatment may include diet and lifestyle changes, supplements, pharmaceutical medications, and talk therapy.

Before drawing up a treatment plan for any psychiatric illness — depression, bipolar disorder, schizophrenia, anxiety disorders, obsessive-compulsive disorder (OCD), or attention deficit hyperactivity disorder (ADHD), for example — consider genetic testing to help predict the effectiveness and side-effect profile of your medication choices. I recommend the Genomind Genecept Assay (www.genomind.com), which identifies the pathways in the brain affected by the illness and sheds light on how your body is likely to *metabolize* (absorb and use) certain medications. The results help your doctor choose the most effective medication and tailor the dose to reduce potentially negative medication side effects.

Don't suddenly stop taking any medications your doctor has prescribed, because stopping cold turkey may cause some nasty side effects. Instead, set realistic goals for managing your medication(s) and illness(es) and transition gradually to other treatments. For example, your initial goal may be to reduce the number of prescription medications you take or how much of a certain medication you take while adopting a healthier diet and implementing new stress-reduction techniques. Take small steps to achieve your goal while maintaining your mental health.

Promoting brain function with diet

Start by adopting a healthy diet and lifestyle, as explained in Chapter 2. In terms of diet, focus on eating foods that are good for your brain and avoiding foods that are bad for it:

✔ **Get tested for food allergies and sensitivities (see Chapter 13).** Gluten sensitivity is often at the root of brain and cognitive dysfunction, including autism, bipolar disorder, depression, and schizophrenia. If testing isn't an option, adopt a gluten-free, casein-free diet for 12 weeks to see whether symptoms improve.

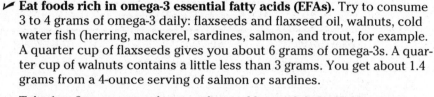

✔ **Eat foods rich in omega-3 essential fatty acids (EFAs).** Try to consume 3 to 4 grams of omega-3 daily: flaxseeds and flaxseed oil, walnuts, cold water fish (herring, mackerel, sardines, salmon, and trout, for example. A quarter cup of flaxseeds gives you about 6 grams of omega-3s. A quarter cup of walnuts contains a little less than 3 grams. You get about 1.4 grams from a 4-ounce serving of salmon or sardines.

Take 1 to 2 teaspoons of top-quality cod liver oil daily. Unlike most fish oils, cod liver oil contains more DHA (docosahexaenoic acid) than EPA (eicosapentaenoic acid); your brain is 75 percent fat, 25 percent of which is DHA.

✔ **Nurture a healthy gut.** What happens in the gut often shows up in the brain. Restore and maintain gut health, as I explain in Chapter 14.

✔ **Avoid foods rich in saturated, hydrogenated, and partially hydrogenated trans fats.** These include baked goods (cakes, cookies, doughnuts, pies, and so on), processed foods, fast foods, fatty cuts of meat (beef, pork, and lamb), butter, margarines, milk, ice cream, cheese, junk food (chips and crackers), mayonnaise, and most salad dressings.

✔ **Eat a colorful variety of vegetables and fruits.** In addition to the vitamins and minerals they contain, vegetables and fruits are full of antioxidants and bioflavonoids, which have neuroprotective properties. Blueberries and pomegranates are usually at the top of the list when it comes to antioxidants that protect neurons from *free radicals,* highly reactive molecules that can damage cells.

✔ **Eat more nuts and seeds.** Although flaxseeds and walnuts capture the headlines when it comes to brain foods, nearly all nuts are high in good fats and other brain-friendly nutrients. They're also a great source of fiber.

✔ **Eliminate glutamate and aspartame from your diet.** These two excitatory neurotransmitters damage brain cells. Glutamate commonly appears on food labeling as monosodium glutamate (MSG) or "natural flavoring," and aspartame is commonly used in diet drinks.

✔ **Limit your alcohol consumption.** A little alcohol is good for you; for example, 1 to 2 ounces with dinner (red wine is best).

✔ **Stay hydrated.** Drink 8 ounces of water every two waking hours.

Supplementing to support brain function

Several nutritional supplements have proven effective in supporting brain function and treating various mental and cognitive dysfunctions, as listed in Table 20-1.

Table 20-1   Nutritional Supplements for Healthy Brain Function

Supplement	Good for	Notes/Risks
Acetyl-L-carnitine	Alzheimer's disease, dementia	Very safe
Alpha-lipoic acid	Alzheimer's disease, dementia	Very safe
Choline	Alzheimer's disease, dementia	Very safe
Chromium	Atypical depression	Generally safe May trigger shift to mania in people with underlying bipolar disorder
DHEA	Depression, bipolar disorder	Take only under medical supervision (see Appendix C for precautions)
Folate	Depression, Alzheimer's disease, dementia	Very safe
Inositol	Depression; panic disorder May be helpful for bipolar disorder, anxiety, OCD, eating disorders, hostility, sadness, tension, and fatigue	Very safe May cause gastrointestinal upset including diarrhea May trigger shift to mania in people with underlying bipolar disorder
Huperzine A	Dementia; depression; memory loss	Take with caution May slow heart rate, increase risk of seizure in people with epilepsy, increase gastrointestinal tract blockage, worsen stomach ulcers, worsen asthma or emphysema symptoms, or increase blockage of the urinary tract or reproductive system
L-theanine	Anxiety	Very safe

Supplement	Good for	Notes/Risks
N-acetyl cysteine	Addiction; bipolar disorder (especially bipolar depression); OCD; hair-pulling, nail biting, skin-picking, and other grooming disorders; schizophrenia; irritability/anger (especially in autism)	Generally safe (see Appendix B for precautions)
Phosphatidylserine	ADHD, Alzheimer's disease, dementia, depression	Generally safe May cause insomnia or digestive upset at doses exceeding 300 mg daily
Rhodiola rosea (golden root or arctic root)	Mild to moderate depression, stress, Alzheimer's disease, dementia, anxiety, bipolar depression, ADHD	Generally safe May cause agitation, insomnia, anxiety, headache, irritability, increased blood pressure, or chest pain May trigger shift to mania in people with underlying bipolar disorder
SAMe	Alzheimer's disease, dementia, depression	Generally safe May worsen underlying agitation, anxiety, irritability, or panic May trigger shift to mania in people with underlying bipolar disorder
St. John's wort	Mild to moderate depression	Consult your healthcare provider before use (see Appendix B for precautions)
Taurine	Anxiety	Very safe Taurine is one of the most abundant amino acids in the brain

(continued)

Table 20-1 *(continued)*		
5-HTP	Anxiety, depression, insomnia	Generally safe, but don't take if you're on an SSRI antidepressant
		May cause nausea, vomiting, diarrhea, sedation, headache, insomnia, or heart palpitations
Vinpocetine	Dementia, memory/cognitive decline, stroke	Take with food; don't take if you have low blood pressure, are taking blood-thinning agents, or are within two weeks before or after undergoing surgery
Vitamins B1 (thiamin), B6, and B12	Depression, hallucinations, memory/cognitive difficulties, paranoia	Very safe
		Have your vitamin B levels tested to determine whether you have a deficiency before supplementing your diet
Vitamin D3	Depression	Very safe at 2,000 IUs daily
		Have your vitamin D level tested to determine whether you have a deficiency before supplementing your diet (see Appendix A for details)

Going beyond diet and supplementation

Several exercise regimens, including mindfulness, yoga, and Qigong, have proven to be effective adjunct treatments for a variety of mental and cognitive conditions. Any discipline that gets you more focused on the moment eases depression, anxiety, and irritability, and sharpens the mind overall. For more about these disciplines, check out *Mindfulness For Dummies,* by Shamash Alidina; *T'ai Chi For Dummies,* by Therese Iknoian; and *Yoga For Dummies,* by Larry Payne and Georg Feuerstein (all published by John Wiley & Sons, Inc.). Other physical activity, especially cardiovascular exercises such as jogging and swimming, alleviates depression and anxiety, too, while improving your overall health and sense of well-being. Talk therapies and related counseling are also very effective nonmedication alternatives for treating depression and other mental health issues.

Overcoming Alcoholism and Substance Abuse

Alcoholism and substance abuse are often caused by underlying mental health conditions and respond best when both the mental health condition (often depression) and the alcoholism or substance abuse are treated concurrently. If you're living with anxiety, depression, post-traumatic stress disorder (PTSD), schizophrenia, or seasonal affective disorder (SAD), skip ahead to the relevant section to determine how to treat that particular dysfunction.

If you have an addiction, don't stop cold turkey. Withdrawal may result in anxiety, nausea or vomiting, headache, insomnia, irritability, confusion, irregular heartbeat, severe confusion, hallucinations, or seizures, which may be life-threatening. Team up with your doctor to draw up a withdrawal schedule and obtain medications that help alleviate withdrawal symptoms, or check yourself into a rehab program that will provide these services.

The natural cures approach of treating alcoholism and substance abuse focuses on making diet and lifestyle changes (see Chapter 2), reducing cravings, and detoxing the body. Here I offer guidance on how to reduce cravings and detox your body.

Reducing cravings

You can do a great deal to reduce cravings by making lifestyle changes. Get involved in healthy activities and distance yourself from activities that involve drinking or substance abuse and from situations and people that act as triggers. Seek counseling and treatment, if necessary. Reach out to friends and family members for help or seek out a support group, such as Alcoholics Anonymous, where people understand the challenges you face and can offer words of advice and encouragement. Engaging in physical activities, such as jogging, swimming, yoga, Qigong, or tai chi, can also help reduce cravings.

To reduce the physical cravings for alcohol or other substances, try the following foods, herbs, and supplements:

- ✔ **To regulate blood sugar levels destabilized by alcohol,** eat rice (in moderation), nuts, and seeds.

- ✔ **To relieve your cravings,** take the following, depending on your addiction:

  - **Alcohol addiction:** Take 1 g of evening primrose oil two to three times daily and eat bananas and sunflower seeds.

  - **Heroin or opiate addictions:** Ask your doctor about taking Kratom as a tea or in capsule form. During the writing of this book, Kratom was legal in every U.S. state except Indiana. Kratom is far less addictive than heroin and even methadone, which is commonly used to help wean users off heroin.

  - **Cocaine addiction:** Take 600 mg of N-acetyl cysteine every 12 hours. N-acetyl cysteine also helps to detox the body and may reduce cravings for alcohol and heroin, as well.

- ✔ **To alleviate anxiety and restlessness that accompany withdrawal,** take 140 mg of a valerian root supplement two to four times daily. For general anxiety relief, take a vitamin B supplement in double or triple doses:

B vitamin	Dosage
Thiamin HCL	20 mg two times daily
Riboflavin 5'-phosphate sodium	20 mg two times daily
Niacin (niacinamide and nictotinic acid)	10 mg nicotinic acid and 130 mg niacinamide two times daily
B6 (pyridoxyl 5'-phosphate)	20 mg two times daily
B12 (methylcobalamin, sublingual fast-dissolving tablet)	400 mcg two times daily
Folate (5-MTHF)	400 mcg two times daily

Get plenty of sleep. Your brain needs to adapt to the changes in chemical stimulants or depressants it's been subjected to for so long. Sleep rejuvenates your brain and body while giving you a break from the battle against addiction.

Detoxing

In respect to alcoholism and substance abuse, *detox* usually refers to abstinence. In the world of natural cures, however, *detox* involves helping your body purge itself of toxins. Detoxing is a whole-body effort that starts at the gut, so the first order of business is to start eating right; see the earlier section "Supporting a Healthy Brain" for dietary recommendations and turn to Chapter 14 for guidance on nurturing a healthy gut.

Fluids and fiber play a key role in detoxing your system, so make sure you're drinking at least 8 ounces of water every two waking hours and consuming 45 to 50 total grams of dietary fiber daily. You may also want to consider taking the following supplements, which are particularly effective in detoxing the liver:

Supplement	Dosage
Milk thistle	100 mg daily
Calcium D-glucarate	250 mg daily
Glutathione (reduced glutathione [GSH])	500 mg daily
N-acetyl cysteine	600 mg daily

Dealing with Alzheimer's Disease, Dementia, and Other Cognitive Disorders

Dementia is a loss of brain function — thinking, memory, reasoning — caused by certain illnesses or injury to the brain. Although dementia has no cure, early detection can slow progression and perhaps improve the course of the illness. The key is to identify and treat the underlying cause of this debilitating symptom. The most common causes of dementia include Alzheimer's disease, nutrient deficiency, brain injury (due to stroke or trauma, for example), and so on, but there are several forms of dementia that haven't been linked to a specific cause. In this section, I explain how you can slow the progression of cognitive decline.

Slowing the progression of Alzheimer's

Alzheimer's disease, which accounts for about 50 to 60 percent of all cases of dementia, is an age-related deterioration of brain function resulting in a decline in cognitive functioning that affects memory, thinking, and behavior. Currently, Alzheimer's disease has no cure, but you may be able to slow its progression and alleviate symptoms by doing the following:

✔ **Nurture a healthy brain.** See "Supporting a Healthy Brain," earlier in this chapter, for guidance. Consuming 8 ounces of oily fish (mackerel, salmon, or sardines, for example) or 4 to 5 grams of pharmaceutical grade fish oil daily is especially important.

Alzheimer's disease is closely linked with diabetes and obesity, so eat a healthy diet (see Chapter 2) with a focus on eliminating sugar, high-fructose corn syrup, and highly processed carbohydrates. (See Chapter 17 for guidance on treating diabetes and related metabolic conditions that likely contribute to Alzheimer's.)

✔ **Exercise regularly.** Exercise, especially cardiovascular exercise, improves circulation throughout the body, including to the brain, while engaging the areas of the brain that govern motor skills.

✔ **Keep your brain active.** Reading, playing games, solving puzzles, and so forth engage your brain in cognitive activities that contribute to forming and creating healthy brain cells.

Several supplements presented in Table 20-1 are effective in slowing the progression of Alzheimer's disease and improving cognitive function, including acetyl-L-carnitine, choline, folate, *Rhodiola rosea,* and SAMe (S-adenosyl-L-methionine).

Looking at other causes of dementia

Other common causes of dementia include the following:

✔ **Stroke:** Stroke — injury to the brain due to blockage of the blood supply to the brain — is the second leading cause of dementia. *Multi-infarct dementia,* also called *vascular dementia,* is caused by multiple small strokes. See Chapter 17 for more about preventing and treating stroke.

✔ **Toxins:** Alcohol and substance abuse, as well as certain prescription medications, may damage or destroy brain cells.

✔ **Diabetes:** Although diabetes is rarely named as a cause of dementia, the role it plays in Alzheimer's disease and other brain illnesses implicates it as an indirect cause of dementia. See Chapter 17 for more about preventing and treating diabetes.

✔ **Nutritional deficiencies:** Deficiencies in B-complex vitamins, folate, magnesium, zinc, and vitamin D are the primary culprits. Nutritional deficiencies may also be caused by problems in the gut that restrict absorption of these key brain nutrients. See "Supporting a Healthy Brain," earlier in this chapter, to find out more about nurturing brain health and function. Head to Chapter 14 for info on digestive health.

✔ **Parkinson's and Huntington's diseases:** Parkinson's and Huntington's diseases are two illnesses that result in neuron loss. (See Chapter 17 for more about preventing and treating Parkinson's disease.)

✔ **Head injuries:** Concussions and other physical brain injuries may cause dementia.

Anger issues, anyone?

Anger isn't generally a mental health issue. In fact, it's often justified. But if you're angry or irritable more frequently or more intensely than is normal for you, take a close look at what you're eating. Several common foods and additives are known to trigger agitation, irritability, and anger, including the following:

✔ Sugar and highly processed carbohydrates

✔ Trans fats (hydrogenated and partially hydrogenated oils)

✔ Glutamate, including monosodium glutamate (MSG)

✔ Food additives, including dyes and preservatives

✔ Caffeine and nicotine

Irritability and anger may be the result of other conditions, including food allergies and sensitivities (see Chapter 13), depression (see "Dealing with Depression," later in this chapter), or vitamin or mineral deficiencies (have your levels tested and adjust or supplement your diet to address any deficiencies).

Herbal remedies, especially valerian root, passionflower, and chamomile, may help alleviate irritability and anger (avoid chamomile if you're allergic to ragweed). In addition, centering disciplines, such as mindfulness mediation and Qigong, can help you cope more effectively with stressful situations. Various talk therapies may also help you restructure your thought processes and build communication and problem-solving skills to address and resolve frustrating issues and interpersonal conflict.

If you can't trace the dementia to a specific cause, focus on diet and lifestyle changes to improve overall brain function, as explained in the earlier section "Supporting a Healthy Brain."

Relieving Anxiety Disorders

People with an anxiety disorder feel excessive fear, distress, or uneasiness in situations that don't merit such reactions. These disorders include obsessive-compulsive disorder (OCD), panic disorder, post-traumatic stress disorder (PTSD), generalized anxiety disorder (GAD), social anxiety disorder, and the various phobias.

The most effective treatments for anxiety disorders involve a combination of healthy diet, exercise, sufficient sleep, and therapy. Cognitive behavioral therapy (CBT) is especially helpful in exploring the connections between thoughts, feelings, and behaviors. The goal is to teach sufferers now to restructure their thought processes so that they can reduce or better control the anxiety they feel in certain situations. Centering disciplines, including mindfulness meditation and Qigong, help calm the mind exposed to stressful conditions.

Taurine is one of the most effective over-the-counter supplements for treating anxiety. L-theanine has also shown promise in alleviating anxiety. Also consider taking a magnesium supplement (specifically magnesium glycinate chelate; see Appendix A). Magnesium helps to modulate the fight-or-flight response and is often depleted as a result of stress.

Herbal remedies for anxiety include kava kava, valerian root, and passion-flower, all of which tend to calm the nerves. Be careful with kava kava, however, because some reports link it to liver damage; take it only with your doctor's permission and supervision.

Overcoming ADHD

Attention deficit hyperactivity disorder (ADHD) is characterized by an inability to focus, sit still, or control one's behavior. ADHD has reached epidemic levels in the United States and other developed countries primarily due to poor diet and an overstimulated lifestyle. Most cases of ADHD can be cured by making the diet and lifestyle changes I recommend in Chapter 2, with an emphasis on eliminating all refined sugars, processed carbohydrates, and trans fats (hydrogenated and partially hydrogenated oils). I also strongly recommend getting tested for food allergies and sensitivities (see Chapter 13); gluten sensitivity is the usual suspect, but numerous other foods, dyes, and additives may worsen symptoms.

Relatively recent research links ADHD, autism, and numerous other chronic health conditions to impaired methylation. *Methylation* is a key biochemical process that helps repair DNA, influences DNA expression, regulates homocysteine (a compound that can damage blood vessels), helps recycle molecules used to detoxify the body, reduces inflammation, produces neurotransmitters that regulate mood, and much more.

To optimize methylation, make sure you're getting sufficient amounts of the following nutrients and digestion-support supplements:

- ✔ **Vitamin B12 (methylcobalamin, in a fast-dissolving tablet):** Take 5,000 mcg one or two times daily. (For maximum bioavailabilty, methylcobalamin may be given by injection or in lipsomal form that's more readily absorbed.)

- ✔ **Vitamin B9, as folate/folic acid (5-MTHF [5-methyltetrahydrofolate]):** 800 mcg one to two times daily. Approximately 30 percent of the population is unable to convert folic acid to the active form of folate, so taking the methylated form of folate is important.

✔ **Zinc, iron, and magnesium:** Have your zinc, iron (ferritin), and magnesium levels tested, and adjust your diet or take supplements to address any deficiencies.

✔ **Digestive enzymes and probiotics:** Improve your digestion to increase absorption of nutrients and prevent leaky gut syndrome, as explained in Chapter 13.

To optimize methylation, consider taking Methyl Protect from XYMOGEN (www.xymogen.com), which contains all of the building blocks required to support the various methylation processes, including methylcobalamin and 5-MTHF. I also like NeuroMethylation Cream from NuMedica (www.numedica.com).

Addressing Autism

Autism spectrum disorder (ASD) is a neurodevelopmental disorder characterized by impaired communication and social interaction along with restricted and repetitive behavior that become apparent before a child turns 3 years old.

As with ADHD, discussed in the preceding section, methylation seems to play a role in the onset and course of autism. I recommend a similar treatment approach for autism and related disorders (such as Asperger syndrome), as I do for ADHD:

✔ **Eliminate wheat/gluten and dairy from your diet.** Leaky gut syndrome is almost always at the root of autism spectrum disorders, and wheat/gluten and dairy often contribute to leaky gut syndrome. Take probiotics and digestive enzymes to improve digestion and increase nutrient absorption. (For more about leaky gut syndrome and details on how to improve digestive and bowel functions, see Chapters 13 and 14.)

✔ **Eat a healthy diet.** Chapter 2 has the details.

✔ **Test for and treat vitamin and mineral deficiencies.** Vitamins B12 and folate play key roles in methylation processes. Omega-3 essential fatty acids provide building blocks for healthy brain cells. Other common deficiencies that may play a role in autism are vitamins B6, A, C, and D, and magnesium, selenium, zinc, and iron.

✔ **Test for and treat heavy-metal toxicity and food allergies and sensitivities.** Talk to your doctor about getting tested for heavy-metal toxicity and see Chapter 13 for more about testing for food allergies and sensitivities.

Pushing Past Bipolar Disorder

Bipolar disorder (formerly referred to as *manic depression*) is characterized by alternating periods of abnormally high and low moods. The single most effective "medication" for treating bipolar disorder is lithium, which happens to be a naturally occurring salt and is one of the few medications that treats both "poles" — depression and mania.

As a first step in treating bipolar disorder naturally, focus on nurturing a healthy brain overall; see "Supporting a Healthy Brain," earlier in this chapter, for details. Adopt a healthy diet and take supplements as necessary to get sufficient amounts of B vitamins, folate, vitamin D, magnesium, and zinc. Other supplements that have shown some promise in treating depression, mania, and the anxiety and sleeplessness that often accompany and may trigger bipolar mood episodes include the following:

- ✔ **Coenzyme Q10** (CoQ10) may help with the depressive side of bipolar disorder.

- ✔ **5-HTP** (5-hydroxytryptophan) supplies the building blocks for *serotonin,* a key mood-related neurotransmitter. 5-HTP may help with depression, anxiety, and sleep.

- ✔ **Inositol** is a sugar, found in cells, that may play a role in depression and mania; lithium affects inositol concentrations within brain cells.

- ✔ **Melatonin** is a hormone your body produces that helps you fall asleep.

- ✔ **N-acetyl cysteine (NAC),** when taken at 1,000 mg twice daily, seems to reduce depression, perhaps by raising levels of glutathione in the brain.

- ✔ **SAMe** (S-adenosyl-L-methionine) has been shown to function as an antidepressant in some studies.

- ✔ **St. John's wort** helps with mild to moderate depression.

- ✔ **Taurine** alleviates anxiety and may help stabilize mood.

- ✔ **Valerian root** helps treat insomnia, which often triggers mood episodes.

Consult your doctor before taking any nutritional supplements for depression or mania. For more about treating bipolar disorder with conventional, alternative, and complementary treatments, check out *Bipolar Disorder For Dummies,* by Candida Fink, MD, and Joe Kraynak. (John Wiley & Sons, Inc.).

Beating Borderline Personality Disorder

Borderline personality disorder (BPD) is a behavioral disorder characterized by patterns of unstable and explosive emotional outbursts. Unlike bipolar disorder, in which mood episodes may have no easily identifiable emotional trigger and typically last for several days or weeks, BPD outbursts are typically in response to upsetting incidents or interpersonal conflicts and often last for only a few minutes or hours. Conventional treatment typically focuses on adjusting thought patterns through talk therapies, such as cognitive behavioral therapy (CBT) and dialectical behavioral therapy (DBT).

If you have BPD, you struggle with anger issues, and many of the natural treatments I recommend for treating anger also help with BPD; see the sidebar "Anger issues, anyone?" earlier in this chapter, for details. Focus on adjusting your diet to avoid spikes and valleys in blood sugar levels. Omega-3 fatty acids have also proven effective, in at least one study, for reducing symptoms of aggression and depression in women with BPD. In addition, a healthy brain is better equipped to handle the emotional stress that commonly triggers anger outbursts. For more about nurturing a healthy brain and brain function, refer to the earlier section "Supporting a Healthy Brain."

Mood irregularities and irritability are commonly connected to sex hormone imbalances (see Chapter 19 for guidance).

Dealing with Depression

Depression (formally referred to as *major depressive disorder,* or *MDD*) is a persistent feeling of intense sadness or fatigue and a lack of interest in activities previously considered enjoyable. When the depression is triggered by a change of seasons, it's referred to as *seasonal affective disorder (SAD).* Although depression can certainly be linked to biochemical irregularities in the brain, treatment doesn't necessarily require pharmaceutical medications.

If you're currently being treated for depression, don't stop taking any medications your doctor prescribed. Suddenly stopping medications, especially selective serotonin reuptake inhibitors (SSRIs), may cause a host of very serious side effects. Consult your doctor regarding treatment options.

The first step in treating depression is to nourish your brain, as explained in the earlier section "Supporting a Healthy Brain," with a focus on eliminating toxins from your body — refined sugar, highly processed carbohydrates, and trans fats — stuff that can make you feel rundown. In addition to adopting a mood-friendly diet, take other steps to alleviate depression, including the following:

- ✔ **Get plenty of fresh air and sunshine.** Spend at least 15 minutes out in the sun daily. Be careful not to get overexposed.

- ✔ **Get enough sleep but not too much.** Experiment with sleeping between seven and ten hours per night to determine the amount of sleep that makes you feel best. Keep a sleep journal. (If you're struggling with sleep issues, head to Chapter 16.)

- ✔ **Establish healthy routines, either alone or with others.** Start by going to bed and waking up at the same times every day. Do something fun. Even if you have to force yourself, engage in an activity that you used to enjoy doing; for example, join a book club or a bowling team.

- ✔ **Set daily goals.** Make a list of things to do each day. As you check items off your list, you develop a sense of accomplishment.

- ✔ **Exercise to release feel-good endorphins.** Even walking a few times a week can boost your mood. Alternate days between centering exercises, such as yoga and Qigong, and cardiovascular exercises, such as walking, biking, and swimming.

The three over-the-counter supplements that have the best track record for treating depression are omega-3, St. John's wort, and SAMe (S-adenosyl-L-methionine), but don't overlook vitamins and minerals, especially the B vitamins, vitamin D, folate, magnesium, and zinc. Consult your doctor before taking St. John's wort or SAMe.

For additional guidance on living well with depression, check out *Depression For Dummies*, by Laura L. Smith and Charles H. Elliott. (John Wiley & Sons, Inc.).

Taking the Bite Out of Eating Disorders

Eating disorders, including *anorexia nervosa* (excessive dieting or exercising) and *bulimia* (binge eating followed by vomiting or abusing laxatives), are characterized by extreme attitudes and behaviors related to food and body image. Anxiety or depression may contribute to these disorders, so be sure to address these issues as well (see the earlier sections "Relieving Anxiety Disorders" and "Dealing with Depression" for guidance).

The natural cures approach to treating eating disorders aligns with conventional treatments — a combination of self-help, psychotherapy, and support from friends and family:

- ✔ **Educate yourself about eating disorders.** Psychoeducation is one of the most powerful tools for changing the way you think about food and eating. Check out *Eating Disorders For Dummies* by Susan Schulherr (John Wiley & Sons, Inc.).

- ✔ **Seek therapy.** Psychotherapy, biofeedback, and centering exercises, such as yoga, Qigong, and mindfulness meditation can all help retool the mind.

- ✔ **Remain engaged.** Get involved in activities that keep your mind occupied with thoughts unrelated to food and weight. Staying engaged with loved ones also provides the support you need to overcome your challenges, although you may want to steer clear of any toxic relationships.

- ✔ **Avoid scales and mirrors.** These devices feed anxiety over body image and weight.

Subduing Schizophrenia

Schizophrenia is a severe brain illness characterized by hallucinations (typically "hearing things"), delusions (false beliefs), social withdrawal, disorganized thinking and speech, abnormal physical movement, and lack of emotion *(flat affect)*. Schizophrenia is thought to be caused by an interplay of genetic susceptibility and exposure to environmental stressors, including toxins, infections, emotional stress, and food allergies or sensitivity (especially gluten sensitivity).

Treatment for schizophrenia almost always requires the use of antipsychotic medication. Instead of trying to avoid medication altogether, work with your doctor to complement treatment with dietary and lifestyle changes, exercise, and therapy.

Although schizophrenia has no cure, you may be able to help prevent it, slow its progress, and improve the course of the illness by doing the following:

- ✔ **If you're planning to have children, make healthy diet and lifestyle choices.** What you eat, drink, or otherwise ingest may influence the way your genes are expressed, and any changes in gene expression may be passed along to your children. Although these changes are especially important for expecting mothers, fathers also need to be careful about what they ingest.

✔ **Get tested and treated for food allergies or sensitivities.** Several studies draw a link between gluten or casein sensitivity and schizophrenia. If you have schizophrenia, try going dairy-free and gluten-free for three months to see whether your symptoms improve. (At the very least, get tested for gluten sensitivity and leaky gut syndrome, as explained in Chapter 13.)

✔ **Nurture a healthy brain.** See the earlier section "Supporting a Healthy Brain" for details. I strongly recommend that you consult with a functional medical practitioner or a naturopath to assess your body's unique chemistry and adjust your diet to address any imbalances. Vitamin B3 (niacin) is often used as a complementary treatment for schizophrenia, and research indicates that a combination of vitamin B12 and folate is helpful. A glycine supplement may also be helpful. Don't expect immediate results; improvement in symptoms may take four to six months.

Schizophrenia responds much better to medical and alternative treatments if the person who has the illness receives support from family members and friends and has the opportunity to contribute to the community, perhaps by returning to work or school. Unfortunately, as with many mental illnesses, schizophrenia tends to drive loved ones away, isolating the person who has the illness. If you have a loved one with schizophrenia, educate yourself and get support through organizations such as the National Alliance on Mental Illness (NAMI; http://www.nami.org), and do what you can to support your loved one on his or her road to recovery.

For more about living well with schizophrenia, check out *Schizophrenia For Dummies* by Jerome Levine and Irene S. Levine. (John Wiley & Sons, Inc.).

Part III
The Part of Tens

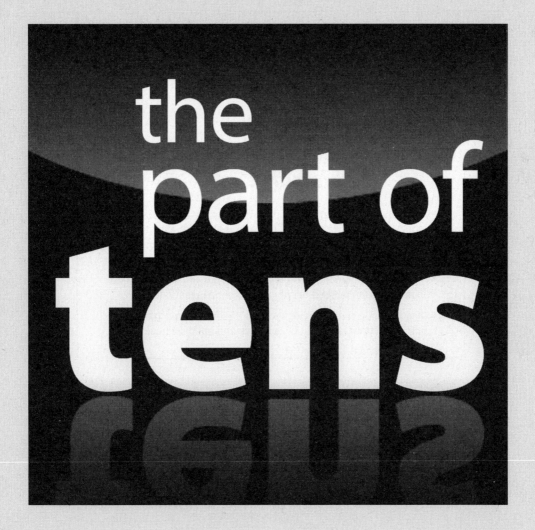

For a list of ten essential supplements to add to your medicine cabinet, head online to www.dummies.com/extras/naturalcures.

In this part . . .

✔ Reap the most benefits from natural medicine by following the suggestions — like getting a professional health evaluation from the start and taking vitamins and minerals in their better forms — outlined here.

✔ Discover ten diet and lifestyle rules that put you on the path to optimal health without burying you in unnecessary details.

✔ Key in on ten simple sayings to help you remember the most important principles that cure illness and optimize health.

Chapter 21

Ten Ways to Get the Most Out of Natural Medicine

*Y*ou can use the natural cures approach to prevent and treat specific illnesses or to become so healthy that any illness has a difficult time establishing a foothold. I strongly encourage you to take the second approach — to adopt a diet and lifestyle that supports optimum health, as I explain in Chapter 2. In this chapter, I offer ten more ways to get the most out of natural cures.

Consulting a Natural Healthcare Provider

To truly get the most out of natural medicine, you should consult a natural healthcare provider — a functional medicine practitioner, naturopath, osteopath, or a chiropractor who's skilled in nutritional medicine. Natural healthcare providers are dedicated to treating patients, not just illnesses. They can order tests and interpret the results to determine what's going on in *your* body and guide you in terms of diet and supplements to address any nutritional deficiencies, food allergies or sensitivities, and other conditions that may be compromising your overall health.

Many natural healthcare providers, especially osteopaths, are covered by health insurance plans, so you may want to start your search by contacting your insurance provider. You may also search for certified practitioners online through the websites of the organizations to which they belong. For example, to find a functional medicine practitioner, conduct your search at www.functionalmedicine.org or visit www.osteopathic.org to find an osteopath.

Targeting Causes, Not Symptoms

Conventional medicine tends to focus on alleviating symptoms rather than treating illness. A conventional doctor is likely to prescribe antacids to treat heartburn and indigestion, decongestants and antihistamines to treat a stuffy nose, and pain relievers to treat a headache. You may feel better for a while, but as soon as you stop the medication, your symptoms return. Even worse, the medicines may actually contribute to the onset of other chronic conditions; for example, taking a proton pump inhibitor to reduce stomach acid restricts the absorption of calcium and magnesium, eventually decreasing bone density and increasing the risk of osteoporosis. The better solution is to go upstream and eliminate whatever is causing the indigestion, which is usually diet, *too little* hydrochloric acid, insufficient amounts of pancreatic enzymes, or unbalanced intestinal microbes.

Just because you feel good doesn't mean you're healthy. In the disease cycle, symptoms are the last to show up and the first to leave. You may be ill long before your know it, so you need to constantly work on optimizing all of the systems that make up your body.

Being Healthy Instead of Not Sick

The goal of conventional medicine is to eliminate illness. The goal of natural medicine is to make you healthy. Although the distinction seems insignificant, the two approaches are worlds apart. When all you're trying to do is eliminate an illness, usually with pharmaceutical medications, radiation, or surgery, you're likely to cause a host of other health conditions. With conventional medication, the cure is often as bad as or worse than the illness. Natural cures strengthen the body's defenses against illness without causing the undesirable side effects that accompany most conventional treatments.

Using Common Sense as Your Guide

Voltaire said, "Common sense is not so common." Case in point? The people who complain about their doctors' inability to cure them are usually couch potatoes who overindulge in sugary foods and drinks, alcohol, tobacco, and processed foods; and eat far more meat and wheat than they do vegetables and fruits. And then they wonder why they feel lousy.

Use your common sense. Like a car, your body runs on the fuel you pump into your tank. Bad fuel leads to poor performance and may permanently damage your body. Here are three commonsense suggestions for improving your overall health:

✔ Eat whole foods low on the glycemic index, diverse in phytonutrients, with plenty of fiber. Most of your diet should be veggies, fruits, nuts (not peanuts), and seeds.

✔ Engage in aerobic exercise for 30 minutes at least every other day with some sort of strength training at least three days a week.

✔ Take a high-quality multivitamin, 4 g of omega-3 essential fatty acids, and 2,000 mg of vitamin D daily.

Steering Clear of Miracle Cures

Salespeople routinely show up at my office to peddle the latest miracle cure — a newly discovered tropical drink from the rain forest that holds the promise of eternal youth or an ingredient extracted from a rare plant that cures everything from colds to cancer. Establishing and maintaining good health requires proper nutrition and exercise, neither of which comes in a bottle.

Taking Vitamins and Minerals in Their Better Forms

Many people take vitamins, minerals, probiotics, and other supplements and give up on these alternative treatments because they don't work. In many cases, supplements don't work because they're low-quality products or are in a form that the body can't absorb or make use of efficiently. To get the most out of nutritional supplements, take them in their better forms from reliable manufacturers. Whenever I recommend a supplement in the chapters in Part II, I indicate the supplement's better form when relevant. For a more comprehensive list, check out Appendixes A and B.

Likewise, high-quality probiotics that contain high levels of many different strains of specific gut microflora are much more effective in maintaining healthy digestion than are cheap products that are processed, shipped, or stored in a way that kills all of the beneficial microorganisms. Buy products only from reputable manufacturers. Visit my website, www.spinelife.com, to view a list of manufacturers I recommend.

Being Skeptical of Expert Advice

Doctors and nutritionists have a long history of leading consumers astray with conflicting advice or incomplete information. For many years, they said that high cholesterol was bad. Then they amended their advice, claiming that LDL was bad, but HDL was good. They advised avoiding saturated fats and taking statin drugs to lower cholesterol but rarely mentioned that lowering your cholesterol increases your risk of depression, dementia, and Parkinson's disease or that it interferes with the production of key hormones and blocks production of CoQ10, which is crucial for production of cellular energy.

Before accepting any expert's health recommendation, test it against what nature tells you and against your own common sense. For example, does it really make sense to take a proton pump inhibitor to reduce the production of stomach acid? How else is your body supposed to fully digest the food you eat?! Earth's many ecosystems have evolved over billions of years, and humans, plants, and animals have evolved side-by-side for at least 2.4 million years. Trust only those recommendations that seek to optimize the body's functions and restore balance. Remain very skeptical of any treatment options designed solely to suppress symptoms.

Making Bold Changes

To become healthy, you need to go all in. Eliminating sugar from your diet without eliminating highly processed carbohydrates does nothing to improve your health. If you have celiac disease or gluten sensitivity, plucking the croutons off of your Caesar salad doesn't help; enough gluten residue remains to trigger an immune response that raises your body's gluten antibodies for several weeks.

Be bold. Develop an exercise routine and stick with it. Dump the junk food in your cabinet and refrigerator and restock with healthy, organic whole foods. Team up with your doctor to explore ways to reduce or eliminate the pharmaceutical medications you're taking. Make a commitment to eliminate stress at home and work and in your relationships.

Eating Organic Foods Whenever Possible

Healthy foods are grown in healthy, nutrient-rich soil. Unfortunately, commercial farming practices often poison the soil or deplete its nutrients, producing foods that are toxic or lower in nutrients than they should be. In addition, many crops, including soybeans and corn, are genetically engineered into foods that human evolution hasn't prepared the human body to process. These genetically engineered foods trigger a variety of illnesses in people — everything from digestive issues to allergies to brain and cognitive disorders.

Whenever possible, buy local and organic vegetables and fruits that are in season. If you eat meat, buy wild fish and game and pastured animal products. Farmer's markets, Amish farms, and whole food grocery stores are a great place to start. You may also want to search online for local organic food buyers' clubs. I buy from a small biodiverse Amish farm in Lancaster, Pennsylvania, where I get to speak with my farmer! How cool is that?

Steering Clear of Food Fights

Healthy eating is an emotional subject. Just look at the heated debates over school lunches. As you set out on your quest to be healthy, I suggest that you not speak about it until you're spoken to. If you choose to go gluten free, for example, don't announce it. When you look and feel better, people will take notice and will ask you what you've been doing. That's when you tell them what you've been doing. They can't argue with that.

The world is filled with gloomy doomers and stinker thinkers. Many people would like to see you fail. Don't give them the satisfaction. Follow my recommendations in this book and let your good health speak for itself. If you feel a need to talk about it, join a group of like-minded people who are looking to share information and support.

Chapter 22

Ten Rules of the Road

*I*f you're not ready to commit to the healthy diet and lifestyle changes I recommend in Chapter 2, here are ten rules to good health that may be easier to follow. You don't have to comply with all the rules, but the more you follow, the greater the benefit.

Eat More Plants

While certain cows may be telling you to "Eat more chickin'," I advise you to eat a rainbow of plant-based foods, organically grown, if possible. By "plant-based," I mean veggies, fruits, nuts (except peanuts), and seeds. By "rainbow," I mean green, yellow, red, orange, and purple. Head to the produce section at the local grocery store, and you'll see a rainbow of colors; select foods from the entire spectrum.

Eating veggies raw or juiced is best, because heating tends to destroy nutrients. If you heat your veggies, steam, bake, or sauté them, and try not to cook them to mush.

Avoid Sugar in All Forms

Processed sugar in all of its many forms is bad for you, so avoid products that contain any sugar (Chapter 2 has a list of the many names sugar goes by):

- ✔ Sugar is addictive.

- ✔ Sugar contributes to *non-alcoholic fatty liver disease (NAFLD)* that's now showing up in kids.

- ✔ Sugar causes insulin resistance, which is the precursor to metabolic syndrome and increases your chances of developing type 2 diabetes. In addition, high levels of insulin dampen the hormone that tells you when you're full, so you just keep eating.

- ✔ Sugar is inflammatory and lowers your immune response, causing chronic pain and frequent illness.

Eat Grains Rarely, If at All

All grains — wheat, corn, oatmeal, quinoa, rye, and so on — are simple carbohydrates that spike your blood glucose levels. If you want to include grains in your diet, I recommend eating no more than one small serving of non-gluten grains daily. For details on gluten and non-gluten grains, see Chapter 2.

Grains are not an essential food. In fact, grains are a relatively new food in the history of human evolution, introduced to the human diet a mere 10,000 years or so ago. Many people feel much better on a totally grain-free diet. Try it, and see how you feel.

Don't Drink Your Calories

Most calories consumed in the U.S. are empty calories in the form of soda pop, fruit juice, energy drinks, and other beverages loaded with some form of sugar, typically high-fructose corn syrup. In addition to spiking your blood glucose and insulin levels, the calories that many of these drinks contain have low or no nutritional value — no fiber, vitamins, minerals, protein, healthy fats, phytonutrients, or other nutrients.

The healthiest beverage you can drink is quality, filtered water. Unsweetened green tea, herbal teas, and even coffee are better than the sugary beverages that have become a staple of the standard American diet.

Don't replace sugary drinks with diet drinks that have artificial sweeteners, such as aspartame. In many ways, diet drinks are worse for you than drinks that contain sugar. And contrary to what many people believe, diet drinks don't help you lose weight.

Drink Plenty of Water

Your body is about 70 percent water, and every cell in your body requires water to function properly, so drink 8 ounces of water every two waking hours. Drink more on days you exercise or are exposed to hotter, drier conditions than normal. (I recommend 8 ounces of water every two hours because it's a good general guideline that's easy to remember, but to be more accurate, drink half your weight in ounces of water daily. For example, if you weigh 200 pounds, then drink 100 ounces of water daily.)

Not all water is created equal. See Chapter 2 for guidance on obtaining quality water.

Exercise Regularly

Exercise is essential for improving every aspect of health, including lung function, circulation, digestion, detoxification, brain function, bone density, and muscle tone. It improves mood, boosts energy, and makes you look and feel younger. Do some form of aerobic exercise for 30 minutes at least every other day along with at least three days a week of strength training — some sort of resistance exercise, such as lifting weights or doing pushups, pull-ups, crunches, burpees, and so on (all of which use your own body weight).

Don't be a weekend warrior. Getting all of your exercise in one or two days a week may actually be harmful, increasing oxidation and free radicals that damage cells. Exercising regularly is the only way to reap the health benefits of exercise.

Stop Eating When You're 80 Percent Full

How you eat is almost as important as what you eat. Follow the Japanese rule of *hara hachi bu* — eat until you are 80 percent full. When you stop eating before you're bursting at the seams, you naturally lose weight and are likely to eliminate any problems related to indigestion, such as gastroesophageal reflux disease (GERD). I also recommend that you chew your food to liquid before swallowing and stop eating three hours before bed.

Healthy living starts in your gut. Proper digestion enables your body to more fully absorb nutrients and prevent a host of autoimmune disorders related to leaky gut and food allergies and sensitivities. Head to Chapters 13 and 14 for details on how to boost your digestive health.

Get an Oil Change

Replace bad fats with good fats:

- ✔ **Bad fats:** Sources of bad fats are margarine; shortening; fried foods; hydrogenated peanut butter; microwaved foods, such as popcorn, that form bad fats during microwaving; commercially prepared cookies, crackers, and chips; chocolate candy; doughnuts and other pastries; and many processed foods. Sources of bad saturated fats include hydrogenated and partially hydrogenated oils, rancid (sharp-smelling) oils, poultry skin, high-temp deep fried foods, cheese, and red meat (beef, pork, and lamb). Avoid fatty cuts of meat and items cooked or prepared with high amounts of saturated fats, such as butter, but keep in mind that butter is better for you than margarine.

- ✔ **Good fats:** Sources of good fats include olive oil, sesame seeds and oil, Brazil nuts, hazelnuts/filberts, avocados, cashews, almonds, macadamia nuts, walnuts, cashews, and pine nuts. Avoid peanuts, canola, and soybean oil. Purchase good quality oils in tinted bottles labeled "cold pressed" and "extra virgin" or "first-pressing." Good sources of omega-3 essential fatty acids (EFAs) are flaxseeds and oil, walnuts, algae, dark leafy green vegetables, cold water fish (cod, salmon, tuna), and pumpkin seeds (avoid soybean and canola, which are mostly genetically modified). Good sources of omega-6 are flaxseed oil (cold pressed); walnuts; safflower, sunflower, and sesame oils (avoid grapeseed oil); and tahini.

Keep in mind that heat and light can change the composition of fats and oils. For medium heat (375 to 449 degrees Fahrenheit [190.6 to 231.7 degrees Celsius]), use olive oil. For high heat, use coconut or palm oil, which are the most stable under higher heat conditions (450 degrees Fahrenheit [232.2 degrees Celsius] or higher).

Don't eat low-fat, fat-free, light, or reduced-fat foods. Manufacturers simply replace the fat with sugar. Healthy fats are good for you. Sugar is bad for you. Low-fat or nonfat foods don't help you lose weight or lower your cholesterol.

Don't Fall Victim to Pharmageddon

Pharmageddon is a common phenomenon in which a patient is prescribed a medication and then must take another medication to treat illnesses caused by the first medication. For example, many antipsychotic medications cause obesity and type 2 diabetes, requiring insulin and medications to treat weight gain. Acid blockers cause anemia. Certain blood pressure medications cause erectile dysfunction. Powerful anti-inflammatory medications to control arthritic pain often cause kidney damage leading to dialysis. Long-term use of ibuprofen may lead to heart attack, stroke, and gastric bleeding. Acetaminophen can cause liver failure. All these adverse reactions require more drugs, and the next thing you know you're on a dozen medications. Welcome to Pharmageddon.

Take the least amount of medication for the shortest period of time. Your doctor has no way of predicting how medications are likely to interact with one another or with your genetic makeup. It's diagnosis by prescription — a trial-by-error approach with you as the guinea pig.

Get Enough Sleep

You need to sleep about one-third of every day to rest your body and give it time to repair itself. Some people need more sleep than others, and you may need a little more or less sleep, depending on what's going on in your life. However, if you're getting less than five hours or more than ten hours, or if you're worn out soon after waking, you have a problem. If you're not getting enough restful sleep, check out Chapter 16 for guidance on addressing sleep issues. If you're sleeping too much and feeling tired all the time, you may be depressed; see Chapter 20 for antidepression remedies.

Chapter 23

Ten Natural Cure Maxims

*N*atural medicine isn't as easy as popping a pill. It's a juggling act that involves diet, lifestyle, nutritional supplements, herbs, body work, and other factors. It requires a great deal of attention to detail. To help keep track of all the details, sometimes it helps to look at the big picture. In this chapter, I present ten principles that drive natural medicine and ease the burden of having to remember all the details.

Community Is the Cure

According to an old African proverb, "If you want to travel swiftly, go alone. If you want to travel far, travel together." As you embark on your journey toward wellness, team up with other like-minded individuals to support one another and hold each other accountable for meeting your goals. Start by getting everyone in your household onboard; living healthy is easier when everyone around you is working to achieve the same goal.

Create your own support group on Facebook, where you can post your progress and celebrate your success with others, but also meet face-to-face every so often. Human contact is healthier than digital communication.

Treat the Patient, Not the Symptoms

For a medical treatment to be effective, it must accommodate the intricate interactions between nature and nurture — an individual patient's unique biological makeup and how it's influenced by diet, lifestyle, and environmental factors. Natural medicine practitioners account for these differences in individual patients and tailor their treatments to meet the unique needs of each patient.

Consult a natural medicine practitioner for a complete health evaluation to identify deficiencies and dysfunctions that you need to address. Although I provide general recommendations on nutrition, supplements, and lifestyle throughout this book, these interventions work best when tailored specifically to meet your individual needs.

You Are What You Eat Has Eaten

Conventional wisdom tells you that you are what you eat, but I go one step further and say, "You are what you eat has eaten." Genetically modified vegetables grown in nutrient-depleted soil that's laced with herbicides and insecticides are obviously not as good for you as those grown organically in rich soil without the use of chemical fertilizers and pesticides. Grass-fed beef from pastured cows is much better for you than beef from corn-fed cows raised on feed lots and pumped full of antibiotics and growth hormones.

Pay the Farmer Instead of the Doctor

Organically grown and raised foods are more expensive than their commercially grown and raised counterparts, but what you'll ultimately save in doctor bills and medications will more than cover the added costs of the healthier food, and you'll feel a whole lot better along the way.

The same is true of nutritional supplements. Although they may be expensive and insurance may not cover their cost, they treat the underlying causes of illness and not just the symptoms. In addition, they're less likely than pharmaceutical medications to cause other serious, chronic, and sometimes irreversible illnesses.

Food Is Your Best Medicine

Food provides your body with much more than just the fuel and building blocks it needs to function; it also conveys information to your genes, flipping microscopic switches on or off that can trigger or protect against serious chronic illnesses, including arthritis, diabetes, and heart disease. Send your genes good information loaded with antioxidants and phytonutrients from plant-based foods. Avoid bathing your genes in highly refined processed fats and sugars that send destructive messages.

Don't let the food industry fool you. Adding fiber to a sugary cereal doesn't make it healthy. Nonfat or low-fat products created by replacing the fats with sugar are often worse for you than the fatty foods. Products advertised as gluten-free are often packed with other starches that are likely to spike your blood glucose and insulin levels.

Dread White Bread

White flour products have been severely processed, bleached, and stripped of their nutritional value. They're essentially another form of sugar. Like sugar, they spike your blood glucose and insulin levels and increase your risk of developing diabetes and cardiovascular illness.

I recommend eliminating all cereal grains, including wheat and corn, from your diet. Until about 10,000 years ago, humans lived perfectly healthy lives without grains as a part of their diet, and you can live perfectly well without them, too. In fact, you'll probably feel better not eating grains. Instead of bread, add another vegetable to your plate, preferably one that's not starchy. If you can't do without grains, consume them in moderation — a small serving a couple times a week — and choose from the least processed of the whole grains: millet, quinoa, rice, amaranth, and tapioca.

Don't Drink Your Calories

Soda, fruit juices, sports drinks, vitamin water, and other high sugar drinks are liquid death. Yet the average person in the U.S. drinks 53 gallons of soda per year. That's almost a gallon per week, and given the fact that I don't drink soda, someone else is consuming my share. High calorie liquid beverages of all kinds increase your risk for obesity, diabetes, cognitive decline, and heart disease. In the meantime, they make you fat, tired, and irritable.

Stop drinking sweetened drinks of all kinds. Artificial sweeteners are no better for you than sugar or high-fructose corn syrup and may actually be worse for you. Drink water or unsweetened green or herbal tea. Plenty of teas are on the market these days. Chances are you can find one you like.

Let Your Genes Be Your Guide

Although your genes alone don't determine your destiny in terms of health, they do influence the structure and function of every cell and every system in your body. Fortunately, through the miracles of modern science, healthcare professionals can now examine an individual's genotype *(genetic constitution)* to gauge the person's risk for contracting certain illnesses and to identify biological deficiencies and dysfunctions that call for adjustments in the person's treatment plan. For example, some people have a genetic mutation that prevents them from converting folic acid to folate. Giving such a person folic acid to treat a folate deficiency does little good; a methylated form of folate solves that problem.

Genetic testing, now available in most states, gives your healthcare provider the information she needs to make informed treatment decisions and tailor your treatment plan to your specific needs. This type of testing is especially useful in determining which supplements or medications are likely to work best for you. If you have a specific illness that's not responding to treatment, ask your natural healthcare provider whether genetic testing may help to shed light on the problem.

Stress Kills

Short-term stress is natural and beneficial. Thanks to the fight-or-flight response, you get a surge of adrenaline and energy that increases your awareness, boosts your strength, and supercharges your reflexes. Long-term stress, on the other hand, kills. It raises your blood pressure, increases the risk of cardiovascular disease, and elevates cortisol, which blocks insulin, contributing to insulin resistance, which leads to metabolic syndrome and ultimately diabetes.

You basically have three options for dealing with a stressful situation or person: resolve it, avoid it, or let it go. By "let it go," I mean let the stress go — sometimes, the only thing within your control is whether you choose to feel stressed about it. Why worry if you can't do anything about it?

Sleep on It

Sleep provides the body with downtime to rest, process information, restore proper function, and repair itself. If you're not getting enough sleep (typically about eight hours a day), you're going to get sick. Your brain will be the first to feel it. If you're having trouble falling asleep or staying asleep, head to Chapter 16 for guidance.

If you need a sleep aid, start with calcium, magnesium, 5-HTP (5-hydroxytryptophan), and melatonin. If these don't do the trick, ask your doctor about adding one of the following prescription medications *for short-term use only*: Ambien, Desyrel, or Klonopin.

Part IV
Appendixes

Vitamins in Their Better Forms

Vitamin	Better Form
A	Retinyl palmitate and beta-carotene
B1 (thiamin)	Benfontamine
B2 (riboflavin)	Riboflavin 5'-phosphate
B3 (niacin)	Nicotinic acid
B5	Pantothenic acid
B6	Pyridoxal 5'-phosphate
B7	Biotin
B9 (folate)	5-MTHF
B12	Methylcobalamin, sublingual fast-dissolving tablet
Choline	Choline dihydrogen citrate
C	Mixed mineral ascorbates
D	D3 (cholecalciferol)
E	Mix of tocopherols and tocotrienols
K	K2 (menaquinone)

To find out why taking vitamins and minerals in their better forms is so important, visit www.dummies.com/extras/naturalcures.

In this part . . .

- Look up scores of vitamins and minerals and take them in their better forms to improve absorption, bioavailability, and safety of these key micronutrients.

- Discover the uses and potential side effects of nearly 100 of the most common nutritional supplements on the market to find out whether a specific supplement is right for you and the health condition you're experiencing.

- Get the facts on several natural occurring hormones that are safer alternatives to the synthetic versions commonly used in hormone replacement therapy (HRT).

- Quickly reference over 100 herbs, from aloe to yerba mate, to find out which conditions each herb is effective in treating.

- Check out a host of homeopathic remedies to discover which illnesses each remedy is commonly used to cure.

- Get the scoop on 65 essential oils most commonly used in aromatherapy, from allspice berry to ylang ylang.

Appendix A

Vitamins and Minerals

• •

*T*o carry out the biological functions necessary to live, breathe, develop, heal, and engage in all the other wonderful activities that make life worth living, your body requires vitamins and minerals. In this appendix, I provide essential information about vitamins (Table A-1) and minerals (Table A-2) and the foods in which they're commonly found. I also specify each vitamin's and mineral's *better form* — the specific chemical compound of the vitamin or mineral that's best for one or more reasons; for example, vitamin C is commonly sold in the form of ascorbic acid, but vitamin C also comes in the form of various mineral ascorbates, which are less acidic and more bioavailable (that is, more readily accessible to the human body). I also include information on electrolytes in Table A-3.

Before buying a product, contact the manufacturer and ask for an independent third-party lab analysis that verifies the product's quality and ingredients. Prior to seeing me, many of my patients had tried poor-quality products and had given up on supplements because they didn't work. They're surprised when the supplements I prescribe are effective. The moral of the story: Buy products only from manufacturers that follow strict quality control procedures and subject their products to rigorous, independent lab tests to ensure that you're getting what's printed on the label.

What you won't find in this appendix are recommended daily allowances (RDAs) for these vitamins and minerals. Functional medicine isn't fond of minimum daily requirements because nutrition isn't a one-size-fits-all approach to health. Instead, it's unique to the individual. I strongly encourage you to consult a functional medical practitioner for a complete workup along with functional testing to identify your unique nutritional needs.

Try to get most of your daily dose of vitamins and minerals from the foods you eat, taking supplements only when necessary. Foods often contain just the right mix of vitamins in a form that's easy for your body to use and may contain other essential micronutrients that are not part of any supplement.

Vitamins

Vitamins are organic compounds or groups of organic compounds that your body needs but either can't make or may not make in sufficient quantities, so you need to consume them. Table A-1 presents the essential vitamins along with a couple other key compounds that play a role similar to that of vitamins.

Table A-1	Essential Vitamins	
Vitamin	**May Help with**	**Food Sources**
A (retinol) *Better form:* Retinyl palmitate and beta-carotene	Cardiovascular health; cancer prevention; eye disease, including cataracts and macular degeneration; skin conditions, including acne and psoriasis; measles; inflammatory bowel disease (IBD) ***Note:*** Don't take an elevated dose of vitamin A as retinol or retinyl esters without your doctor's approval. If you're pregnant, don't take vitamin A beyond your prenatal vitamins. Supplement vitamin A in children only as a last resort and only at low dosages.	Yellow, orange, and green vegetables and fruits, including carrots, pumpkins, sweet potatoes, winter squash, broccoli, peas, kale, spinach, apricots, peaches, tangerines
B1 (thiamin) *Better form:* Benfontamine	Brain and nervous system support, cardiovascular health, beriberi, Wernicke-Korsakoff syndrome, cataracts, Alzheimer's disease, heart failure	Sunflower seeds, navy beans, black beans, barley, green peas
B2 (riboflavin) *Better form:* Riboflavin 5'-phosphate	Cardiovascular health, migraine headaches, cataracts, glaucoma, cervical cancer	Soybeans, beet greens, spinach, tempeh, yogurt
B3 (niacin) *Better form:* Nicotinic acid, not niacinamide (nicotinamide) or inositol hexanicotinate	Cardiovascular health, high cholesterol, atherosclerosis, diabetes, osteoarthritis ***Note:*** Don't take niacin if you have gout, and don't take more than 1.5 grams daily without medical supervision and monitoring of liver enzymes.	Tuna, chicken, turkey, salmon, lamb

Vitamin	May Help with	Food Sources
B5 (pantothenic acid)	Adrenal system support, nervous system support, high cholesterol, high triglycerides, wound healing, rheumatoid arthritis	Whole grain cereals, eggs, meat, legumes, shitake mushrooms
B6 (pyridoxine) *Better form:* Pyridoxal 5'-phosphate	Heart disease, morning sickness, macular degeneration, depression, premenstrual syndrome (PMS), carpal tunnel syndrome, rheumatoid arthritis, tardive dyskinesia ***Note:*** Compromised liver function may prevent the liver from converting other forms of B6 into pyridoxal 5'-phosphate, which the body can use.	Tuna, turkey, beef, chicken, salmon
B7 (biotin)	Blood glucose regulation, hair and nail problems, seborrheic dermatitis, diabetes, peripheral neuropathy	Organ meats, peanuts, almonds, barley, brewer's yeast
B9 (folate) *Better form:* 5-MTHF (5-methyl-tetrahydrofolate)	Brain and nervous system health, neural tube defect prevention in pregnancy, heart disease, age-related hearing loss, macular degeneration, depression, cancer	Leafy green vegetables, legumes and lentils, avocado, broccoli, mango
B12 (cobalamin) *Better form:* Methylcobalamin, sublingual, fast-dissolving tablet	Pernicious anemia, heart disease, macular degeneration, fatigue, breast cancer, male infertility	Fish and shellfish, dairy products, organ meats (especially liver and kidney), eggs
Choline *Better form:* Choline dihydrogen citrate	Brain and nervous system health, neural development in pregnancy, liver and kidney health, asthma	Eggs, brussels sprouts, broccoli, cauliflower, collard greens
C *Better form:* Mineral ascorbates	Heart disease, high blood pressure, common cold, cancer, osteoarthritis, macular degeneration, pre-eclampsia, asthma, immune support ***Note:*** Avoid vitamin C as ascorbic acid and any products that contain sugar or artificial sweeteners.	Papaya, bell peppers, broccoli, pineapple, citrus fruits and juices

(continued)

Table A-1 (*continued*)

Vitamin	May Help with	Food Sources
D *Better form:* D3 (cholecalciferol)	Osteoporosis and other bone disorders, immune support, autoimmune disorders, neurological brain disorders, Alzheimer's disease, dementia, balance, parathyroid problems, high blood pressure, cancer, seasonal affective disorder (SAD), diabetes, heart disease, multiple sclerosis (MS), obesity, overall longevity ***Note:*** If you're taking a vitamin D supplement, adequate calcium and magnesium intake are also required. See note following this table for dosage information.	Sunlight, beef liver, cheese, egg yolks, fatty fish
E *Better form:* Mix of tocopherols and tocotrienols	Heart disease, cancer, photodermatitis, Alzheimer's disease, eye health, menstrual pain, diabetes, pre-eclampsia, tardive dyskinesia, rheumatoid arthritis, lipid production	Liver, eggs, nuts (especially almonds, hazelnuts, and walnuts), sunflower seeds, green leafy vegetables
K *Better form:* K2 (menaquinone)	Excessive bleeding; osteoporosis ***Note:*** Don't supplement with vitamin K if you're on blood-thinning medications.	Kale, spinach, greens (mustard, collard, and beet)

Have your vitamin D levels checked yearly and try to maintain an optimal level of 50 to 80 ng/ml. If your level is less than 50 ng/ml, increase exposure to sunlight or take a vitamin D3 supplement. Without sunblock and with arms and legs exposed, your skin makes 10,000 to 15,000 units of vitamin D. Here's how much additional vitamin D you need based on your vitamin D level:

Vitamin D Level	*Additional Vitamin D Needed*
<10 ng/mL	10,000 units per day
10–20 ng/mL	10,000 units per day
20–30 ng/mL	8,000 units per day
30–40 ng/mL	5,000 units per day
40–50 ng/mL	2,000 units per day

Minerals

Several essential minerals work together along with vitamins and other nutrients to produce tissue, bones, blood, and various chemicals used in biological processes; to promote proper blood circulation; to support fluid regulation, nerve transmission, muscle contraction, and energy production; and much more. Table A-2 presents the essential minerals along with the better form of each, a list of health conditions each mineral may be helpful in treating, and a list of foods high in that particular mineral.

All mineral chelates are not created equal. As much as possible, choose supplements from manufacturers and suppliers that use Albion Advanced Nutrition's patented mineral technology to provide the highest quality minerals for optimal absorption and utilization.

Table A-2	Essential Minerals	
Mineral	*May Help With*	*Foods Sources*
Calcium *Better form for bone:* MCHC (microcrystalline hydroxyapatite concentrate) *For sleep:* Calcium lactate *For detox of estrogens, xenobiotics:* Calcium D-glucarate *For other uses:* Calcium gylcinate chelate	Osteoporosis prevention and treatment, hypoparathyroidism, PMS, high blood pressure, obesity, high cholesterol, rickets, stroke, colon cancer, detox	Tofu, dairy products, green leafy vegetables, soft bones (sardines and canned salmon), calcium-fortified foods
Chromium *Better form:* Chromium picolinate	Diabetes, weight loss, strength training, heart health, atypical depression	Broccoli, barley, oats, green beans, tomatoes
Copper *Better form:* Copper bis-glycinate chelate	Anemia, osteoarthritis, osteoporosis	Seafood, organ meats, nuts, legumes, chocolate

Table A-2 (*continued*)

Mineral	May Help With	Foods Sources
Iodine *Better form:* Potassium iodine	Autoimmune thyroid issues, oral inflammation, fibrocystic breast changes, vaginitis, wounds, radiation exposure, goiter prevention	Iodized salt, seafood (plant and animal), garlic, cod, yogurt
Iron *Better form:* Iron bis-glycinate	Anemia, exercise capacity, cough associated with ACE inhibitor use, ADHD *Note:* Get your blood levels checked and supplement only if deficient in iron.	Red meat (especially liver), egg yolks, leafy green vegetables, dried fruit, fortified cereals and grains
Magnesium *Better form for constipation, cognition, muscle support, and sleep:* Magnesium citrate *For general health:* Magnesium malate and magnesium glycinate chelate	Asthma, depression, diabetes, fibromyalgia, noise-related hearing loss, arrhythmia, high blood pressure, migraine headache, osteoporosis, pre-eclampsia and eclampsia, PMS; restless legs syndrome *Note:* Make sure your doctor checks your red blood cell (RBC) magnesium level and not your serum level and that your level is 4.2 to 5.9 ng/mil RBC. (To maintain serum levels sufficient to keep your heart beating, your body may extract magnesium from cells, making your serum level look normal while your RBC level shows a deficiency.)	Pumpkin seeds, spinach, Swiss chard, soybeans, sesame seeds
Manganese *Better form:* Manganese bis-glycinate chelate	Osteoporosis, arthritis. PMS, diabetes, epilepsy	Cloves, oats, brown rice, garbanzo beans, spinach
Molybdenum *Better form:* Molybdenum bis-glycinate chelate	Fat and carbohydrate metabolism	Legumes; nuts, especially almonds; soybeans; dairy products; whole grains

Mineral	*May Help With*	*Foods Sources*
Phosphorus *Better form:* Phosphoric acid	Hypophosphatemia (low phosphate levels), hypercalcemia (high calcium levels), calcium-based kidney stones, muscle pain and fatigue, constipation	Meat, poultry, fish, eggs, dairy products
Selenium *Better form:* Selenium glycinate complex	Heart disease, cancer, immune function, asthma, HIV, male infertility, rheumatoid arthritis	Brewer's yeast; wheat germ; liver; butter; fish, especially mackerel, tuna, halibut, flounder, herring, and smelt
Zinc *Better form:* Zinc glycinate chelate	Acne, macular degeneration, common cold, sickle cell disease, stomach ulcers, ADHD, cold sores, HIV/AIDS, Wilson's disease **Note:** Take up to 40 mg daily for acute illness only for a few days and then reduce to 20 mg daily. For long-term use, take 1 mg copper for every 20 mg zinc.	Oysters and shellfish, red meats, poultry, cheese

Electrolytes

Electrolytes and water are essential to keeping the body hydrated and supporting electrochemical activity in the body. You typically get plenty of electrolytes in your daily diet, but they can be depleted with exercise, fever, diarrhea, and the use of diuretics. Table A-3 presents the electrolytes along with basic information about each of them.

Table A-3	Electrolytes		
Electrolyte	*Function*	*Deficiency Symptoms*	*Toxicity Symptoms*
Chloride	Supports electro-chemical activity and digestion	Muscle weakness, loss of appetite, irritability, dehydration, severe fatigue	pH imbalance, fluid retention, high blood pressure
Potassium	Helps build proteins and muscle, break down and use carbohydrates, control electrical activity of the heart, and maintain pH balance	Weak muscles, abnormal heart rhythm, slight rise in blood pressure	Dangerous heart rhythms; supplement with potassium only under close medical supervision
Sodium	Helps maintain fluid balance, supports nerve transmission and muscle contraction	Nausea, vomiting, headache, short-term memory loss, confusion, lethargy, loss of appetite, restlessness, irritability, muscle weakness, spasms, cramps, seizures, coma	Fluid retention, high blood pressure

Appendix B

Nutritional Supplements

••

*E*ven though nutritious foods supply the vitamins and minerals the body needs to function normally, they don't contain everything the body needs to prevent and cure disease. Table B-1 lists numerous nutritional supplements that are useful in preventing and treating a host of common health issues. I list the common uses for each supplement and what you need to watch out for. Note that, unless otherwise noted, the supplement is taken orally.

Table B-1	Nutritional Supplements	
Supplement	*Used For*	*Precautions/Potential Side Effects*
5-HTP (5-hydroxytryptophan)	Appetite suppression, depression, sleep disorders, anxiety, headaches (including migraines), fibromyalgia, attention deficit hyperactivity disorder (ADHD), seizure disorders, Parkinson's disease	Consult a doctor before taking if you're being treated for depression or Parkinson's disease
Acetyl-L-carnitine	Heart and blood vessel conditions, including angina, arrhythmias, congestive heart failure, cardiomyopathy, chest pain, and high blood pressure; high cholesterol; chronic fatigue syndrome; Down syndrome; kidney and liver disease; male infertility; anorexia; HIV; intermittent claudication; Alzheimer's disease and memory loss; depression; alcoholism-related thinking problems; diabetes-related nerve pain. Also helps burn fat	May cause anxiety, restlessness, overstimulation, insomnia, nausea Don't take if you're taking pentylenetetrazol, a circulatory and respiratory stimulant; may stimulate *atherogenesis,* plaque formation in the arteries

(continued)

Table B-1 (*continued*)

Supplement	Used For	Precautions/Potential Side Effects
Adrenal extract	Low adrenal function, fatigue, stress, allergies, asthma, skin conditions, rheumatoid arthritis	Potential contamination from diseased animals; may cause anxiety, irritability, headache, insomnia
Alpha-linolenic acid	Heart disease, high cholesterol, high blood pressure, asthma	Increased risk of bleeding; stop taking before surgery
Alpha-lipoic acid	Metabolic syndrome; diabetes-related nerve pain, memory loss, chronic fatigue syndrome, HIV/AIDS, cancer, liver disease, heart disease, cataracts, glaucoma, lowering blood glucose levels (possibly) *Topical application for* aging skin	Generally safe
Beta glucan	High cholesterol, high blood sugar, immune system support *Topical application for* eczema, dermatitis, wrinkles, wounds, and burns	Avoid when taking medications to suppress the immune system
Betaine hydrochloride	Hypokalemia, anemia, asthma, atherosclerosis, candidiasis, allergies, gallstones, inner ear infections, rheumatoid arthritis, thyroid disorders, IBS, inflammatory bowel disease (IBD)	May cause heartburn and increase risk of ulcer
Boric acid	*As suppository for* vaginal yeast infections; *topically to* prevent infection and as eye wash in a highly diluted form	Don't take internally or apply to the skin of infants or young children or to open wounds
Bovine cartilage	*Taken by mouth or injected* for rheumatoid and osteoarthritis and certain cancers; *topical application for* acne, anal pruritus, and sore gums. *Suppository for* hemorrhoids	May cause diarrhea, nausea, swelling, local redness, and itching

Supplement	*Used For*	*Precautions/Potential Side Effects*
Branched-chain amino acids	Amyotrophic lateral sclerosis (ALS), hepatic encephalopathy, tardive dyskinesia, athletic performance, muscle development, nerve function	Take only up to 6 months. May cause fatigue and loss of coordination; consult your doctor before taking to treat ALS or if you have kidney or liver disease
Brewer's yeast	Diabetes, diarrhea, fatigue, high cholesterol, cold, upper respiratory tract infection, flu, loss of appetite, acne, recurring boils, PMS	May cause allergic reaction in sensitive individuals; consult doctor if you're taking medicine for diabetes
Bromelain	Inflammation, osteoarthritis, hay fever, sinusitis, colitis	May increase bleeding; don't use bromelain if you have gastritis or ulcers or are taking a blood thinner, such as warfarin or Coumadin
Carnosine	*H. pylori* infection; diabetes complications, including nerve damage, cataracts, and kidney problems; hepatitis C (zinc-carnosine); peptic ulcer (zinc-carnosine); liver damage caused by anesthesia *Topical application for* wound healing	Generally safe
Chondroitin sulfate	Osteoarthritis, osteoporosis, sprains, strains, heart disease, high cholesterol, anemia *In eye drop form for* dry eyes; *in cream or ointment form for* joint pain	May cause nausea; creams and ointments may not penetrate skin
Colloidal silver	Bacterial, viral, and fungal infections; conjunctivitis; emphysema; bronchitis; skin conditions *Topical application for* acne, burns, and as an antibiotic	Possible irreversible skin discoloration (possibly turning your skin blue) if silver builds up in vital organs

(continued)

Table B-1 (*continued*)

Supplement	Used For	Precautions/Potential Side Effects
Colostrum	Immune support, injuries healing, build up of stamina and muscle, mood enhancement, colitis *Note:* Use pure bovine colostrum collected within the first 16 hours after birth.	Generally safe; may cause nausea, vomiting, abnormal liver function tests, and decreased red blood cell count in HIV-positive people
Coenzyme Q10	Congestive heart failure, chest pain, high blood pressure, diabetes, Huntington's disease, Parkinson's disease, muscular dystrophy, chronic fatigue syndrome, warfarin-related hair loss, immune system support *Topical application for* gum disease	Generally very safe
Conjugated linoleic acid (CLA)	Atherosclerosis, cancer prevention, weight loss	Generally safe; may cause upset stomach, diarrhea, nausea, and fatigue
D-glucarate	Breast, prostate, and colon cancers; detox; fibrocystic breast syndrome; PMS	No known adverse side effects
Diindolylmethane (DIM)	Breast, uterine, and prostate health; healthy testosterone levels in men; premenstrual syndrome (PMS) symptoms	Don't take if you're pregnant or breastfeeding May act as estrogen in the body or block the effects of estrogen, so it can be good or bad for use in treating estrogen-related conditions, such as breast, uterine, or ovarian cancers; endometriosis; or uterine fibroids; or in treating prostate cancer Until more research is available, use DIM with caution and consult your healthcare provider

Supplement	Used For	Precautions/Potential Side Effects
D-ribose	Supports mitochondrial energy production	Possible adverse effects include hypoglycemia, gout exacerbation, and diarrhea
Evening primrose oil	Rheumatoid arthritis, osteoporosis, Raynaud's syndrome, multiple sclerosis, Sjogren's syndrome, cancer, high cholesterol, heart disease, alcoholism, Alzheimer's disease, schizophrenia, chronic fatigue syndrome, asthma, ADHD *Topical application for* eczema, psoriasis, acne, menopausal symptoms, and skin conditions	May cause upset stomach and headache. Consult doctor before taking if you have epilepsy
Fish oil	Heart disease and stroke prevention, atrial fibrillation, cancer, high blood pressure, high triglycerides, depression, bipolar disorder, psychosis, ADHD, Alzheimer's disease, glaucoma, macular degeneration, diabetes, asthma, arthritis, chronic obstructive pulmonary disease (COPD), IBD, lupus, osteoporosis, preeclampsia	May cause acid reflux, burping, fishy aftertaste, loose stools, nosebleeds, mild blood thinning, potential rise in LDL (bad cholesterol); may impair immune system response at high doses
Flaxseed oil	Arthritis, high cholesterol, anxiety, depression, bipolar disorder, enlarged prostate, vaginal infections, atherosclerosis, high blood pressure, heart disease, diabetes, ADHD, constipation, COPD, asthma, high triglycerides, IBD, lupus, osteoporosis, preeclampsia, schizophrenia	May cause diarrhea or mild blood thinning Men with prostate cancer should use ground flaxseeds instead of flaxseed oil

(continued)

Table B-1 (*continued*)

Supplement	Used For	Precautions/Potential Side Effects
Fructooligosac-charides (FOS)	Constipation, traveler's diarrhea, high cholesterol	May cause flatulence initially due to alterations in gut flora and diarrhea at high doses
GABA (gamma-amino butyric acid)	Anxiety, mood enhancement, PMS, ADHD, blood pressure stabilization, epilepsy, muscle tightness, muscle growth, fat burning	Consult doctor before taking with any psychiatric and anticonvulsant medication
Gamma linolenic acid (GLA)	Supports healthy skin, nerve health and function, and cardiovascular health; helps to balance the body's normal response to inflammation; is a potent antioxidant	Safe, non-toxic, and generally well-tolerated with no serious adverse side effects at doses up to 2.8 grams daily for 12 months Do not take if you're pregnant
Glucosamine	Arthritis, knee pain, back pain, strains, sprains, glaucoma	May cause upset stomach, diarrhea
Glutamic acid or glutamine	Stomach ulcers, ulcerative colitis, Crohn's disease, depression, irritability, anxiety, insomnia, recovery from medical procedures	Don't take if you have liver or kidney disease; don't take more than 40 grams daily or 0.65 grams per kilogram of body weight for children
Glutathione	Cataracts, glaucoma, alcoholism, asthma, cancer, heart disease, atherosclerosis, high cholesterol, hepatitis, liver disease, AIDS, chronic fatigue syndrome, memory loss, Alzheimer's disease, osteoarthritis, Parkinson's disease, immune system support	Generally very safe

Supplement	Used For	Precautions/Potential Side Effects
Glycine	Detox, enlarged prostate, schizophrenia, stroke	Consult doctor before taking if you have kidney or liver disease
Grapeseed extract	Varicose veins, hemorrhoids, macular degeneration, bruising, atherosclerosis, high blood pressure, swelling after injury, heart attack, stroke, detox	May cause upset stomach, nausea, vomiting, or diarrhea
Grapefruit seed extract	High cholesterol; atherosclerosis; cancer; psoriasis; bacterial, viral, and fungal infections, including yeast infections and the flu *Topical application for* muscle fatigue, skin tone, acne, oily skin	Don't take internally if you're pregnant or breastfeeding Check with doctor or pharmacist about any prescription medication interactions
Green tea	Mental alertness, weight loss, digestive health, headaches, human papillomavirus (HPV), high cholesterol, tooth decay, gingivitis, detox, cardiovascular disease, cervical dysplasia, Crohn's disease, chronic fatigue syndrome *Topical application for* sunburn and puffiness under eyes	Contains caffeine, which may cause headache, nervousness, sleep problems, irritability, irregular heartbeat, and heartburn
Huperzine A	Alzheimer's disease, memory impairment	Don't take if you're taking prescription medication for Alzheimer's disease
Indole-3-carbinol	Cancer prevention, fibromyalgia, cervical dysplasia, lupus	Generally safe; may cause skin rashes and slightly elevated liver enzyme levels
Kelp	Thyroid disorders, including enlarged thyroid (goiter); obesity; arthritis and joint pain; atherosclerosis; constipation; bronchitis; emphysema; anxiety	Consult doctor before taking if you're being treated for a thyroid disorder

(continued)

Table B-1 (*continued*)

Supplement	Used For	Precautions/Potential Side Effects
L-arginine	Heart and blood vessel conditions, including angina, congestive heart failure, chest pain, and high blood pressure; age-related cognitive impairment; erectile dysfunction; male infertility; immune support	Don't take if you have oral or genital herpes, because it can trigger herpes flare-ups; don't take if you have asthma, because it increases pulmonary inflammation Consult your doctor before taking if you're being treated for kidney or liver disease
L-theanine	Anxiety, insomnia, high blood pressure, Alzheimer's disease; also taken to optimize effects of cancer medication	Generally safe, but consult doctor if you're taking any anti-anxiety medications
Lutein	Macular degeneration, cataracts, retinitis pigmentosa, colon cancer, breast cancer, type 2 diabetes, heart disease	Generally very safe
Lycopene	Heart disease prevention; atherosclerosis; cancers of the prostate, breast, lung, bladder, ovaries, colon, and pancreas; HPV; cataracts; asthma	Generally very safe
Lysine	Cold sores, genital herpes, osteoporosis, shingles	May cause upset stomach at high doses Can be applied topically or taken orally
Malic acid	Aluminum detox *Taken with magnesium for* fibromyalgia-related pain and tenderness; *topical application for* skin conditions, including dry skin, acne, skin darkening, and removing old skin cells	No known adverse side effects

Supplement	Used For	Precautions/Potential Side Effects
Medium-chain triglycerides	Athletic performance, diabetes, hypothyroidism	May cause upset stomach; consult doctor before using if you're being treated for kidney or liver disease
Methionine	Detox for acetaminophen poisoning, increasing urine acidity, liver disorders, wound healing, alcoholism, allergies, asthma, Parkinson's disease	Consult doctor before using if you're being treated for kidney or liver disease; supplement with B vitamins to prevent high levels of homocysteine, which increases risk of cardiovascular disease
MSM (methyl sulfonylmethane)	Chronic pain, arthritis, osteoporosis, bursitis, tendonitis, tenosynovitis, muscle cramps, scleroderma, stretch marks, wrinkles, allergies, asthma, autoimmune disorders, fibromyalgia, hair and nail health, headaches, heartburn	Generally safe, but at high doses may cause upset stomach, diarrhea, and cramping; consult doctor before using if you're currently taking blood thinning medication
N-acetyl cysteine (NAC)	ALS, Alzheimer's disease, angina; bile duct blockage in infants, bronchitis, bipolar depression, chelation of heavy metals, lung function, COPD, cystic fibrosis, detox for acetaminophen and carbon monoxide poisoning, flu prevention, gastritis, HIV, pneumonia, postnasal drip, to reduce risk of heart attack and stroke **Note:** N-acetyl cysteine is the precursor to glutathione, the body's principle defense against reactive oxygen molecules and the detoxification of drugs, metabolites, and other compounds.	Generally safe; may increase risk of bronchospasms in people with asthma

(continued)

Table B-1 (*continued*)

Supplement	Used For	Precautions/Potential Side Effects
Pectin	Diabetes, high cholesterol, high triglycerides, acid reflux (GERD), prevention of colon and prostate cancers	May cause stomach upset, diarrhea, or cramping
Perilla oil	Asthma, nausea, sunstroke, to induce sweating, alleviate muscle spasms	Consult doctor before using if you're taking blood thinning medication
Phenylalanine	Depression, ADHD, Parkinson's disease, chronic pain, arthritis, alcohol withdrawal, vitiligo (lost skin pigmentation)	Generally safe; may cause heartburn, headaches, and nausea
Phosphatidyl-choline	Alzheimer's disease, memory loss, anxiety, bipolar disorder, tardive dyskinesia, hepatitis, eczema, gallbladder disease, circulation problems, high cholesterol, PMS, immune system support, detox, optimizing kidney dialysis	At high doses, may cause upset stomach, diarrhea, and nausea
Phosphatidyl-serine	Alzheimer's disease, age-related cognitive decline, memory loss, dementia, ADHD, depression, exercise-induced stress, athletic performance	Generally very safe
Proline-rich polypeptides (PRPs)	Prevention and treatment of bacterial and viral infections ***Note:*** Proline-rich polypeptides support and regulate the body's immune response, stimulating an underactive immune system and dampening an overactive immune system. They also promote production and balancing of cytokines, which play a key role in communication between cells.	Generally very safe Do not use if you're pregnant or have received an organ transplant

Supplement	Used For	Precautions/Potential Side Effects
Propolis	Bacterial, viral, and fungal infections; cancer of the nose and throat; immune system support; gastrointestinal conditions, including *H. pylori* infection *Topical application for* cold sores and herpes outbreaks (as a mouth rinse)	Don't take if you have asthma or are allergic to bee byproducts
Psyllium	Constipation, diabetes, diarrhea, diverticulitis, hemorrhoids, high cholesterol, IBS	May cause diarrhea or loose stools; take two or three hours before or after medications or other supplements
Pycnogenol	Circulation, allergies, asthma, tinnitus, high blood pressure, muscle soreness, osteoarthritis, diabetes, ADHD, endometriosis, menopause, erectile dysfunction, retinopathy, heart disease and stroke prevention, healthy skin, aging	Consult doctor before using if you're taking blood thinning medication
Pyruvate	Obesity, high cholesterol, cataracts, cancer, athletic performance	May cause upset stomach, gas, bloating, and diarrhea at higher levels
Red yeast rice	High cholesterol, indigestion, diarrhea, circulation, spleen and stomach health	Can have the same side effects as statins, so ask your doctor to monitor your creatine phosphokinase (CPK) level and liver enzymes and watch out for myopathy (muscle weakness) and myositis (muscle inflammation) Take with CoQ10 10 to 200 mg daily, as red yeast may reduce levels of CoQ10

(continued)

Table B-1 (*continued*)

Supplement	Used For	Precautions/Potential Side Effects
Resveratrol	Atherosclerosis, lowering of LDL (bad) cholesterol, increasing of HDL (good) cholesterol, cancer prevention, diabetes, weight loss; prevention of accelerated aging	Generally very safe
Royal jelly	Asthma, hay fever, liver and kidney disease, pancreatitis, insomnia, PMS, stomach ulcers, bone fractures, menopause, skin disorders, high cholesterol, immune system support *Topical application* to scalp to encourage hair growth	Don't take if you have asthma or are allergic to bee byproducts
SAMe (S-adenosyl-L-methionine)	Depression, anxiety, heart disease, fibromyalgia, osteoarthritis, bursitis, tendonitis, lower back pain, dementia, Alzheimer's disease, chronic fatigue syndrome, liver disease, Parkinson's disease, ADHD, multiple sclerosis, seizures, migraines, PMS SAMe is a potent methyl donor (needed for the synthesis of neurotransmitters, proteins, nucleic acids, and phospholipids) and supports healthy homocysteine levels	May cause gas, vomiting, constipation, dry mouth, headache, insomnia, anorexia, dizziness, and nervousness; consult doctor before taking if you're being treated for depression or bipolar disorder
Soy isoflavones	High cholesterol; high blood pressure; heart and blood vessel disease prevention; type 2 diabetes; asthma; lung, endometrial, prostate, and thyroid cancers; osteoporosis; constipation; diarrhea; PMS; menopause, vaginitis; enlarged prostate	May cause constipation, bloating, and nausea or rash and itching; consult doctor before taking if you have a history of breast or uterine cancer

Supplement	Used For	Precautions/Potential Side Effects
Sulforaphane	Cancer prevention, detox	Generally very safe
Taurine	Congestive heart failure, high blood pressure, hepatitis, high cholesterol, cystic fibrosis, epilepsy, autism, ADHD, eye problems, diabetes, alcoholism	Consult doctor before using if you're being treated for kidney or liver disease
Trimethylglycine (TMG) betaine anhydrous	Elevated homocysteine levels, liver disease (detox), hepatitis, depression, congestive heart failure, obesity, immune system support *Topical application for* dry mouth (in toothpaste)	No record of adverse side effects
Tyrosine	Phenylketonuria (PKU), depression, ADD, ADHD, narcolepsy, stress, PMS, Parkinson's, Alzheimer's, chronic fatigue syndrome, cocaine withdrawal, heart disease, stroke, erectile dysfunction, schizophrenia, appetite suppression	Consult doctor before using if you're being treated for kidney or liver disease, hyperthyroidism, or Graves' disease
Vinpocetine	Alzheimer's, impaired memory or cognition, dementia, hearing loss, tinnitus, stroke prevention and treatment, menopause, chronic fatigue syndrome, seizures	Don't take if you're pregnant, nursing or taking blood pressure medication
Whey protein	Milk alternative for lactose intolerance, allergies, asthma, high cholesterol, obesity, late-stage cancer, colon cancer, athletic performance	Don't take if you're allergic to milk; consult doctor before using if you're being treated for kidney or liver disease
Xylitol	Natural sweetener, cavity prevention, ear infection prevention, bone density support *Intranasal application for* sinusitis and allergies	A natural sweetener At higher doses, may cause diarrhea or loose stools; increase dosage slowly to reduce the risk of this common side effect

Appendix C

Natural Hormones

• •

*Y*our body manufactures and uses hormones as part of its internal communication system to regulate all of your body's biological processes, including those related to growth and development, digestion, heart rate, immune response, sexual function, reproduction, mood, and much more. Too much or too little of a hormone can result in major disturbances in these biological processes, leading to illness.

Throughout this book, I point out conditions that may be related to hormonal imbalances. Treating these conditions may require supplementing your diet with one or more of the over-the-counter hormones or hormone precursors (building blocks) presented in Table C-1.

Too much of any given hormone may cause serious adverse side effects. Therefore, before beginning any hormone supplementation, get tested first and supplement your body's production of hormones only if the tests show that you have a deficiency. Take hormones only under the careful supervision of a qualified medical practitioner. Your doctor can test and monitor your hormone levels to ensure that your levels are healthy.

Opt for hormone supplements in topical (applied to the skin) or sublingual (taken under the tongue) forms instead of capsules you swallow. Hormone supplements in capsule form are broken down in the liver and therefore require higher doses.

Table C-1	**Natural Hormones**	
Hormone	**Used For**	**Precautions and Potential Side Effects**
DHEA (dehydroepiandrosterone)	Lupus, adrenal insufficiency, depression, osteoporosis, obesity, erectile dysfunction, improved libido in women, aging, HIV, menopause, inflammatory bowel disease (IBD), infertility, schizophrenia, dementia	Test first and supplement only under medical supervision. DHEA is the precursor to testosterone and estrogen. It may increase the risk of hormone-affected cancers (prostate, breast, ovarian, uterine, and cervical); skin conditions, including acne; hair loss; unwanted hair growth, such as facial hair on women; increased sweating; weight gain; agitation, irritability, or mania; abnormal heartbeat; bleeding or blood clotting; and other hormonal side effects.
Melatonin	Insomnia (especially in helping you fall asleep, not in staying asleep), menopause, breast cancer, prostate cancer, attention deficit hyperactivity disorder (ADHD), autism, fibromyalgia **Note:** Don't take more than about 3 mg of melatonin per night. Excessive amounts of melatonin may disrupt your sleep or make you feel groggy in the morning.	Don't take if you're pregnant, planning to get pregnant, are nursing, or have an autoimmune condition, such as multiple sclerosis (MS). Avoid driving or operating machinery for a few hours after taking it; alcohol may magnify the sedative effect. May cause headache, dizziness, stomach cramps, irritability, decreased libido, vivid dreams or nightmares, and in men decreased sperm count and breast enlargement.

Hormone	Used For	Precautions and Potential Side Effects
Pregnenolone	Fatigue, Alzheimer's disease, memory enhancement, immune system support, psoriasis, scleroderma, menopause, premenstrual syndrome (PMS), arthritis, depression, heart disease, allergic reactions, lupus, MS, prostate problems, seizures	Take in low doses (5 to 10 mg daily), skipping a day or two each week. Don't take if you're pregnant, planning to get pregnant, or nursing, or if you have prostate problems, heart disease, or low HDL. May cause acne, hair loss, facial hair in women, aggressiveness, irritability, and increased levels of estrogen.
Progesterone	Hot flashes, uterine bleeding, PMS, inducing menstrual periods, hormone replacement therapy (HRT), osteoporosis, infertility	Don't take if you're pregnant, are breastfeeding, or have arterial or liver disease. Consult a doctor if you're being treated for depression or breast cancer. If menstruating, use during the second half of your cycle.

Appendix D
Herbs

• •

*F*or as long as humans have walked the earth, plants have been used to treat a host of common ailments, from allergies to headaches to heart disease and even cancer. In fact, many modern medicines have been developed by extracting the active ingredients of various plants. Table D-1 lists more than 100 of the most common and helpful herbs still in use today.

Just because herbs are plants and serve as natural cures doesn't mean that all herbs are completely safe. Some herbs, even medicinal herbs, may be toxic. Obtain herbal remedies from reputable suppliers and carefully read and follow label instructions and warnings. If you're pregnant, planning to get pregnant, or nursing, consult your doctor before using any herbal remedies.

Table D-1	Herbal Remedies
Herb	**Commonly Used For**
Aloe	Burns, wounds, skin irritations, constipation, ulcers
American ginseng	Weakness, fever, cough, wheezing, increasing stress tolerance
Andrographis	Cold, flu, diarrhea
Angelica	Indigestion, gas, colic, circulation, cough, congestion
Anise	Indigestion, nausea, gas, bloating, colic, cough (expectorant), menstrual pain, asthma, whooping cough, bronchitis, scabies, lice
Arnica	Bruises, sprains, strains, muscle pain
Artichoke	Liver and gallbladder health, stomach upset, digestion, colon conditions
	May help with atherosclerosis and high cholesterol
Ashwagandha root (mild sedative)	Chronic stress, rheumatoid arthritis, lupus, low sex drive

(continued)

Table D-1 (*continued*)

Herb	Commonly Used For
Asian ginseng	Cold, flu, heart health, physical and mental performance, stress, erectile dysfunction, menopausal symptoms
	May help reduce the risk of certain types of cancer and lower blood sugar for those with type 2 diabetes
Astragalus	Stress, bacterial and viral infection, inflammation
	May help prevent cancer and diabetes, improve heart function, and protect the liver and kidneys
Barberry	Upset stomach, diarrhea, fever
	May be useful for gallbladder conditions and heartburn
Basil	Stomach upset, cuts and scrapes (antibacterial agent), insect repellent
	May help treat colds, headaches, and heart disease
Bilberry	Venous insufficiency, atherosclerosis, diabetes, diarrhea, eye/vision conditions
Bitter melon	High blood glucose levels, diabetes
Black cohosh	Cramps, hot flashes, irritability, mood swings, sleep disturbances, other menopausal symptoms
	May help with arthritis and osteoporosis
Bladderwrack	May help prevent cancer, reduce cellulite, and support weight loss
Black walnut	Depression, heart disease, cancer, rheumatoid arthritis, *Candida*/yeast infection, ringworm, other fungal/yeast infections of the skin
	May be used as a deworming agent to rid the system of parasites
Blessed thistle	Detox, gas, bloating
	May have antitumor and anticancer effects and may help alleviate menopausal symptoms
Blue cohosh	Menstrual issues (to stimulate menstruation and improve menstrual symptoms), inducing labor
Boswellia (anti-inflammatory analgesic)	Arthritis pain, high blood pressure, heart disease, gastritis, bronchitis

Herb	Commonly Used For
Bromelain (pineapple extract)	Inflammation caused by a variety of conditions, including arthritis, inflammatory bowel disease (IBD), asthma, lupus
Bugleweed	Hyperthyroidism (overactive thyroid)
Burdock (diuretic)	Digestion, detox, cancer, diabetes, HIV/AIDS
	May help treat acne, eczema, and psoriasis
Butcher's broom	Circulation, heart problems, varicose veins, hemorrhoids
Calendula (anti-inflammatory, antiviral, antibacterial agent)	Stomach upset, ulcers, menstrual cramps, burns, bruises, cuts (speeds healing)
	May help with ear infections and prevent dermatitis
Camphor	Back pain, sore muscles, arthritis pain, congestion
Cascara (laxative)	Chronic constipation
	Note: Stop using if it causes diarrhea
Castor oil	Constipation, sore muscles, arthritis, nerve damage, lower back pain
Catnip (mild sedative)	Sleep, digestion, menstrual cramps
	May help treat colds and flu by making you sweat
Cat's claw	Inflammation
	May help treat arthritis and stomach ulcers and reduce fever
Cayenne	Pain associated with arthritis, shingles (after blisters disappear), and peripheral neuropathy; lower back pain
	May be useful in treating psoriasis, improving digestion, suppressing appetite, and improving overall circulation
Celery seed (diuretic)	Arthritis, gout, muscle spasms, inflammation, to calm the nerves
Chamomile	Bruises, sprains, strains, fractures, osteoarthritis, wounds
Chickweed	Detox, obesity, minor burns, skin irritation, rashes
	Can also be used as a gentle laxative
Cinnamon	Stabilizes blood glucose levels in people with type 2 diabetes, strengthens immune system response, treats yeast and fungal infections, improves digestion

(continued)

Table D-1 (*continued*)

Herb	Commonly Used For
Clove	Dental pain, gum disease, bad breath, pain from sore muscles and arthritis, indigestion, stomach upset, nausea Sometimes used as an antiperspirant/deodorant
Coconut oil	Weight loss, high cholesterol, internal fungal infections, skin and hair revitalization
Comfrey	Sore throat, cough, respiratory illness, pain, skin irritations, ulcerations, abrasions, cuts, burns
Cornsilk	Urinary tract or kidney inflammation
Corydalis (central nervous system suppressant)	Pain, high blood pressure
Cranberry	Urinary tract infections (UTIs), bladder and kidney conditions
Damiana (mild stimulant)	Prostate issues (often combined with saw palmetto) May be helpful in boosting libido
Dandelion (diuretic and mild laxative)	Bladder, liver, and kidney conditions; detox; certain skin conditions, including acne May help with diabetes, high cholesterol, high blood pressure, rheumatoid arthritis
Devil's claw	Pain, inflammation, arthritis, muscle pain, gout
Dong quai	Hot flashes, cramps, night sweats, mood swings, and other menopausal symptoms; circulation; liver health; immune system function
Echinacea	Immune system function (shortening the duration of a cold, flu, cough, sore throat, and fever), wound care (speeding healing and preventing infection of cuts and abrasions) May help treat UTIs, vaginal yeast infections, and ear and sinus infections
Elderberry	Cold, flu, sinus infection, wound healing
Elecampane	Improving breathing (in cases of asthma and bronchitis) and digestion
Ephedra, or ma huang (decongestant)	Asthma, bronchitis, cough, cold, hay fever, sinus infection

Herb	*Commonly Used For*
Eucalyptus (decongestant)	Asthma, bronchitis, cough, cold, hay fever, sinus infection, muscle and joint pain, or as a mouthwash
	May also be useful, when applied topically, for healing wounds and fungal infections and as an insect repellant
Evening primrose oil	Bruises
	May also be useful in treating eczema, rheumatoid arthritis, premenstrual and menopausal symptoms, breast pain, diabetic neuropathy
Eyebright	Conjunctivitis, bloodshot eyes, tired eyes, and other eye and vision problems
Fennel	Digestion, abdominal cramps, gas, bloating
	Also useful as an expectorant to make coughs more productive and clear lung infections; may also promote weight loss
Fenugreek	High blood pressure, high cholesterol, digestive upset, liver and pancreas health
Feverfew	Tension headaches, migraines, inflammation, arthritis, fever, menstrual cramps
Flaxseed (laxative)	Colon health, high cholesterol, heart disease, diabetes, cancer (especially breast, colon, and prostate cancers), and a host of other conditions; good for overall health
Garlic (antioxidant, decongestant)	Heart disease, atherosclerosis, high cholesterol, high blood pressure, cancer, enlarged prostate, asthma, bronchitis, cold, fungal infections (ringworm, jock itch, and athlete's foot)
Gentian	Digestive health, gastrointestinal inflammation, gallbladder problems
	May also help treat internal parasites and help with smoking cessation
Ginger root	Cold, flu, stomach upset, diarrhea, nausea, arthritis, colic, heart conditions, headache, motion sickness
	May help lower cholesterol
Ginkgo biloba	Circulation, memory, Alzheimer's disease, dementia, glaucoma, macular degeneration, pain caused by reduced blood flow to the legs, anxiety, premenstrual symptoms, Raynaud's disease

(continued)

Table D-1 (*continued*)

Herb	*Commonly Used For*
Ginseng	Immune system health, heart health, physical and mental performance, stress, low libido, erectile dysfunction, menopausal symptoms
	May lower blood sugar for those with type 2 diabetes and help reduce the risk of certain types of cancer
Goldenrod	Arthritis, gout, allergies, asthma, cold, flu, inflammation of the bladder or urinary tract, kidney stones, hemorrhoids, minor wounds, eczema, inflammation of the mouth and throat
Goldenseal (antibiotic, often combined with Echinacea)	Cold, flu, upper respiratory infections, cold sores, minor wounds, pink eye and other eye infections
	May help treat diarrhea, UTIs, vaginitis
Gotu kola	Circulation to the legs, varicose veins, syphilis, hepatitis, stomach ulcers, epilepsy, diarrhea, fever, asthma, cold, upper respiratory infections, anxiety, insomnia, minor wounds, burns, eczema, psoriasis, scleroderma, scar prevention, stretch mark reduction
Grapeseed (antioxidant)	Heart disease, diabetes, high blood pressure, high cholesterol, cancer, blood circulation in the legs, edema (swelling from an injury or surgery)
	May be helpful in treating Alzheimer's disease and hemorrhoids and improving vision (especially night vision)
Green tea	Atherosclerosis, high cholesterol, heart disease, cancer, IBD, diabetes, arthritis, liver disease
	May promote weight loss by boosting metabolism
Hawthorn	Angina (chest pain), arrhythmia (irregular heartbeat), high blood pressure, atherosclerosis, heart failure, circulatory conditions
Hops	Digestion, anxiety, insomnia, bladder infections and irritation, bruises
	A special extract called *hops bract polyphenols* may help prevent periodontal disease
Horehound	Cough, cold, flu, sore throat, bronchitis, digestion, gas, bloating, heart rhythm problems, pain

Herb	Commonly Used For
Horse chestnut	Circulation, vein and capillary health (which helps with bruising, varicose veins, and hemorrhoids), varicose veins, cellulite, wrinkles, cough, congestion
Horsetail (diuretic)	UTIs, kidney stones, osteoporosis, brittle nails, minor wounds and burns
Jamaican dogwood	Pain relief, muscle spasms, cough, fever, inflammation, sleep aid
	Warning: Is potentially toxic and used in insecticides to control lice and flea infestations; use only under a doctor's close supervision
Kava	Anxiety, insomnia
	Warning: May cause liver damage; use only under a doctor's close supervision
Lavender (sedative)	Anxiety, agitation, headaches, exhaustion, muscle and joint pain, insomnia
	When applied to scalp, may help regrow hair in people with alopecia areata (an autoimmune disorder that causes hair loss)
Lemon balm	Gas, bloating, colic, anxiety, sleep aid, minor wounds, insect bites and stings, cold sores from herpes simplex
Licorice	Digestion (helping with acid reflux and stomach ulcers), cough, cold, bronchitis, asthma, eczema, cold sores
	May help promote weight loss
Linden	Cough, cold, sore throat, fever, anxiety, indigestion, arrhythmia, nausea, vomiting, skin health
	May be helpful in treating high blood pressure
Lobelia	Respiratory conditions (including asthma, bronchitis, and cough), skin infections, insect bites and stings, poison ivy, and ringworm
	Warning: Potentially toxic in high doses
Maca root	Libido, menstrual irregularities
	May also help in the treatment of chronic fatigue syndrome
Maitake (mushroom)	Immune system function, liver function
	May help lower blood pressure and prevent cancer

(continued)

Table D-1 (*continued*)

Herb	*Commonly Used For*
Marshmallow	Asthma, bronchitis, cough, sore throat, indigestion, stomach ulcers, Crohn's disease, ulcerative colitis, chapped skin, skin inflammation
Milk thistle	Detox; liver, kidney, and gallbladder function; damage caused by alcohol abuse, acetaminophen toxicity, and mushroom poisoning; viral hepatitis (especially hepatitis C); tumors; cancer
Motherwort	Heart health, circulation, high cholesterol, high blood pressure, nervous system health, anxiety, menstrual problems (delayed menstruation, menstrual cramps, and premenstrual and menstrual symptoms)
Mullein (antibacterial pain reliever)	Earache (when combined with garlic), sore throat, cough, irritated lungs, damage caused by smoking May also help relieve pain and swelling of rheumatoid arthritis
Mustard	Digestion, circulation, congestion, respiratory system infection
Myrrh	Gingivitis, mouth ulcers, periodontal disease, laryngitis, thrush; cough, cold, and bronchitis (as an expectorant); minor wounds, abrasions, and fungal infections (applied topically)
Oregano (antioxidant, antibacterial, and anti-inflammatory)	Cancer and heart disease prevention, respiratory health, diabetes
Oregon grape root	Stomach cramps, diarrhea, internal parasites, eye infections, psoriasis, skin irritation, itching, inflammation; protection against bacterial, viral, and fungal infection
Passionflower	Anxiety, sleep aid Often combined with valerian root or kava and lemon balm
Pau d'Arco (antifungal, antiviral)	*candida* yeast infections, cold, flu, arthritis, fever, dysentery, boils, ulcers, cancer, inflammation of the prostate, herpes simplex, internal parasites, bacterial infections, psoriasis
Peppermint	Indigestion, irritable bowel syndrome (IBS); cough, sore throat, minor skin irritations and itching, tension headaches May also be helpful in treating headaches, anxiety, nausea, diarrhea, menstrual cramps, flatulence, bloating

Herb	Commonly Used For
Plantain	Insect bites and stings, skin irritations, minor burns, minor cuts (to stop bleeding)
Pomegranate (antioxidant)	May help prevent and treat cancer, diabetes, and heart disease, and treat osteoarthritis; applied topically, may help with eczema, psoriasis, and dry skin
Pygeum	Enlarged prostate (often combined with saw palmetto), libido, hair loss
Raspberry leaf	Diarrhea, cold, stomach upset, menstrual cramps, reduction of menstrual bleeding
Red clover	Menopausal symptoms; eczema, psoriasis, and other chronic skin conditions; respiratory conditions; as protection against osteoporosis and breast cancer
Reishi (mushroom)	Anxiety, high blood pressure, bronchitis, asthma, insomnia, liver diseases (including hepatitis and to prevent alcohol-related cirrhosis) May boost immune system function
Rosemary	Digestion, protection against foodborne pathogens, stress, memory function, concentration, joint pain, alopecia (an autoimmune disorder that causes hair loss)
Sage	Digestion, cold, fever, sore throat, gingivitis, sore gums, hot flashes, reduction of menstrual bleeding, wound care; also useful as a deodorant
Sarsaparilla (anti-inflammatory)	Gout, arthritis, psoriasis
Saw palmetto	Enlarged prostate, UTIs, sperm production, libido, hair loss associated with male pattern baldness May help treat prostate cancer
Senna (laxative)	Constipation
Shiitake (mushroom)	Immune system function, cardiovascular health, high cholesterol, cancer prevention and treatment, lessening the side effects of chemotherapy
Siberian ginseng (immune system booster)	Preventing and reducing the severity and duration of colds and flu, reducing the frequency, severity, and duration of herpes outbreaks; improving physical and mental performance

(continued)

Table D-1 (*continued*)

Herb	Commonly Used For
Skullcap (sedative)	*American skullcap:* Anxiety, insomnia, convulsions *Chinese skullcap:* Inflammation, allergies, cancer, headaches; may also have antifungal properties
Slippery elm	Cough, sore throat, cold, Crohn's disease, ulcerative colitis, IBS, acid reflux, diarrhea, wound healing, boils, burns, psoriasis, other skin conditions
Spirulina (highly nutritious algae)	Immune system function; also used to supplement the diet during detox fasts
St. John's wort	Depression, premenstrual and menopausal symptoms, seasonal affective disorder (SAD), anxiety disorders (obsessive compulsive disorder and social phobia, for example); fibromyalgia, lupus, wounds, minor burns, eczema, hemorrhoids May cause loose stools and increased sun sensitivity and may trigger a shift to mania in people with underlying bipolar disorder; consult your healthcare provider before use and avoid exposure to sunlight and other sources of UV radiation
Stevia (natural, low-calorie sweetener)	Type 2 diabetes, weight loss
Stinging nettle (antihistamine and anti-inflammatory)	Sinus allergies, asthma, constricted bronchial and nasal passages, adrenal and kidney health, gout, enlarged prostate (often combined with saw palmetto), nighttime incontinence, arthritis pain and inflammation May help with osteoporosis and female reproductive health
Tea tree oil (antibacterial, antiviral, antifungal)	Fungal infections (athlete's foot, ringworm, and jock itch), insect bites and stings May also be useful in treating acne
Thuja	Common skin ailments (including psoriasis, scabies, athlete's foot, and ringworm); pain from arthritis, rheumatism, and sore muscles and joints; bronchitis, cold, and other respiratory conditions
Thyme	Congestion, sleep aid, sore throat, cough, digestion, oral health

Herb	Commonly Used For
Turmeric (anti-inflammatory, antibacterial, and antifungal)	Indigestion, stomach ulcers, ulcerative colitis, osteoarthritis, heart disease, cancer, bacterial and viral infections, uveitis (infected iris) **Note:** Often taken in the form of curcumin (the active ingredient in turmeric) or with black pepper to increase availability and absorption of curcumin
Uva ursi (antibacterial)	Cystitis (bladder inflammation), UTIs
Valerian (sedative)	Anxiety, insomnia **Note:** Avoid driving or operating machinery for a few hours after taking valerian; alcohol may magnify sedation
Vitex	Hormone balance in women, premenopausal and menopausal symptoms, painful and irregular periods **Note:** Best when taken long-term; don't take if you're using oral contraceptives
Wild cherry	Cough, cold, bronchitis May be helpful as a sleep agent to treat insomnia
Wild yam (phytoestrogen)	Premenopausal and menopausal symptoms, nausea, morning sickness, osteoporosis, high cholesterol, stomach upset, cramps
Willow bark (anti-inflammatory)	General pain relief, bursitis, tendonitis, osteoarthritis, menstrual cramps, headache, lower back pain May help to reduce fever
Witch hazel (astringent)	Hemorrhoids, acne, abrasions, minor burns, insect bites, varicose veins, puffy eyes
Wormwood (bitter herb)	Digestion, heartburn and gas prevention May be helpful in cleansing formulations to purge internal parasites **Warning:** May be toxic at high doses
Yarrow	Digestion, stomach and menstrual cramps, anxiety, insomnia, fever, wound care (slows bleeding when applied to cuts)
Yellow dock	Itchy skin conditions, stimulation of digestion and bowel movements
Yerba mate (stimulant)	Reduction of inflammation in gout and arthritis, lowering cholesterol

Appendix E

Homeopathic Remedies

• •

*H*omeopathy is based on the law of familiars or treating like with like —
using a substance that causes certain symptoms in a healthy person
to alleviate those same symptoms in someone who's ill. For example, coffee
keeps most people awake, but for some people who have trouble sleeping,
a homeopathic preparation of coffee helps them sleep. (See Chapter 3 for
more about homeopathy.) Table E-1 lists many of the more common substances used as homeopathic remedies and the ailments those treatments
are used for.

Table E-1	Common Homeopathic Treatments
Homeopathic Remedy	**Ailments It Treats**
Aconitum napellus (aconite)	Angina, anxiety, arrhythmia, asthma, heart failure, postoperative pain
Allium cepa	Allergies, colds, cough, ear infection, hay fever, headache, laryngitis, sore throat
Antimonium tartaricum	Acne, asthma, bronchitis, chicken pox, cold, cough, respiratory conditions
Apis mellifica	Bee stings, hives, insect bites, urinary conditions
Arnica montana	Arthritis, bruises, black eyes, muscle pain, physical trauma, pulled muscles or tendons, shin splits, shock from trauma, tinnitus following injury
Arsenicum album	Anxiety; asthma; cold and flu; diarrhea; eye pain, burning, or itching; food poisoning; skin conditions, including eczema, psoriasis, dry skin, rashes; sore throat; indigestion
Belladonna	Chicken pox and shingles; cold; colic; delirium; earache; eye pain, burning, or itching; dry, hot nose; fever; headache; measles and mumps; sore throat; stomachache with loss of appetite; tonsillitis; toothache

(continued)

Table E-1 *(continued)*

Homeopathic Remedy	Ailments It Treats
Bryonia alba	Abdominal pain, arthritis, back spasms, colic, constipation, cough, diarrhea, fever with chills, flu, gas, headache, heartburn, indigestion, mood disorders, sciatica, sprains and strains
Calcarea carbonica	Anxiety and phobias, bone and joint pain, chronic fatigue, dental problems, digestive disorders, headache, menstrual issues, muscle weakness, osteoarthritis, teething discomfort
Calcarea phosphorica	Fractures that are slow to heal, growing pains, headache, joint pain, rheumatism, tooth decay, teething discomfort
Cantharis	Acid reflux, attention deficit and attention deficit hyperactivity disorders (ADD and ADHD), bladder infections, bleeding/hemorrhaging, burns, digestion issues, insect bites and stings, sunburn
Carbo vegetabilis	Chronic, unexplained illness; cough; heartburn and other digestion conditions; tinnitus
Chamomilla	Colic, diarrhea during teething, earache, fever, insomnia, toothache, irritability (especially in children), menstrual issues (including cramping and breast pain), swollen glands, teething discomfort
Cocculus indicus	Dizziness, motion sickness, nausea, vertigo, menstrual issues
Coffea cruda	Anxiety, depression, headaches, insomnia
Colocynthis	Colic, neuralgia (nerve pain), sciatica
Euphrasia (eyebright)	Eye conditions, including inflammation, injuries, irritation, conjunctivitis, and watery eyes; nasal allergies and excessive discharge
Ferrum phosphoricum	Diarrhea with fever; fever; headache; earache that doesn't respond to belladonna; hemorrhaging, especially nose bleeds; sore throat; cough that's better at night; sleeplessness and restless dreams
Gelsemium	Cold, flu, headache, heat exhaustion, anxiety, neuralgia, sore throat, vertigo
Hepar sulphuris	Abscesses, acne, cold, ear infection, gingivitis, hay fever, cough, croup, hoarseness, sore throat, skin infection, night sweats

Homeopathic Remedy	Ailments It Treats
Hypericum (St. John's wort)	Anxiety, bee stings, dental pain related to dental procedures such as tooth extraction or root canal, depression, headache, insect bites, nerve injury, postoperative pain, puncture wounds (to prevent lockjaw), skin conditions including corns and varicose ulcers; splinters; tailbone injury Also useful as a topical treatment for all sorts of injuries and burns
Ignatia amara	Emotional disorders, including depression, grief, and anxiety; headache; sore throat; cough; menstrual problems
Ipecacuanha (ipecac)	Asthma, bronchitis, heavy bleeding (nasal or menstrual), headache, migraine, morning sickness, motion sickness, nausea, recurrent fevers, whooping cough
Kali bichromicum	Bronchitis; cold with thick, gooey mucus; earache and ear infection; localized pain (especially with headache); migraines; nasal allergies and sinusitis; vaginitis
Kali carbonicum	Asthma, backache, bronchitis, cold, congestion, pneumonia, respiratory infections
Lachesis	Acne, circulatory problems (characterized by bluish, purplish, or blotchy skin), hemorrhoids, high blood pressure, migraines, painful periods, Raynaud's syndrome, rosacea
Ledum	Alcoholism, bee stings, black eyes, bruises, gout, insect bites, puncture wounds, rheumatism, sprains and strains
Lycopodium	Anxiety; constipation; digestive issues related to the liver, gallbladder, urinary, and digestive tracts; flatulence; irritable bowel syndrome (IBS); nausea and vomiting; panic attacks
Magnesia phosphorica	Abdominal and menstrual cramps, colic, muscle spasms
Mercurius vivus	Bad breath, boils, colds, cystitis, earache, gingivitis, diarrhea, sore throat, sweating, tonsillitis, trembling, weakness
Natrum muriaticum	Eye conditions, including dry eyes, itchy eyes, poor eyesight, and glaucoma; water imbalances that may cause sinusitis, hay fever, edema, puffy eyes, circles under eyes, water retention, and perspiration problems; fatigue

(continued)

Table E-1 *(continued)*

Homeopathic Remedy	Ailments It Treats
Nux vomica	Digestion issues, including acid reflux, gas, heartburn, indigestion, nausea, and vomiting; constipation alternating with diarrhea; hemorrhoids; flu
Phosphorus	Anxiety, bleeding, cold, constipation, cough, dark circles under eyes, diarrhea, flu, hoarseness, indigestion, nausea, pallor, vomiting
Podophyllum	Diarrhea, heartburn, indigestion, IBS
Pulsatilla	Bedwetting, chicken pox, cold with heavy yellow discharge, cough, cystitis, earache, fainting, indigestion, insomnia, menstrual problems, sties, varicose veins
Rhus toxicodendron	Aches and pains, back pain, chicken pox, cold sores, cough, flu, hives, hoarseness, poison ivy, sore muscles, rheumatoid arthritis, sciatica, sprains and strains
Ruta graveolens	Back pain, bone injuries, dental problems (dry socket), eye strain, headache, joint pain, sciatica, sprains and strains
Sepia	Depression, exhaustion, female hormone imbalance, hair thinning, hot flashes, irritability, mood swings, seasonal affective disorder (SAD)
Silica	Hair, skin, and nail issues; nutritional deficiencies
Spongia tosta	Asthma, colds, cough, croup, exhaustion, goiter, hoarseness, laryngitis, sore throat, thyroid problems
Staphysagria	Anxiety, bladder infection, cystitis, depression, emotional distress, menopause symptoms, posttraumatic stress disorder (PTSD), urinary urgency
Sulfur	Acne, cold, conjunctivitis, constipation, diarrhea, digestive disorders, eczema, hemorrhoids, nausea, shortness of breath, skin conditions, sties
Tabacum	Anxiety, morning sickness, motion sickness, nausea, vomiting
Urtica urens (stinging nettle)	Allergies, anemia, bee stings, burns, hives, insect bites, poison ivy, rheumatism, skin irritations
Veratrum album	Cough, constipation, cramps, diarrhea, headache, heat exhaustion, menstrual disorders, nausea, vomiting

Appendix F

Aromatic Essential Oils

A romatherapy is the practice of using aromatic essential oils extracted from plants to improve mental and physical health. Table F-1 highlights the most commonly used essential oils and lists the ailments that each is most often used to treat.

Don't take essential oils internally. Essential oils are commonly combined with salts to be used in baths, mixed with a carrier oil to be used in massage or applied topically, or used with a diffuser to spread the aroma throughout a room. For details on the various ways to use essential oils, see Chapter 3.

Table F-1	Essential Oils
Essential Oil	*Used For*
Allspice berry	Arthritis, bronchitis, cough, depression, exhaustion, indigestion, muscle cramps, muscle tone, nausea, rheumatism, stiffness, stomach cramps
	Also used as an aphrodisiac
Amyris	Anxiety, depression, insomnia, stress
	Also used as an antiseptic, sedative, and fixative (for stabilizing oil mixtures)
Anise	Bronchitis, cold, cough, colic, flu, indigestion, rheumatism, stomach cramps
Atlas cedar	Acne, arthritis, bronchitis, cough, cystitis, dandruff, dermatitis, stress
Basil	Bronchitis, cold, cough, depression, infection, insect bites, muscle fatigue
	Also used as an insect repellant
Bay	Circulation issues, dandruff, hair care, neuralgia, oily skin, sprains and strains

(continued)

Table F-1 (*continued*)

Essential Oil	*Used For*
Bergamot	Acne, bad breath, depression, eczema, fever, infection, tension
	Note: Increases sensitivity to sunlight
Black pepper	Arthritis, circulatory problems, heartburn, indigestion, infections, loss of appetite, nausea
Camphor	Acne, arthritis, bronchitis, cold, cough, fever, flu, inflammation, muscle aches and pains, nervous depression, rheumatism, sprains and strains
Cardamom	Colic, flatulence, heartburn, indigestion, nausea, impotence, low sexual response
	Also used as a laxative and expectorant
Carrot seed	Arthritis, bronchitis, cold, edema, flu, gout, rheumatism, and skin conditions, including dermatitis, eczema, and rashes
	Also used as a detox agent for liver and digestive system and to strengthen mucus membranes in the nose, throat, and lungs
Cassia bark	Cold, diabetes, diarrhea, gas, infection, nausea
	Note: May be very irritating to the skin
Chamomile	Abscesses, allergies, arthritis, boils, colic, cuts, cystitis, dermatitis, earache, flatulence, headache, insect bites, insomnia, nausea, neuralgia, premenstrual syndrome (PMS), rashes, rheumatism, skin irritations, sprains and strains, stress, teething, wound care
	Also used as an anti-allergenic, antiseptic, sedative, and digestive tonic
Cinnamon	Anxiety, bladder infections, cardiovascular health, circulation problems, cold, depression, diarrhea, flu, gas, indigestion, infections, low libido
	Also used as an antioxidant and to support the immune system and metabolism
Citronella	Cold, flu, minor infections
	Used most frequently as an insect repellant
Clary sage	Cramps, dandruff, depression, hot flashes, infection, menstrual problems, oily hair or skin, painful periods, stress

Essential Oil	*Used For*
Clove	Acne, arthritis, asthma, bad breath, bronchitis, bruises, burns, cuts, diarrhea, exhaustion, flatulence, respiratory conditions, toothache, tuberculosis, ulcers, vomiting
Coriander	Arthritis, cold, digestive problems, fatigue, flu, low blood glucose, nausea, muscle spasms, rheumatism, stomach cramps
Cypress	Arthritis, bronchitis, circulation issues, hemorrhoids, menopause symptoms, insect bites, oily skin, relaxation, rheumatism, varicose veins, water retention, wound care Also used as an antibacterial, antimicrobial, and antiseptic agent, and as an astringent, deodorant, and diuretic
Eucalyptus	Bruises, burns, colds, concentration, fever, headache, wound care Also used as a disinfectant
Fennel	Aging skin, water retention, indigestion, lymphatic system
Frankincense	Anxiety, blemishes, dry skin, ganglion cyst, wound care Also used as an anti-aging agent
Geranium	Bruises, burns, diarrhea, insect bites
Ginger	Constipation, cramps, indigestion, motion sickness, muscle aches, nausea, sore throat, toothache, vomiting
Grapefruit	Cold, detoxification, stiffness, stress, water retention
Helichrysum	Burns, bruises, colds, lethargy, scars, stretch marks, sunburn, wound care
Hyssop	Anxiety, asthma, bronchitis, bruises, nasal congestion, cold, cough, low blood pressure, fatigue, flu, respiratory conditions, sore throat, tonsillitis, viral infections, water retention
Jasmine	Depression; sexual issues, including impotence, premature ejaculation, and low libido; respiratory issues, including cough, hoarseness, and laryngitis; skin issues, including dry, greasy, irritated skin, stretch marks, and scars; muscle pain, sprains, and strains Also used to induce labor
Juniper berry	Acne, anxiety, arthritis, cellulite, cystitis, dandruff, eczema, gout, kidney stones, menstrual cycle regulation, mental exhaustion, obesity, painful periods, psoriasis, rheumatism

(continued)

Table F-1 (*continued*)

Essential Oil	*Used For*
Lavandin	Muscle stiffness, aches, and pains; respiratory issues, including cold, cough, and flu
Lavender	Abscesses, acne, anxiety, arthritis, asthma, boils, bronchitis, bruises, burns, cold, colic, flatulence, headache, insect bites and stings, insomnia, laryngitis, lice, migraines, nausea, oily skin, psoriasis, rheumatism, sunburn, vomiting, whooping cough, wound care Also used as an antibacterial agent and antiseptic and as an insect repellent
Lemon	Arthritis, asthma, bronchitis, cellulite, circulatory conditions, constipation, flu, high blood pressure, nose bleeds, oily skin, rheumatism Also used as an astringent, diuretic, and laxative
Lemon eucalyptus	Insect repellant
Lemongrass	Digestive disorders, dry skin, excessive sweat, hair care, headache, jet lag, stress
Lemon verbena	Digestive disorders, cramps, indigestion, liver detox, stress
Lime	Boils, cold, corns, cramps, cuts, fever, nosebleed, oily skin, warts
Marjoram	Constipation, cough, cramps, migraines, muscle aches, nervous system disorders, rheumatism
Melissa	Cold, cough, cramps, menstrual pain, nausea, stress Also used as an insect repellant
Myrrh	Amnesia, bleeding gums, cracked and dry skin, dysentery, gingivitis, hyperthyroidism, memory loss, mouth ulcers, sore throat
Myrtle	Acne, asthma, bladder infection, bronchitis, diarrhea, hormone imbalances, hypothyroidism, insomnia, lung infection, oily skin Also used as an astringent, sedative, and expectorant
Neroli	Anxiety, colitis, depression, diarrhea, insomnia, post-traumatic stress disorder, shock, stomach cramps, stress
Nutmeg	Arthritis, circulatory issues, constipation, digestive issues, fatigue, muscle aches, nausea, neuralgia, rheumatism

Essential Oil	Used For
Orange	Cold, constipation, digestive issues, flatulence, flu, gingivitis, stress Also used as an antidepressant, antiseptic, and detox agent, and in household cleaners
Oregano	Boils, bronchitis, *Candida* yeast overgrowth, cold, digestion, fungal infections (such as athlete's foot and jock itch), insect bites, pancreatitis, parasites, plantar warts, respiratory ailments, ringworm, staph infection, strep throat Also used as an antimicrobial and antifungal agent, and as a muscle relaxant
Palmarosa	Acne, anorexia, dermatitis, digestion issues, exhaustion, fever, gastrointestinal infection, scarring, sore muscles
Patchouli	Acne, anxiety, burns, clogged pores, depression, dermatitis, eczema, fatigue, fungal infections (athlete's foot, jock itch, ringworm), insect bites, substance abuse/addiction, water retention, wrinkles, wound healing Also used as an antifungal and antibacterial agent, a diuretic, and as a uterine tonic and insect repellent
Peppermint	Acne, asthma, bronchitis, colic, congestion, depression, dermatitis, flatulence, gallbladder issues, headache, indigestion, insect bites, migraines, motion sickness, muscle aches and pains, nausea, painful periods, pneumonia, pruritus (anal itching), ringworm, scabies, spastic colon, stomach cramps, stress, sunburn, tuberculosis
Peru balsam	Bronchitis, chapped skin, circulatory issues, cold, cough, eczema, flu, rash, respiratory conditions, rheumatism, sensitive skin, stress
Petitgrain	Anger, insomnia, muscle spasms, panic disorders, stomach pains
Pine	Asthma, bronchitis, catarrh, circulatory issues, cold, cough, cuts, cystitis, excessive perspiration, fatigue (mental, physical, sexual), flu, gout, laryngitis, lice, muscle aches and pains, neuralgia, prostate problems, rheumatism, scabies, sinusitis, sores, urinary tract infections (UTIs)
Red cedarwood	Acne, congestion, dandruff, respiratory conditions, UTIs Also used as an antiseptic and astringent

(continued)

Table F-1 (*continued*)

Essential Oil	Used For
Rose absolute	Anger, anxiety, arrhythmia, depression, eczema, fear, grief, dry wrinkled skin, menopause, menstrual conditions, stress
Rose otto	Anger, arrhythmia, depression, eczema, fear, grief, dry wrinkled skin, menopause, menstrual conditions, stress
	Note: Preferred over rose absolute for topical applications
Rosemary	Arthritis, circulatory issues, dandruff, gout, greasy hair, hair loss, headache, memory loss, migraines, muscle cramps and aches and pains, nervous disorders, rheumatism, wound care
Rosewood	Acne, cold, dry skin, fever, flu, headache, oily skin, scarring, sensitive skin, stress, stretch marks
	Also used as an aphrodisiac
Sandalwood	Asthma, bronchitis, chapped skin, congestion, cystitis, depression, diarrhea, dry skin, laryngitis, nausea, oily skin, scarring, sensitive skin, stress, stretch marks, UTIs, vomiting
Spearmint	Acne, asthma, bronchitis, catarrh, constipation, dermatitis, diarrhea, exhaustion, fever, flatulence, headache, hiccups, migraines, nausea, pruritus, scabies, sinusitis, sore gums, teething, vertigo
Tangerine	Constipation, diarrhea, flatulence, stretch marks, water retention
Tea tree	Acne, asthma, bronchitis, blisters, catarrh, chicken pox, cold, cold sores, congestion, corns, cough, cuts, cystitis, diaper rash, fever, flu, fungal infections (athlete's foot, jock itch, ringworm), gingivitis, insect bites, itching, migraine, oily skin, sinusitis, sores, tuberculosis, warts, whooping cough, yeast infections (*Candida* yeast infection and vaginal thrush)
	Also used as an antiseptic, antibacterial, antifungal, and antiviral agent
Thyme	Atherosclerosis, bacterial infections (including MRSA), blood clots, bronchitis, cold, cough, croup, diarrhea, dry skin, fungal infections, hair loss, oily skin, pneumonia, psoriasis, sciatica, scoliosis, snoring, sore throats, tuberculosis, whooping cough
	Also used as an antiseptic and antifungal agent

Essential Oil	Used For
Vanilla	Depression, fever, high blood pressure, cancer prevention, inflammation, insomnia, low sex drive, menstrual regulation
	Also used as an antidepressant, an antioxidant, an aphrodisiac, and a sedative
Vetiver	Anger, anxiety, arthritis, exhaustion, insomnia, muscle aches and pains, scars, stings, stress, wound care
White fir	Anxiety, arthritis, asthma, bronchial obstructions, cough, fever, flu, rheumatism, sinusitis, sore muscles, UTIs, wound care
	Also used as an anti-inflammatory, anti-arthritic, anticatarrhal agent, and as an expectorant and stimulant
Wintergreen	Arthritis, bleeding gums, bronchitis, circulation disorders, insect bites, itching, joint stiffness, migraine, toothache
Ylang ylang	Anger, anxiety, arrhythmia, depression, hypertension, insomnia, stress
	Also used as an aphrodisiac

Index

• T •

tachycardia, 252
talk therapy, 317
tangerine, 394
tannin, 77
tar shampoos, 126
taurine, 311, 317, 367
tea
    black, treating burns with, 68
    fenugreek, 161
    green, 111, 160, 291, 362, 379
    herbal, 51–52, 54–55
    oolong, 113
tea tree oil
    blisters, treating, 111
    boils, treating, 108
    as cleaning agent, 34
    general discussion, 383, 394
    for jock itch, 110
    oral care with, 160
    ringworm, treating, 122
    steam room with, 101
Technical Stuff icon, 3
teething, 186
temporomandibular joint dysfunction (TMJ or TMD), 165–166
tension headaches, treating, 72
Terry's nails, 131
testosterone, low, 296–297
thuja, 383
thyme, 383, 394
thyroid disorders
    general discussion, 272–274
    Graves' disease, 274–276
    Hashimoto's thyroiditis, 278
    hyperthyroidism, 275
    hypothyroidism, 276–278
    overview, 271
    thyroid screening, 274
    toxic adenomas, 276
tick bites, 77
tinctures, herbal, 55–56
tinea pedis, 169–171
tinnitus, 141–142
Tip icon, 3
TMG (trimethylglycine) betaine anhydrous, 367
TMJ (temporomandibular joint dysfunction), 165–166
toenails, ingrown, 175–176
toothaches, 167
toothpaste, 160

tourniquets, 70
toxic adenomas, 276
toxins, removing from homes, 33–36
trans fats, 24, 113–114, 249, 261, 309
trichomoniasis, 290, 305–306
trimethylglycine (TMG) betaine anhydrous, 367
triphala eye wash, 150
Truvia, 23
trypsin, 81
turmeric, 83, 88, 108, 122, 383
type 1 diabetes, 260, 264
type 2 diabetes, 260
tyrosine, 368

• U •

ulcers, gastric, 211–212
upper respiratory tract conditions
    coughs, 86–87
    laryngitis, 87–88
    overview, 85
    postnasal drip, 88–89
    sinus congestion, 88–89
    sneezing, 89
    sore throats, 90
urinary tract infections (UTIs), 222–224
uterine fibroids, 285–286
uticaria, treating, 117–118
uva ursi, 383

• V •

vaccinations
    and autism, 320
    benefits and risks, 189–192
    chicken pox, 188
vaginal depletion packs (vag packs), 283
vaginal suppository treatment, 283
vaginitis, 290–291
valerian, 383
vanilla, 395
varicose veins, 181
vascular laser, 123
vegan diet, 229
vegetables, 19, 26, 333
veins, varicose, 181
Verified Non-GMO seal, 25
vertebral subluxation, 60, 75
vertigo, treating, 142–144
vetiver, 395
vibration, whole body, 266
villous atrophy, 229

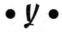

● **𝒴** ●

● **𝒵** ●

About the Author

Scott J. Banks, DC, IFMCP, CGP, PC, holds a Bachelor of Science degree from Farleigh Dickinson University and a Doctor of Chiropractic from New York Chiropractic College, and is an Institute for Functional Medicine Certified Practitioner. As an adjunct professor at Nassau Community College in Garden City, New York, Dr. Banks teaches anatomy and physiology. He has been in clinical practice for more than 33 years with offices in Long Island, New York.

In 2013, Dr. Banks joined an elite group of Institute for Functional Medicine Certified Practitioners, uniquely trained to identify and treat the root causes of illness, disease, and chronic disorders. By shifting the traditional disease-centered focus of medical practice to a systems-oriented, patient-centered methodology, Dr. Banks concentrates on the whole person, not just an isolated set of symptoms. As a functional medicine practitioner, he spends time with his patients, listening to their histories and looking at the interactions among genetic, environmental, and lifestyle factors that can influence long-term health and complex, chronic disease.

Always striving to further his medicinal knowledge and offer additional health-oriented solutions for his patients, Dr. Banks is also a Certified Gluten Practitioner with the expertise to identify and treat gluten-related disorders, such as celiac disease and nonceliac gluten sensitivity (NCGS).

Recognized among thousands of wellness practitioners, Dr. Banks was awarded the distinguished honor of America's Greatest Healer by the Navel Expo 2009. He has appeared on *Dr. Phil* as a clinical nutrition expert and regularly speaks nationally to students, doctors, and the public on the natural approach to health and well-being. Dr. Banks has delivered many lectures to physicians for XYMOGEN, Metagenics, and Designs for Health nutritional companies. In addition, he has conducted webinars involving physicians worldwide for the Institute for Functional Medicine. Sign up for a free newsletter and receive other health information at his website, www.spinelife.com.

Dedication

To my Dad, Bernard Banks. At the young age of 90, he is a testament to living life to its fullest every day. He has been eating well and following my nutritional advice for well over 20 years. He is a living example of what natural cures can do for you as you move through life. He is as sharp as a tack and continues to be my inspiration and what I aspire to be when I finally grow up. He has always encouraged me to be the best and to learn, love, and play, and I will always be grateful to the greatest man on earth. I would also like to dedicate this book to my patients, who have blessed me with the opportunity to help them through their health challenges. I have learned so much from them, and I have been humbled by their daily reminders that when it comes to healthcare one size does not fit all.

Author's Acknowledgments

Writing this book has been a dream come true, a dream that took a team of talented individuals to make possible.

First I'd like to thank my agent, P. J. Campbell, for bringing this opportunity my way and for her positive reinforcement and relentless drive in promoting me as the right person to author this book. You breathed the first breath of life into this book, and for that I thank you.

Thanks also to Tracy Boggier, Senior Acquisitions Editor at Wiley, who ultimately chose me to write this book and worked tirelessly in the early stages to get it on the right track. Her input on the table of contents, audience, and vision of the book set the course for this book.

Thanks to Joe Kraynak, my writing partner and wordsmith, whose insight and guidance made this project easier than I could've imagined. Without his patience, persistence, and whatever-it-takes attitude, I'd probably still be writing this book. Thank you so much, Joe!

Special thanks also to Tracy Barr, who has a collection of talents perfectly tailored to producing top-notch guides *For Dummies*. Tracy was instrumental in the formulating the book's vision during its initial stages, offering sage advice on how to cram 800 pages of wisdom into a 400-page book, and ensuring the consistency and quality of the manuscript from start to finish.

My deep appreciation also goes out to Geri Brewster, RD, MPH, CDN, for checking the manuscript meticulously for technical errors and offering a much appreciated second opinion regarding recommended treatments.

I would not be here if it were not for the inspiration and education that I have received from the Institute for Functional Medicine over the last 20 years. Special thanks to my mentors, including Drs. Jeffrey Bland, David Jones, Mark Hyman, David Perlmutter, and Tom O'Bryan; JJ Virgin, CNS, CHFS; and the entire staff at IFM.

Finally, I want to thank my family — Jane, Dane, and Joseph — for allowing me the space and giving me the support I needed to complete this project. Thank you to my staff for taking over everything else so I could focus on this book.

Publisher's Acknowledgments

Senior Acquisitions Editor: Tracy Boggier

Editor: Tracy L. Barr

Technical Editor: Geri Brewster, RDN, MPH, CDN

Project Coordinator: Erin Zeltner

Cover Image: ©iStock.com/Dimitris66